AF688455

Endocrinology: A Collection of Cases

Endocrinology: A Collection of Cases

Editor: Alberto Lewis

AMERICAN
MEDICAL PUBLISHERS
www.americanmedicalpublishers.com

AMERICAN
MEDICAL PUBLISHERS
www.americanmedicalpublishers.com

Cataloging-in-Publication Data

Endocrinology: a collection of cases / edited by Alberto Lewis.
p. cm.
Includes bibliographical references and index.
ISBN 979-8-88740-636-7
1. Endocrinology. 2. Endocrinology, Comparative. 3. Endocrinology, Experimental.
4. Developmental endocrinology. 5. Hormones. I. Lewis, Alberto.
RC648 .A38 2023
6164--dc23

© American Medical Publishers, 2023

American Medical Publishers,
41 Flatbush Avenue,
1st Floor, New York,
NY 11217, USA

ISBN 979-8-88740-636-7 (Hardback)

This book contains information obtained from authentic and highly regarded sources. Copyright for all individual chapters remain with the respective authors as indicated. All chapters are published with permission under the Creative Commons Attribution License or equivalent. A wide variety of references are listed. Permission and sources are indicated; for detailed attributions, please refer to the permissions page and list of contributors. Reasonable efforts have been made to publish reliable data and information, but the authors, editors and publisher cannot assume any responsibility for the validity of all materials or the consequences of their use.

Trademark Notice: Registered trademark of products or corporate names are used only for explanation and identification without intent to infringe.

Contents

Preface

Every book is a source of knowledge and this one is no exception. The idea that led to the conceptualization of this book was the fact that the world is advancing rapidly; which makes it crucial to document the progress in every field. I am aware that a lot of data is already available, yet, there is a lot more to learn. Hence, I accepted the responsibility of editing this book and contributing my knowledge to the community.

Endocrinology is an area of medical science that focuses on the study and treatment of disorders related to the endocrine system. The endocrine system consists of glands that produce hormones, which are essential for regulating various bodily functions. There can be several causes of endocrine disorders. They can arise from hormone-producing glands, such as the thyroid, adrenal glands, pituitary gland, pancreas, or the ovaries and testes. The symptoms of endocrine disorders vary depending on the specific gland and hormones involved. A few of the common symptoms include fatigue, weight changes, mood swings, abnormal growth patterns, changes in sexual function, excessive thirst or urination, and changes in appetite. Diagnosing endocrine disorders involves a thorough review of medical history, physical examination, and laboratory tests. Imaging techniques such as ultrasounds, CT scans, or MRIs may also be used to visualize the affected glands or detect tumors. This book is a compilation of case studies that discuss the most vital concepts and emerging trends in the field of endocrinology. Those in search of information to further their knowledge will be greatly assisted by it.

While editing this book, I had multiple visions for it. Then I finally narrowed down to make every chapter a sole standing text explaining a particular topic, so that they can be used independently. However, the umbrella subject sinews them into a common theme. This makes the book a unique platform of knowledge.

I would like to give the major credit of this book to the experts from every corner of the world, who took the time to share their expertise with us. Also, I owe the completion of this book to the never-ending support of my family, who supported me throughout the project.

Editor

1

Diabetes Mellitus, Extreme Insulin Resistance and Hypothalamic-Pituitary Langerhans Cells Histiocytosis

Mathilde Sollier,[1] Marine Halbron,[1] Jean Donadieu,[2] Ahmed Idbaih,[3] Fleur Cohen Aubart,[4] Corinne Vigouroux,[5] Martine Auclair,[5] Olivier Bourron,[1] Marie Bastin,[1] Géraldine Béra,[6] Philippe Touraine,[7,8] Jacques Young,[9] Héléna Mosbah,[1] Agnès Hartemann,[1] Fabrizio Andreelli,[1] and Chloé Amouyal[1]

[1] *Diabetology-Metabolism Dpt, Sorbonne Université, APHP, Institut Hospitalo-Universitaire de Cardiometabolisme et Nutrition (ICAN), Pitié-Salpêtrière-Charles Foix Hospital, 75013 Paris, France*
[2] *Hemato-Oncology Dpt, Trousseau Hospital, APHP, 75012 Paris, France*
[3] *Sorbonne Université, Inserm, CNRS, UMRS 1127, Institut du Cerveau et de la Moelle épinière, ICM, AP-HP, Hôpitaux Universitaires La Pitié Salpêtrière -Charles Foix, Service de Neurologie 2, Mazarin, 75013 Paris, France*
[4] *Department of Internal Medicine 2, Sorbonne Université, APHP, Institut Hospitalo-Universitaire de Cardiometabolisme et Nutrition (ICAN), Pitié-Salpêtrière-Charles Foix Hospital, 75013 Paris, France*
[5] *Inserm UMRS 938, Centre de Recherche Saint-Antoine, Sorbonne Université, Reference Center for Rare Diseases of Insulin Secretion and Insulin Sensitivity, Institut Hospitalo-Universitaire de Cardiometabolisme et Nutrition (ICAN), Paris, APHP, Saint Antoine Hospital, Paris, France*
[6] *Nuclear Medicine Dpt, Sorbonne Université, APHP, Pitié-Salpêtrière-Charles Foix Hospital, 75013 Paris, France*
[7] *Department of Endocrinology and Reproductive Medicine, Pitié-Salpêtrière Hospital, APHP, Reference Center for Rare Endocrine Diseases of Growth, Reference Center for Rare Gynecological Pathologies, Institut Hospitalo-Universitaire de Cardiometabolisme et Nutrition (ICAN), Sorbonne University, 75013 Paris, France*
[8] *Pitié-Salpêtrière-Charles Foix Hospital, 75013 Paris, France*
[9] *Reproductive Endocrinology Department, Paris Sud University, APHP, Le Kremlin-Bicêtre, 94275, France*

Correspondence should be addressed to Fabrizio Andreelli; fabrizio.andreelli@aphp.fr

Academic Editor: Lucy Mastrandrea

Background. Langerhans Cell Histiocytosis (LCH) is a rare inflammatory neoplasm characterized by an infiltration of organs by Langerin + (CD207+) and CD1a+ histiocytes. Diabetes insipidus is a frequent manifestation of the disease, while diabetes mellitus is very rare. We report the first case of a 20-year-old man suffering from hypothalamopituitary histiocytosis and diabetes mellitus with serum anti-insulin receptor antibodies. *Case Presentation.* A 20-year-old patient was admitted for the evaluation of growth delay and hyperphagia. HbA1c level and fasting blood glucose were in the normal range. The diagnosis of hypothalamopituitary histiocytosis was based on histological features after biopsy of a large suprachiasmatic lesion identified on magnetic resonance imaging (MRI). Association of vinblastine and purinethol was started followed by a second-line therapy by cladribine. During the follow-up, the patient was admitted for recurrence of hyperglycemic states and extreme insulin resistance. The screening for serum anti-insulin receptor antibodies was positive. Each episode of hyperglycemia appeared to be correlated with tumoral activity and increase in serum anti-insulin receptor antibodies and appeared to be improved when the disease was controlled by chemotherapy. *Conclusion.* We report the first description of a hypothalamopituitary histiocytosis associated with serum anti-insulin receptor antibodies, extreme insulin resistance, and diabetes. Parallel evolution of glucose levels and serum anti-insulin receptor antibodies seemed to be the consequence of immune suppressive properties of cladribine.

1. Background

Langerhans Cell Histiocytosis (LCH) is a rare disease characterized by an infiltration of organs by Langerin+ (CD207+) and CD1a+ histiocytes [1, 2]. Although it can occur at any time of life with an incidence of 4.6 cases per million habitants, LCH is more frequent in children (with onset at a peak age of 1-3 years) [3]. The pathogenesis of LCH is not clear but is likely linked to an inflammatory neoplasm. The definitive diagnosis relies on histology with expression of CD1a antigen or CD207 antigen according to the revised criteria of the Histiocyte Society [1]. Multiple tissues can be concerned by LCH but the most frequent are bones, skin, and pituitary [4]. Indeed, a recent review of endocrine manifestations showed that pituitary deficiency associated with diabetes insipidus (DI) is one of the most frequent endocrine diseases observed at onset of LCH [5]. Endocrine pancreas is rarely concerned and to our knowledge only five cases of pancreatic infiltration by LCH cells have been reported in the literature [6–10]. In addition, association between LCH and diabetes mellitus with or without hypothalamopituitary involvement has been published [11–15]. We report for the first time the case of a 20-year-old man presenting a hypothalamopituitary histiocytosis and positive for serum anti-insulin receptor antibodies with a follow-up characterized by alternating periods of diabetes mellitus with extreme insulin resistance and periods of normoglycemia.

2. Case Presentation

The patient #1509232 is a young male with a history of polyuria and polydipsia since he was 11 years old. This symptom was neglected. The patient had a normal academic progression and medical work-up (at age of 14 years and 17 years) excluding several times the diagnosis of diabetes mellitus, as no hyperglycemia has been detected. At the age of 20 years and 5 months he became polyphagic and his weight increased from 60 to 90 kg without any other complaint. Finally, 5 months later, a brain MRI was performed and a large hypothalamus mass (20x20mm) with thickening of the pituitary stalk and compression of the third ventricle was observed. A strong contrast enhancement was observed after administration of gadolinium (Figures 1(a), 1(b), and 1(c)).

The patient was admitted in the department of endocrinology and the biological explorations concluded to a panhypopituitarism associated with diabetes insipidus. At the initial assessment, the following was also discovered: (i) the patient presented stage I obesity (BMI=26.6 kg/m2), (ii) delayed bone age relative to chronological age (resp., 16 years for a chronological age of 20), and (iii) a growth delay with a deceleration of linear growth at age of 15 years.

A stereotactic biopsy of the brain mass was performed at age of 21 years (Table 1, M1) and immunohistochemistry showed positive staining for CD1a and PS100, supporting the diagnosis of LCH. Presence of BRAF V600E mutation was explored because this mutation in LCH is associated with more severe disease than did those with wild-type BRAF and irreversible damage, such as neurologic and pituitary injuries [16]. In addition, presence of BRAF V600E mutation may offer the possibility of a targeted therapy by BRAF inhibitor (vemurafenib or PLX8394, a second-generation BRAF inhibitor) [17]. Unfortunately, the mutation was not observed and this has limited the possibility to use BRAF inhibitors). Disease work-up failed to find any extra pituitary-hypothalamic extension.

The patient was referred to the oncology department to start vinblastine (one infusion of 10mg per week) and purinethol (100mg per day) according to the French guidelines HL2010 protocol [18]. He did not receive corticosteroids. The patient signed an informed consent to be enrolled in the French LCH registry according to regulation [19].

One month after, the patient was admitted to the emergency room for altered consciousness (Table 1, M0). The blood tests showed hypernatremia at 164mmol/l and hyperglycemia at 25.8mmol/l without ketosis. Importantly, blood glucose levels were in the normal range 6 months before and at the time of the brain biopsy. After continuous administration of fluids and rapid acting insulin analogue (124UI/24hr), he was admitted to the diabetology department.

The search for type 1 diabetes (anti-GAD and anti-IA2 antibodies) was negative. C-peptide level was 9μg/l in the fasting state (normal range: 0.8-4.2 μg/l). The lipid profile showed hypertriglyceridemia at 5.7mmol/l (5,4g/l) and low HDL-cholesterol level at 0.41 mmol/l (0.16g/l). Blood pressure was normal at 125/68mmHg. The abdominal CT-scan found liver steatosis without any pancreatic abnormalities. The weight gain of 19kg during the last 3 months (body mass index: 32kg/m^2) was linked to eating disorder (especially binge-eating disorder). It was decided to continue the first-line therapy up to 6 infusions of vinblastine.

Intriguingly, soon after the diagnosis of diabetes mellitus, daily insulin needs grew up to 400UI per day (4.2UI/kg), indicating a significant insulin resistance state. We did not observe acanthosis nigricans or loss of subcutaneous tissue and we excluded hypersecretion of hyperglycemic hormones. We tested the hypothesis of antibodies against insulin receptors as a cause of insulin resistance. The screening for serum anti-insulin receptor antibodies was performed using a radioreceptor assay as described [20, 21]. In summary, Chinese Hamster Ovary cells overexpressing insulin receptor (CHO-IR) were incubated or not for 90 min at 22°C with control and patient's serum at different dilutions, washed, and then incubated for 90 min at 22°C with a tracer concentration of ^{125}I-insulin with or without unlabeled insulin.

The ability of patient's serum to inhibit binding of [^{125}I] insulin was expressed as a percent decrease of insulin binding at 1:3 dilution as compared to the reference value. At the diabetes diagnosis, insulin receptor antibodies were positive (42% decrease in insulin binding) (Table 1), allowing the diagnosis of type B insulin resistance, a disease often associated with autoimmune disorders or hematological diseases. We then excluded systemic lupus erythematous, multiple myeloma, and Hodgkin's disease. Interestingly, insulin receptor antibodies levels decreased when first-line therapy was achieved (19% decrease in insulin binding) in parallel to a spectacular decrease in daily insulin needs (Table 1).

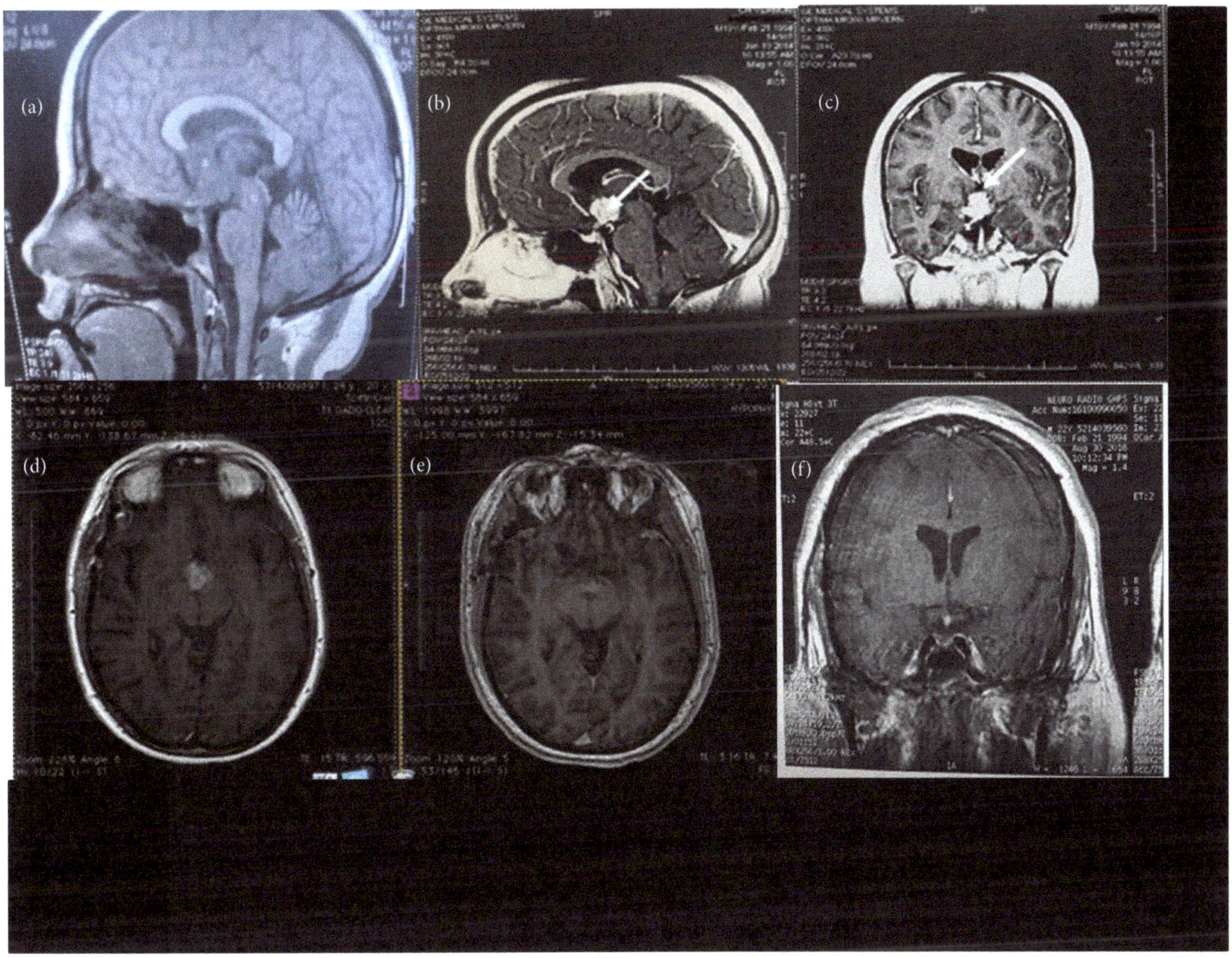

FIGURE 1: *Evolution of brain MRI during follow-up.* At diagnosis, the normal T1-weighted hyperintense signal of the posterior pituitary has disappeared (a). Contrast-enhanced hypothalamic mass after gadolinium infusion ((b) and (c)); compression of third ventricle and thickening of pituitary stalk (b). Comparison of brain MRI (T1 with gadolinium) at diagnosis (M0) (d) and at the end of the first-line therapy (e). MRI showed a significant decrease of the hypothalamic mass but the persistence of contrast enhancement after gadolinium. Brain MRI (T1 after gadolinium infusion) at M30 showing a hypothalamic lesion stable in size and with decreased hypersignal compared to previous MRI (f).

Insulin therapy could be discontinued and replaced by a monotherapy with metformin (850mg twice a day). HbA1c remained stable at 6.5% (48 mmol/mol) until M8. In contrast, no improvement of binge-eating disorder was observed and body mass index kept increasing significantly during this period (Table 1).

Seven months after initial diagnosis of diabetes mellitus, intensification of hypoglycemic therapy with sulfonylurea and liraglutide LAR added to metformin was needed because glucose levels increased. The change in glucose levels was observed at the same time as a further increase of serum insulin receptor autoantibodies at M8 and M10 (43 and 42 percent decrease of insulin binding to its receptor upon incubation of CHO-IR cells with patient's serum at 1:3 dilution, resp.) (Table 1). Although a significant decrease of the size of the brain mass was observed when compared to initial evaluation, persistence of contrast enhancement after gadolinium administration suggested an incomplete response to therapy (Figures 1(d) and 1(e)).

A second-line therapy was started, consisting in 6 cycles of cladribine (5mg/m2/24h, 5 days/week, each month) from month 12 to month 18 after the diagnosis. At M30, brain MRI showed a decrease of both tumor volume and contrast enhancement (Figure 1(f)). In addition, glucose levels were controlled with the association of metformin and liraglutide (HbA1c level decreased to 7.5% or 58mmol/mol). Diabetes improvement was associated with a decrease of insulin receptor antibodies levels until M31. Unfortunately, a new recurrence of uncontrolled diabetes (HbA1c: 11.2%, 99 mmol/mol) occurred at M32 needing insulin therapy. Insulin receptor antibodies were once again positive (36% inhibition of insulin binding by patient's serum at 1:3 dilution), while brain MRI did not reveal tumor recurrence.

It was decided to initiate new cycles of cladribine. The patient received a first cycle at M32 after diagnosis and a second one month later. During this period, insulin daily doses decreased from 300UI to 36UI at the end of cladribine cycles. Additionally, HbA1c level decreased from 11.2% to 8.6% (from

TABLE 1: *Evolution of blood glucose levels, BMI, and anti-insulin receptor antibodies in blood.* Evolution of fasting blood venous glycemia (measured at each administration of chemotherapy or at each assessment of anti-insulin receptor antibodies) and the ability of patient's serum to inhibit insulin binding to its receptor. The reduction of [^{125}I]insulin binding in the presence of patient's serum (used at 1:3 dilution) was measured on CHO cells overexpressing insulin receptor as described (18-20). Ins: insulin. Met: metformin.

	IMC (kg/m2)	Anti-insulin receptor antibodies	Blood glucose levels (mM)	Admissions	Therapy for diabetes	Therapy for histiocytosis
M-1	24		4,4	Stereotactic biopsy		
M0	31,5		25,8	Hyperosmolar hyperglycemic coma	Ins	Vinblastine + purinethol
M1	32		15		Ins + Met + sulfamides	Vinblastine + purinethol
M2	31	42	13		Ins + Met + sulfamides	Vinblastine + purinethol
M2	32,1	35	8,2		Ins + Met + sulfamides	Vinblastine + purinethol
M2	32,1	19	5,5		Met	Vinblastine + purinethol
M8	33,8	43	13,7	Relapse of hyperglycemia	Met + sulfamides + GLP-1 analog	Vinblastine + purinethol
M10	35,2	42	11		Met + sulfamides + GLP-1 analog	Cladribine
M20	35,2	49	11		Met + sulfamides + GLP-1 analog	Cladribine
M28	37,6	30	14,3		Met + sulfamides + GLP-1 analog	
M31	37,6	2	5,5		Met + GLP-1 analog	
M32	39	36	22	Relapse of hyperglycemia	Ins	Cladribine
M33	39	32	17		Ins	Cladribine

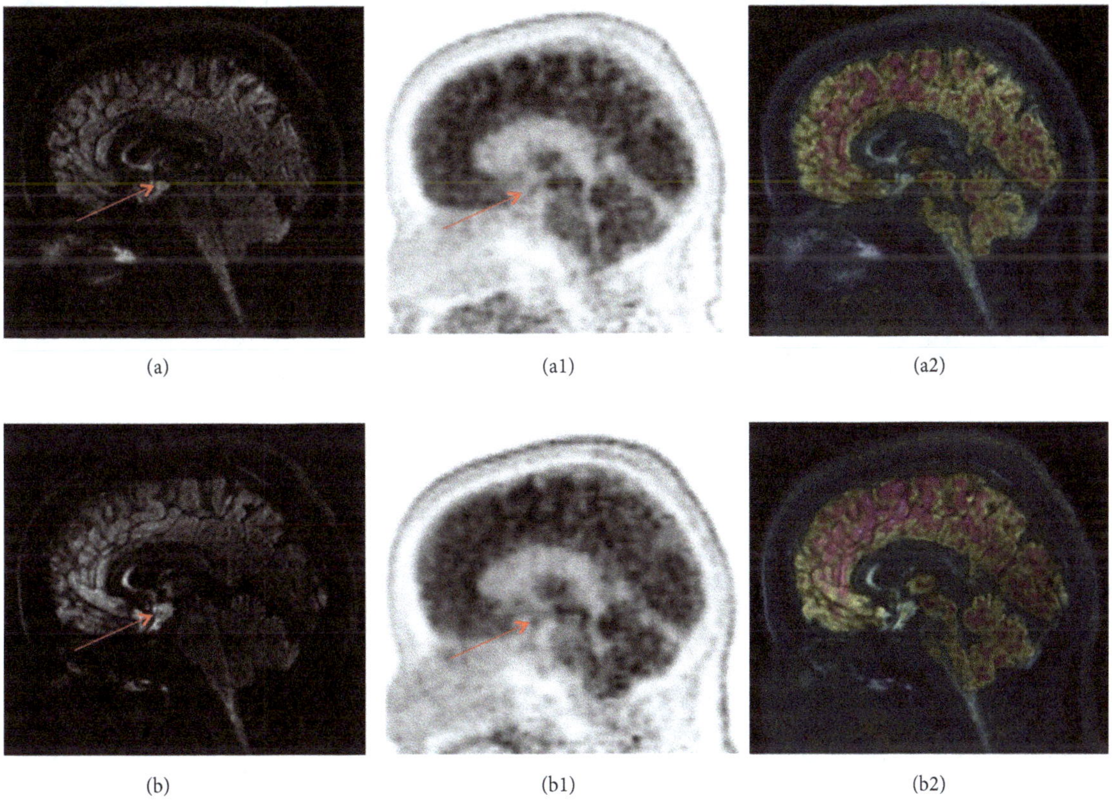

FIGURE 2: *Sagittal PET-MRI brain imaging.* Sagittal PET-MRI brain imaging with [18F]FDG at M32 (a, a1, a2) and at M35 (b, b1, b2) of follow-up. Nodular thickening of the floor of the third ventricle and pituitary infundibulum, in hyperintense FLAIR, without [18F]FDG-uptake, measuring 7 mm in height x 13 mm in the axial plane, without significant enhancement, globally unchanged from the previous MRI. Linear and fine enhancement of the pituitary infundibulum with stable appearance.

99 to 70 mmol/mol). The PET-MRI made during the relapse of diabetes at M32 showed a nodular thickening of the floor of the third ventricle and pituitary infundibulum with no [18F]-FDG-uptake (Figures 2 and 3). Control of diabetes was maintained until M35 and PET-MRI was unchanged at that time (Figures 2 and 3). The follow-up was marked by a very complex clinical disorder, with behavioural difficulties, polyphagy and agressivity; neurological difficulties, loss of memory; and very instable basal metabolic situation, hyperglycemia, and recurrent hypernatremia episodes. Four years after the diagnosis of LCH, the patients is actually frequently hospitalized in a psychiatric hospital.

3. Case Discussion

We reported a case of isolated hypothalamic-pituitary LCH and panhypopituitarism, with multiple episodes of extreme insulin resistance and diabetes mellitus. Each episode appeared to be associated with tumoral activity and appeared to be improved when brain tumor was controlled by chemotherapy.

Each period of hyperglycemia was characterized by important specificities. First, blood glucose levels were extremely high at each recurrence of diabetes and induced massive dehydration and hypernatremia in a context of diabetes insipidus. A second major characteristic was the insulin resistance state. Important doses of insulin (4UI/kg/D) were necessary to maintain glycemia around 11 mmol/l, regardless of how insulin was administered, intravenously or subcutaneously. The hyperglycemia periods alternated with periods of improvement of glucose homeostasis; oral hypoglycemic monotherapy with metformin was then sufficient to achieve the target of HbA1c (< 6.5% or 48 mmol/mol). Such fluctuations in glucose homeostasis and insulin resistance raise the question of the etiology of this diabetes. Low levels of ketone bodies and negativity of islet antibodies contributed to excluding the diagnosis of type 1 diabetes. The most frequent etiologies of insulin resistance (such as infectious disease, lipodystrophy, excessive secretion of hyperglycemic hormone, or corticosteroids therapy) were absent. In addition, the increase in body weight observed before onset of diabetes was not sufficient to explain by itself such an important level of insulin resistance at the discovery of diabetes.

Thus, we hypothesized that insulin resistance could be triggered by serum anti-insulin receptor antibodies. Indeed, in this condition (known as type B insulin resistance), such antibodies are known to reduce insulin (exogenous or endogenous) transduction signaling in insulin target

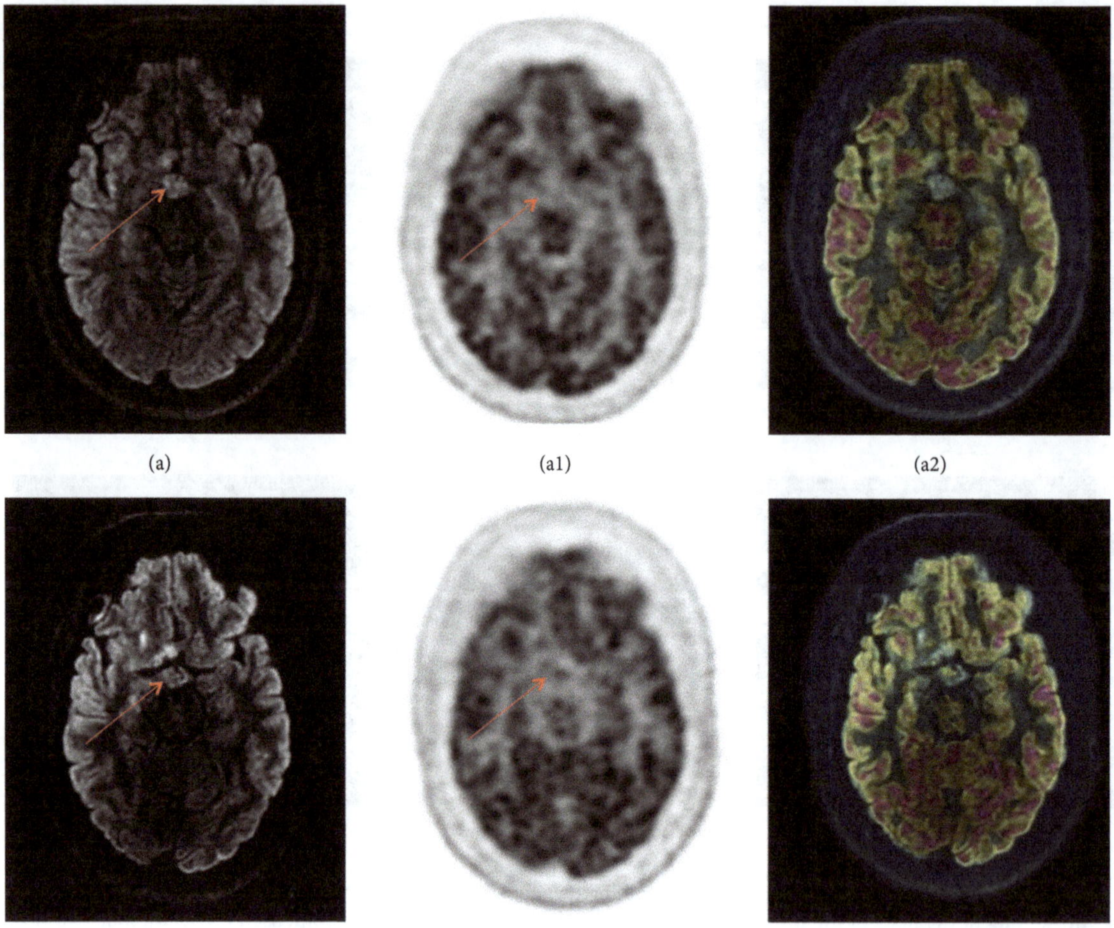

(a) (a1) (a2)

(b) (b1) (b2)

FIGURE 3: *Axial PET-MRI brain imaging.* Axial PET-MRI brain imaging with [18F]FDG at M32 (a, a1, a2) and at M35 (b, b1, b2) of follow-up.

tissues [22]. Arioglu et al. compared 24 patients with type B insulin resistance and admitted in their clinical center with representative case reports gathered from the literature [23]. Most type B insulin resistance was described in patients with systemic autoimmune diseases (especially systemic lupus erythematous) or associated with multiple myeloma and with Hodgkin's disease. All of these diseases were absent in our patient.

In our case, the positivity of anti-insulin receptor antibodies in blood and the observation of resistant hyperglycemic state despite intravenous or subcutaneous insulin therapy strongly suggested a possible causal link between these antibodies and the pathophysiology of diabetes. Accordingly, during the follow-up, we established a parallel evolution of serum insulin receptor antibodies and glucose homeostasis. In contrast, no correlation was found between serum insulin receptor antibodies (or control of diabetes) and body weight.

Whether positivity of insulin receptor antibodies and LCH is a direct relationship or a fortuitous association is not clear. Indeed, cases of diabetes mellitus associated with LCH are rare if we except a transient glycemic intolerance during corticoid steroid therapy. Among the 3200 cases in the national French LCH registry, which enrolled 56 cases of hypothalamic tumor, we failed to find any similar conditions [19, 24, 25]. In the literature, only nine cases with diabetes and LCH have been so far reported and summarized in Table 2.

As in our case, seven of these five observations have in common a diabetes insipidus as first symptom of LCH in the hypothalamic-pituitary region [7, 11–13, 15]. The onset of diabetes mellitus was described as a hyperglycemic hyperosmolar syndrome in three previously published observations [11, 12, 14]. As for our patient, hyperosmolarity was probably the consequence of massive glycosuria and polyuria, which leads to massive dehydration in a context of diabetes insipidus. In few observations, onset of diabetes was observed after a body weight gain in relation with hyperphagia when histiocytosis developed in the infundibulum as in our case [7, 11, 13, 15]. Only one publication reported massive insulin needs as observed in our case [12]. Lastly, localization of LCH in pancreas has been exceptionally observed in two cases without diabetes. Yu RC et al. reported the postmortem findings in an 18-month-old boy with infiltration of pancreas by cells with the characteristic features of LCH [9]. However, the islets of Langerhans were preserved. Muwakkit et al. published a case of disseminated LCH in a 4-week-old infant with a cystic lesion in the pancreas discovered at abdominal CT [10]. This lesion improved with systemic therapy of LCH.

TABLE 2: Characteristics and specific organ involvement of cases of diabetes mellitus associated with LCH.

Age at diagnosis of histiocytosis (years)	Sex	Diagnosis of histiocytosis	Diabetes insipidus	Delay between diagnosis of histiocytosis and diabetes	Pathophysiology of diabetes	Daily insulin needs	Reference
31	M	Bone biopsy	+	2 years	Central obesity, insulin resistance	NA	[11]
60	F	Autopsy (histiocytes cells in vertebral marrow, pituitary, lung	+	3 years	Central obesity, insulin resistance	3300 UI/day	[12]
26	M	Autopsy (histiocytes cells in pancreas)	+	2 years	Destruction of pancreatic islets by pancreas infiltration of histiocytosis	80UI/day	[7]
28	F	Lymph node biopsy	+	Few months	Central obesity, insulin resistance	NA	[13]
NA	M	Autopsy (histiocytes cells in skin, liver, bones)	-	6 months	NA	NA	[14]
54		Central nervous system, bones	+	NA	Glucocorticoids, overweight	NA	[15]
60	F	Central nervous system, bones	+	NA	Overweight	NA	[15]
54	M	Gengives	+	NA	Glucocorticoids, overweight	NA	[15]
45	F	Bones, lung, lymph nodes	-	NA	Obesity	NA	[15]

The first-line treatment used for LCH remains empirically derived chemotherapy [18], whereas cladribine has been proposed as a second-line therapy [26]. In contrast with the other cases published, we showed that therapy of LCH had beneficial effect on diabetes mellitus. The patient first received vinblastine and then cladribine as a second-line treatment because vinblastine cycles had only partial effect on brain mass volume. Cladribine therapy provided an excellent effect on brain mass volume. Improvement of glucose homeostasis (in parallel to decline of anti-insulin receptor antibodies in blood) was observed during first- and second-line therapy of LCH. Thus, it could be postulated that reduction of the brain mass volume and/or LCH activity will explain almost in part the improvement of glucose homeostasis. Nevertheless, it is difficult to determine if metabolic amelioration was a consequence of tumor shrinkage or an immune-suppressive effect but some arguments seemed to favor the latter. Indeed, recurrence of hyperglycemia exacerbation at M32 was not associated with changes of volume of the brain mass or its metabolic activity assessed by PET-MRI brain imaging with [18F]FDG. In contrast, this episode was closely correlated with the level of antibodies. Furthermore, at our knowledge, there is no publication about hypothalamic syndrome and anti-insulin receptor antibodies.

4. Conclusion

For the first time, we describe a case of LCH and diabetes and anti-insulin receptor antibodies. In this unique case, insulin resistance could be explained by presence of serum anti-insulin receptor antibodies with a direct link between anti-insulin receptor antibodies and LCH. We hypothesized that recurrent insulin resistant states can be assimilated to a paraneoplastic syndrome. We observed a positive effect of vinblastine and cladribine on glycemic control, probably explained by immune control independent of tumor size evolution.

Consent

Consent for publication has been obtained from the patient and a copy can be transferred to the editor upon request.

Authors' Contributions

Mathilde Sollier and Fabrizio Andreelli wrote the manuscript. Marine Halbron, Jean Donadieu, Ahmed Idbaih, Fleur Cohen Aubart, Marie Bastin, and Corinne Vigouroux provided critical revisions to the manuscript. Mathilde Sollier, Marine Halbron, Jean Donadieu, Ahmed Idbaih, Fleur Cohen

Aubart, Olivier Bourron, Philippe Touraine, Jacques Young, Héléna Mosbah, Agnès Hartemann, Fabrizio Andreelli, and Chloé Amouyal have been involved in the management of the patient. Jacques Young played a crucial role in the diagnosis of hypothalamic-pituitary Langerhans cells histiocytosis. Corinne Vigouroux and Martine Auclair carried out all determinations of serum anti-insulin receptor antibodies. Géraldine Béra performed PET-MRI brain imaging with [18F]FDG. All authors read and approved the final manuscript.

References

[1] J.-F. Emile, O. Abla, S. Fraitag et al., "Revised classification of histiocytoses and neoplasms of the macrophage-dendritic cell lineages," *Blood*, vol. 127, no. 22, pp. 2672–2681, 2016.

[2] J. Haroche, F. Cohen-Aubart, B. J. Rollins et al., "Histiocytoses: emerging neoplasia behind inflammation," *The Lancet Oncology*, vol. 18, no. 2, pp. e113–e125, 2017.

[3] A. Guyot-Goubin, J. Donadieu, M. Barkaoui, S. Bellec, C. Thomas, and J. Clavel, "Descriptive epidemiology of childhood Langerhans cell histiocytosis in France, 2000-2004," *Pediatric Blood & Cancer*, vol. 51, no. 1, pp. 71–75, 2008.

[4] The Writing Group of the Histiocyte Society, "Histiocytosis syndromes in children," *The Lancet*, vol. 329, no. 8526, pp. 208-209, 1987.

[5] P. Makras, K. I. Alexandraki, G. P. Chrousos, A. B. Grossman, and G. A. Kaltsas, "Endocrine manifestations in Langerhans cell histiocytosis," *Trends in Endocrinology & Metabolism*, vol. 18, no. 6, pp. 252–257, 2007.

[6] R. Goyal, A. Das, R. Nijhawan, D. Bansal, and R. K. Marwaha, "Langerhans cell histiocytosis infiltration into pancreas and kidney," *Pediatric Blood & Cancer*, vol. 49, no. 5, pp. 748–750, 2007.

[7] P. J. Hurley, G. C. Hitchcock, and J. D. Wilson, "Histiocytosis x and double diabetes," *Australasian Annals of Medicine*, vol. 16, no. 3, pp. 250–254, 1967.

[8] J. Sananes, F. Laurent, M. Joullie, B. Vergier, B. Damoo, and J. Drouillard, "Histiocytosis X revealed by pancreatic and pulmonary localisations," *European Radiology*, vol. 3, no. 5, pp. 468–470, 1993.

[9] R. C. Yu, A. Attra, C. M. Quinn, T. Krausz, and A. C. Chu, "Multisystem Langerhans' cell histiocytosis with pancreatic involvement.," *Gut*, vol. 34, no. 4, pp. 570–572, 1993.

[10] S. Muwakkit, A. Gharagozloo, A. K. Souid, and B. A. Spirt, "The sonographic appearance of lesions of the spleen and pancreas in an infant with Langerhans' cell histiocytosis," *Pediatric Radiology*, vol. 24, no. 3, pp. 222-223, 1994.

[11] I. Ben Ghorbel, M. Houman, S. B'chir, S. Chamakhi, and M. Miled, "Une forme disséminée d'histiocytose langerhansienne associant un diabète insipide et un diabète sucré," *La Revue de Médecine Interne*, vol. 22, no. 5, pp. 469–474, 2001.

[12] L. G. Rowntree and R. J. Poppiti, "Diabetes insipidus, diabetes mellitus, and insulin resistance with histiocytosis," *Journal of the American Medical Association*, vol. 156, no. 4, pp. 310–312, 1954.

[13] A. C. Thai, I. Sng, R. Suri, and J. S. Cheah, "Disseminated histiocytosis X with diabetes insipidus and diabetes mellitus in an adult female (histiocytosis with DI and DM)," *Annals, Academy of Medicine, Singapore*, vol. 17, no. 2, pp. 294–298, 1988.

[14] D. S. Trochtenberg and E. N. Dessypris, "Reversible hepatomegaly and diabetes mellitus in an adult with disseminated histiocytosis X," *The American Journal of the Medical Sciences*, vol. 299, no. 3, pp. 179–184, 1990.

[15] K. Alexandraki, P. Makras, A. Protogerou et al., "Cardiovascular risk factors in adult patients with multisystem Langerhans-cell histiocytosis: evidence of glucose metabolism abnormalities," *QJM: An International Journal of Medicine*, vol. 101, no. 1, pp. 31–40, 2007.

[16] S. Héritier, J. Emile, M. Barkaoui et al., "*BRAF* mutation correlates with high-risk langerhans cell histiocytosis and increased resistance to first-line therapy," *Journal of Clinical Oncology*, vol. 34, no. 25, pp. 3023–3030, 2016.

[17] S. Héritier, Z. Hélias-Rodzewicz, R. Chakraborty et al., "New somatic BRAF splicing mutation in Langerhans cell histiocytosis," *Molecular Cancer*, vol. 16, no. 1, p. 115, 2017.

[18] R. Haupt, M. Minkov, I. Astigarraga et al., "Langerhans cell histiocytosis (LCH): Guidelines for diagnosis, clinical work-up, and treatment for patients till the age of 18 years," *Pediatric Blood & Cancer*, vol. 60, no. 2, pp. 175–184, 2013.

[19] C. Rigaud, M. A. Barkaoui, C. Thomas et al., "Langerhans cell histiocytosis: therapeutic strategy and outcome in a 30-year nationwide cohort of 1478 patients under 18 years of age," *British Journal of Haematology*, vol. 174, no. 6, pp. 887–898, 2016.

[20] J. Maiza, M. Caron-Debarle, C. Vigouroux, and S. Schneebeli, "Anti-insulin receptor antibodies related to hypoglycemia in a previously diabetic patient," *Diabetes Care*, vol. 36, no. 6, p. e77, 2013.

[21] M. Auclair, C. Vigouroux, C. Desbois-Mouthon et al., "Anti-insulin receptor autoantibodies induce insulin receptors to constitutively associate with insulin receptor substrate-1 and -2 and cause severe cell resistance to both insulin and insulin-like growth factor I," *The Journal of Clinical Endocrinology & Metabolism*, vol. 84, no. 9, pp. 3197–3206, 1999.

[22] O. Bourron, M. Caron-Debarle, M. Hie et al., "Type B Insulin-resistance syndrome: a cause of reversible autoimmune hypoglycaemia," *The Lancet*, vol. 384, no. 9953, p. 1548, 2014.

[23] E. Arioglu, A. Andewelt, C. Diabo, M. Bell, S. I. Taylor, and P. Gorden, "Clinical course of the syndrome of autoantibodies to the insulin receptor (type b insulin resistance)," *Medicine*, vol. 81, no. 2, pp. 87–100, 2002.

[24] I. Marchand, M. A. Barkaoui, C. Garel, M. Polak, and J. Donadieu, "Central diabetes insipidus as the inaugural manifestation of langerhans cell histiocytosis: natural history and medical evaluation of 26 children and adolescents," *The Journal of Clinical Endocrinology & Metabolism*, vol. 96, no. 9, pp. E1352–E1360, 2011.

[25] S. Ng Wing Tin, N. Martin-Duverneuil, A. Idbaih et al., "Efficacy of vinblastine in central nervous system Langerhans cell histiocytosis: A nationwide retrospective study," *Orphanet Journal of Rare Diseases*, vol. 6, no. 1, p. 83, 2011.

[26] J. Donadieu, F. Bernard, M. Van Noesel et al., "Cladribine and cytarabine in refractory multisystem Langerhans cell histiocytosis: Results of an international phase 2 study," *Blood*, vol. 126, no. 12, pp. 1415–1423, 2015.

2

Asymptomatic COVID-19 as a Risk Factor of Diabetic Ketoacidosis and Mucormycosis: A Case Report and Review of the Literature

Soheila Torabiyan, Behnam Dalfardi, and Mojgan Sanjari

Endocrinology and Metabolism Research Center, Institute of Basic and Clinical Physiology Sciences, Kerman University of Medical Sciences, Kerman, Iran

Correspondence should be addressed to Mojgan Sanjari; msanjari@kmu.ac.ir

Academic Editor: Osamu Isozaki

Mucormycosis is a lethal and life-threatening fungal infection. Several cases describing the association of COVID-19 and mucormycosis have been reported. In this article, we report a 58-year-old female with a history of diabetes mellitus type 2 who presented by diabetic ketoacidosis, rhino-orbital mucormycosis, and COVID-19. The patient was treated with liposomal amphotericin B and debridement of necrotic tissue of the rhino-orbital area and paranasal sinuses. Unfortunately, she passed away a few days after orbital surgery. We also conducted a review of the literature and reported 3 other similar cases that suffered from mucormycosis in association with COVID-19 and diabetic ketoacidosis and discussed the importance of this association.

1. Introduction

Mucormycosis is an invasive and fatal fungal infection that is caused by Mucorales, an order of zygomycete fungi [1, 2]. This infection is very rare and opportunistic and most commonly seen in underlying compromising conditions such as diabetes mellitus (DM), extensive corticosteroid use, iron overload, hematologic malignancies, neutropenia, primary immunodeficiency, and treatment with immunosuppressants [1–3]. The most common forms of involvement are rhino-orbital-cerebral, pulmonary, and cutaneous [1]. Based on the site of infection and the patient's underlying predisposing condition, the all-cause mortality rate of mucormycosis may reach up to about 80%, particularly in patients with central nervous system involvement [2].

Here, we describe a type 2 DM patient who was involved with diabetic ketoacidosis (DKA), rhino-orbital mucormycosis, and COVID-19 to emphasize the point that development of opportunistic bacterial and fungal infections is a considerable event in patients with SARS-CoV-2 infection and can affect their length of hospital stay and outcome.

2. Case Presentation

A 58-year-old woman presented to the emergency department with a 4-day history of right-sided face swelling, nausea, and intractable vomiting since 2 days before hospitalization. Her past medical history included hypertension and poorly controlled insulin-dependent type 2 DM. On admission, physical examination showed a body temperature of 37.5°c (orally), pulse rate of 90 beats/minute, respiratory rate of 25 breaths/minute, blood pressure of 140/90 mmHg, and a room-air arterial oxygen saturation of 94% (by finger pulse-oximetry). In addition, unilateral swelling, erythema, and facial tenderness in the right side together with right eye proptosis were detected. The patient's right eye had no light perception and no pupillary light reflex. Neurologic examination was also suggestive of the involvement of the 3rd, 4th, and 6th cranial nerves. On admission, laboratory investigations resulted in the following values: white blood cell count ($\times10^3/\mu l$): 15; creatinine (mg/dl): 2.1; blood sugar (mg/d): 350; hemoglobin A1C (%): 8.4; C-reactive protein (mg/l): 36; urine ketone: 3+; and venous

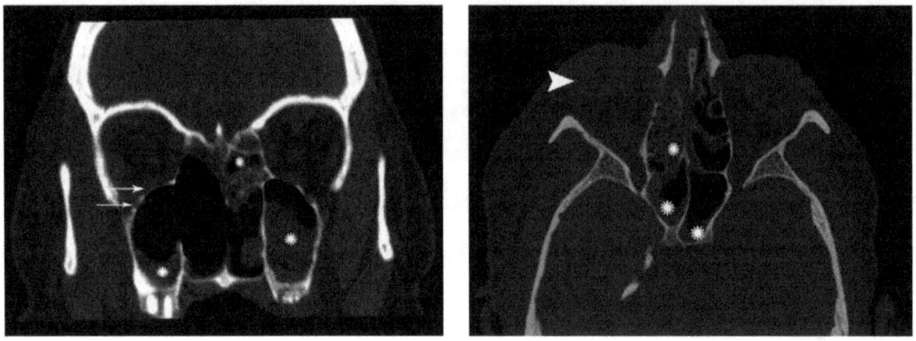

(a) (b)

FIGURE 1: (a) Destruction of orbital bone (white arrows) and sinus involvement (white asterisk). Destruction of the nasal septum is also seen. (b) Proptosis secondary to eye involvement by mucor (white arrowhead) and sinus involvement (white asterisk).

blood gas study: PH: 7.22; HCO3 (mmol/l): 11.7; PCO2 (mmHg): 27.

According to the patient's clinical scenario and the presence of hyperglycemia and metabolic acidosis, she was diagnosed as a case of diabetic ketoacidosis, and treatment with intravenous fluid and insulin was started.

Regarding the possibility of sinusitis, she underwent a noncontrast paranasal sinus and orbit computed tomographic scan (CT) (Figure 1). CT imaging revealed mucosal thickening of all paranasal sinuses, erosive bone lesions involving right-side lamina papyracea, middle and inferior turbinates, and right-side ethmoidal air-cells. All the findings were suggestive of erosive fungal sinusitis (Figure 1). For this reason, she was prepared for endoscopic sinus surgery.

Although the patient had no clinical manifestation, a screen SARS-Cov-2 PCR assay (nasopharyngeal swab test) was performed before surgery that yielded a positive result. We repeated this test for confirmation which was positive again. Noncontrast imaging of the chest was performed (Figure 2).

The patient underwent endoscopic sinus evaluation and surgery. The findings were the presence of necrotic tissue in right-side nasal cavity and paranasal sinuses, necrosis of soft palate, and involvement of the orbital wall. Therefore, debridement of necrotic tissues was carried out. Histopathological evaluation of tissue samples confirmed mucormycosis (Figure 3). Treatment with amphotericin B liposomal (6 mg/kg/day) was started, hyperglycemia was managed, and orbital exenteration surgery was performed. The patient's SARS-Cov-2 infection was asymptomatic, and her oxygen saturation was normal; therefore, according to the available guidelines, she did not receive any specific treatment for this infection.

Despite complete surgical debridement, antifungal therapy, and aggressive management of DKA, the patient showed no treatment response and unfortunately passed away two days after surgery.

Of note, informed consent was obtained from the patient's next of kin. This work was approved by the Ethical Committee of Kerman University of Medical Sciences (Code: IR.KMU.REC.1400.207).

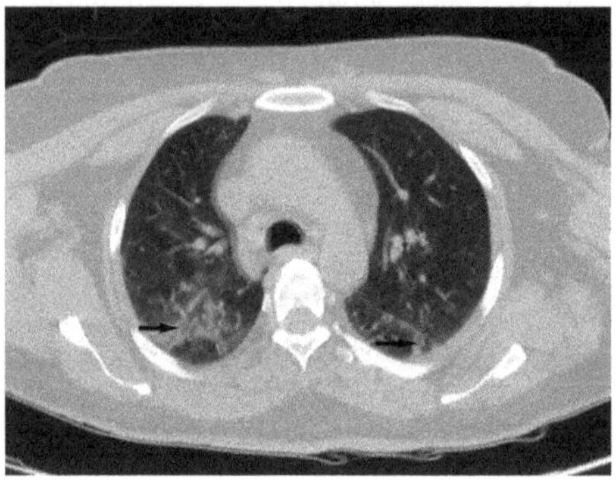

FIGURE 2: Noncontrast thoracic CT scan (axial view) showing bilateral lung infiltrations (black arrows).

3. Discussion

We presented a case of DKA and destructive sinusitis due to mucormycosis, accompanied by an asymptomatic SARS-CoV-2 infection.

More than one year passed from the emergence of COVID-19, and yet, there is no definitive and specific treatment against it [3]. Glucocorticoids and probably remdesivir are the only drugs that have efficacy in COVID-19. Glucocorticoids are inexpensive drugs and reduce mortality in hypoxemic COVID-19 patients [4, 5]. The immune suppression caused by glucocorticoids can increase the risk of different opportunistic fungal infections in cases with COVID-19. The use of other immunomodulatory drugs such as tocilizumab and immune dysregulation induced by SARS-CoV-2 virus are the other causes [4–7].

Invasive fungal infections have been reported increasingly in COVID-19 patients. We identified more than 60 cases of COVID-19 in association with mucormycosis. Mucormycosis is an invasive and life-threatening fungal infection [1]. Mucorales require iron for growth, must evade host phagocytic defense mechanisms, and access the vasculature to disseminate. In the hyperglycemic state of DKA, phagocytic activities are disturbed. In addition, due to impaired transferrin binding in hyperglycemic acidosis, free serum iron increases. Mucorales have a ketone reductase system that allows them to thrive in hyperglycemic and

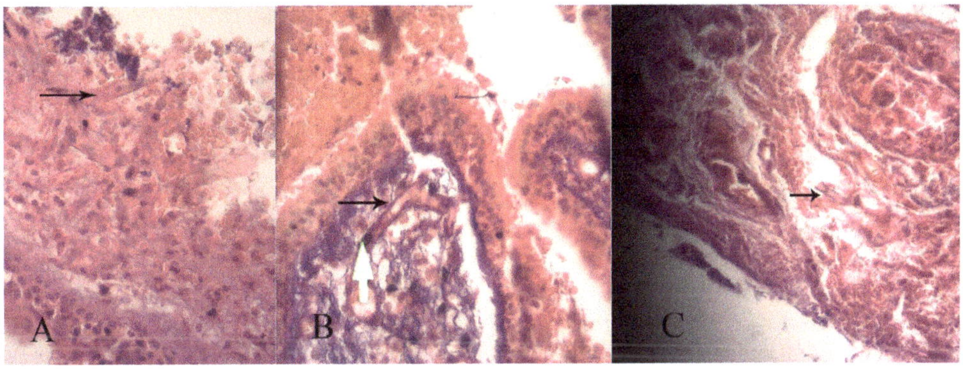

FIGURE 3: (a–c) Tissue biopsy of sinonasal tissue showing infiltration of inflammatory cells and broad-based fungal hyphae (black arrows), diagnostic for mucomycosis.

TABLE 1: Summary of reports on the four cases with COVID-19, DKA, and mucormycosis.

Author	Age in years/ sex	Comorbid illness	Clinical presentation	Treatment for COVID-19	Treatment for mucormycosis	Organ involved by mucormycosis	Outcome
Werthman Ehrenreih/ USA [9]	33/ female	HTN; asthma; undiagnosed DM	Altered mentation; proptosis; DKA; and rhino-orbital mucormycosis	Remdesivir; convalescent plasma	Amphotericin B; DKA management	Rhino-orbito-cerebral mucormycosis	Died
Waizel Haiat et al./Mexico city [10]	24/ female	Obesity	Rhino-orbital mucormycosis; DKA; COVID-19; and ARDS	No treatment	Amphotericin B; mechanical ventilation; DKA management; Imipenem; and linezolid	Rhino-orbital mucormycosis	Died
Alekseyev et al./USA [11]	41/ male	DM type 1	COVID-19 pneumonia; DKA; and rhinocerebral mucormycosis	Hydroxy chloroquine; steroid	Amphotericin B; cefepime; DKA management; and surgical debridement	Rhino-orbito-cerebral mucormycosis	Alive
Torabian et al./Iran (index case)	58/ female	DM type 2; HTN	Rhino-orbital mucormycosis DKA COVID-19 infection	No treatment	Liposomal amphotericin B; debridement of necrotic tissue; and DKA management	Rhino-orbital mucormycosis	Died

acidotic conditions, a capacity that may the higher incidence of mucormycosis in patients with diabetic ketoacidosis [8].

In our literature review, we found that, in more than 85% of these cases, mucormycosis infection occurred after COVID-19 treatment with glucocorticoids. But, only in our case and three other cases, patients had association of COVID-19 and mucormycosis in the absence of taking any treatment, including glucocorticoids, for COVID-19 (Table 1) [9–11]. In the absence of receiving any treatment for COVID-19, occurrence of mucormycosis may be due to immune dysregulation caused by SARS-CoV-2 virus or immunodeficiency related to DM that was aggravated by COVID-19 [5].

DM is a common comorbidity with COVID-19. This combination increases the possibility of complications of DM (including acute complications such as DKA), risk of secondary infections (such as mucormycosis), and patients mortality [12]. DKA is a potential lethal acute complication of DM that occurs as a result of insulin deficiency and production of ketone bodies [12, 13]. Insulin deficiency occurs more often in DM type 1 [12]. Our literature review showed several cases of DKA that were precipitated by COVID-19. Some of them reported no prior history of DM [13], and some others had a history of type 2 DM [12]. The serum level of interleukin 6 (IL6) increases in both DKA and COVID-19 and can be used as a prognostic factor [13, 14]. The interaction between COVID-19 and the rennin-angiotensin-aldosterone system (RAAS) might be another mechanism that induces DKA in COVID-19 patients [13, 15]. Angiotensin-converting enzyme 2 (ACE2) is an important and necessary enzyme in RAAS that catalyzes angiotensin type 2 to angiotensin type 1 and is highly expressed in the pancreas and lungs. It works as an entry point for COVID-19, and after endocytosis of the SARS-CoV-2 virus complex, the expression of ACE2 is reduced [13, 15, 16].

Two mechanisms may cause insulin deficiency in patients with COVID-19. First, direct invasion of SARS-CoV-2 virus may cause pancreatic damage [17]. On the other hand, reduced expression of ACE2 after virus entry can prevent insulin secretion [13, 18]. These two factors might have a role in worsening of pancreatic beta cell function and the presence of DKA in our patient.

Of the four cases reported thus far (including the index case), two cases were from the United States, one was from Mexico, and the other one (index case) was from Iran. The median age was 38.5 (24 to 58) years. Two of the cases had previously diagnosed DM, but in two other cases, DM was previously undiagnosed. Three of the cases were female, and only one was male. Acute respiratory distress syndrome (ARDS) due to COVID-19 was present in only one case. DKA was present in all of these cases. Three cases died, and one case survived.

In summary, infection with SARS-CoV-2 virus may play a triggering role for predisposing patients to DKA, particularly due to its impact on pancreatic tissue. COVID-19 and its treatment regimens may finally predispose patients to mucormycosis. Physicians should consider COVID-19 and its therapies not only as a risk factor of DKA but also for concomitant mucormycosis infection.

References

[1] A. Kanwar, A. Jordan, S. Olewiler, K. Wehberg, M. Cortes, and B. R. Jackson, "A fatal case of rhizopus azygosporus pneumonia following COVID-19," *Journal of Fungi*, vol. 7, no. 3, p. 174, 2021.

[2] O. A. Cornely, A Alastruey-Izquierdo, D Arenz et al., "Global guideline for the diagnosis and management of mucormycosis: an initiative of the European confederation of medical mycology in cooperation with the mycoses study group education and Research consortium," *The Lancet Infectious Diseases*, vol. 19, no. 12, pp. e405–421, 2019.

[3] M. Shakir, M. H. A. Maan, and S. Waheed, "Mucormycosis in a patient with COVID-19 with uncontrolled diabetes," *BMJ Case Reports*, vol. 14, no. 7, Article ID 34326123, 2021.

[4] M. Salehi, K. Ahmadikia, H. Badali, and S. Khodavaisy, "Opportunistic fungal infections in the epidemic area of COVID-19: a clinical and diagnostic perspective from Iran," *Mycopathologia*, vol. 185, no. 4, pp. 607–611, 2020.

[5] D. Garg, V. Muthu, I. S. Sehgal et al., "Coronavirus disease (Covid-19) associated mucormycosis (CAM): case report and systematic review of literature," *Mycopathologia*, vol. 186, no. 2, pp. 289–298, 2021.

[6] G. Kumar, A. Adams, M. Hererra et al., "Predictors and outcomes of healthcare-associated infections in COVID-19 patients," *International Journal of Infectious Diseases*, vol. 104, pp. 287–292, 2021.

[7] L. M. Kimmig, D. Wu, M. Gold et al., "IL-6 inhibition in critically ill COVID-19 patients is associated with increased secondary infections," *Frontiers of Medicine*, vol. 7, Article ID 583897, 2020.

[8] L. Thomas, S. Y. Tay, D. Howard, and H. Falhammar, "Mucormycosis in a 40-year-old woman with diabetic ketoacidosis," *Canadian Medical Association Journal*, vol. 192, no. 16, pp. E431–E433, 2020.

[9] A. Werthman-Ehrenreich, "Mucormycosis with orbital compartment syndrome in a patient with covid 19," *The American journal of emergency medicine*, vol. 42, pp. 264-265, 2021.

[10] S. Waizel-Haiat, A. Guerrero-Paz, L. Sanchez-Hurtado, S. Callejo-Alarcon, and L. Romero-Gutierrez, "A case of fatal rhino orbital mucormycosis associated with new onset diabetic ketoacidosis and covid 19," *Cureus*, vol. 13, no. 2, 2021.

[11] K. Alekseyev, L. Didenko, and B. Chaudhry, "Rhinocerebral mucormycosis and COVID-19 pneumonia," *Journal of Medical Cases*, vol. 12, no. 3, pp. 85–89, 2021.

[12] N. E. Palermo, A. R. Sadhu, and M. E. McDonnell, "Diabetic ketoacidosis in COVID-19: unique concerns and considerations," *Journal of Clinical Endocrinology & Metabolism*, vol. 105, no. 8, p. 360, 2020.

[13] P. K. Reddy, M. S. Kuchay, Y. Mehta, and S. K. Mishra, "Diabetic ketoacidosis precipitated by COVID-19: a report of two cases and review of literature," *Diabetes & Metabolic Syndrome: Clinical Research Reviews*, vol. 14, no. 5, pp. 1459–1462, 2020.

[14] M. Vaduganathan, O. Vardeny, T. Michel, J. J. V. McMurray, M. A. Pfeffer, and S. D. Solomon, "Renin-angiotensin-aldosterone system inhibitors in patients with covid-19," *New England Journal of Medicine*, vol. 382, no. 17, pp. 1653–1659, 2020.

[15] S. R. Bornstein, R. Dalan, D. Hopkins, G. Mingrone, and B. O. Boehm, "Endocrine and metabolic link to coronavirus infection," *Nature Reviews Endocrinology*, vol. 16, no. 6, pp. 297-298, 2020.

[16] J.-K. Yang, S.-S. Lin, X.-J. Ji, and L.-M. Guo, "Binding of SARS coronavirus to its receptor damages islets and causes acute diabetes," *Acta Diabetologica*, vol. 47, no. 3, pp. 193–199, 2010.

[17] P.-O. Carlsson, C. Berne, and L. Jansson, "Angiotensin II and the endocrine pancreas: effects on islet blood flow and insulin secretion in rats," *Diabetologia*, vol. 41, no. 2, pp. 127–133, 1998.

[18] Y. J. Chee, S. J. H. Ng, and E. Yeoh, "Diabetic Ketoacidosis precipitated by COVID-19 in a patient with newly diagnosed diabetes mellitus," *Diabetes Research and Clinical Practice*, vol. 164, Article ID 108166, 2020.

3

Prolonged Honeymoon Period in a Thai Patient with Adult-Onset Type 1 Diabetes Mellitus

Yotsapon Thewjitcharoen,[1] Ekgaluck Wanothayaroj,[1] Haruethai Jaita,[1] Soontaree Nakasatien,[1] Siriwan Butadej,[1] Ishant Khurana,[2] Scott Maxwell,[2] Assam El-Osta,[2,3,4] Waralee Chatchomchuan,[1] Sirinate Krittiyawong,[1] and Thep Himathongkam[1]

[1]*Diabetes and Thyroid Center, Theptarin Hospital, Bangkok, Thailand*
[2]*Epigenetics in Human Health and Disease Laboratory, Department of Diabetes, Central Clinical School, Faculty of Medicine Nursing and Health Sciences, Monash University, Melbourne, Australia*
[3]*Hong Kong Institute of Diabetes and Obesity, Prince of Wales Hospital, The Chinese University of Hong Kong, Hong Kong, China*
[4]*University College Copenhagen, Faculty of Health, Department of Technology, Biomedical Laboratory Science, Copenhagen, Denmark*

Correspondence should be addressed to Yotsapon Thewjitcharoen; kamijoa@hotmail.com

Academic Editor: Toshihiro Kita

Context. The "honeymoon" phase among people with type 1 diabetes mellitus (T1DM) refers to the period (mostly less than 1 year) in which beta-cells remain functional and are able to produce insulin to maintain good glycemic control shortly following the development of diabetes. This phenomenon is still not completely understood. Previous studies have shown that the absence of diabetic ketoacidosis (DKA) at initial presentation, short duration of symptoms, older age at presentation, and strenuous exercise could be potential factors that influence the honeymoon phase. *Objective.* To describe a usual case of adult-onset T1DM with prolonged honeymoon period for more than 5 years. *Methods.* Repeated mixed meal stimulation tests for a period of 6–12 months together with monitoring pancreatic autoantibodies and laboratory data were followed following the onset of diagnosis. *Results.* We report a 24-year-old Thai patient with T1DM with sustained remission without antidiabetic medication for more than 5 years while maintaining low-carbohydrate intake and regular exercise. Repeated mixed meal stimulation tests for a period of 6–12 months revealed preserved beta-cell functions. Interestingly, repeated pancreatic autoantibodies at 5 years after diagnosis still showed positive anti-GAD, anti-IA2, and anti-ZnT8. *Conclusion.* Restored beta-cell function with complete insulin withdrawal in new-onset T1DM has been reported in very few cases with some common factors as in our patient (low-carbohydrate intake with regular exercise). Delaying autoimmune activity by reducing metabolic load in newly diagnosed T1DM might play a role in maintaining the honeymoon period and could lead to an innovative therapeutic option in new-onset T1DM.

1. Introduction

Type 1 diabetes mellitus (T1DM) is heterogeneous in its presentation and progression [1]. The rate of beta-cell deterioration varies among individuals. After diagnosis, there may be a period of temporary restoration of beta-cell function that can last up to 1 year called the "honeymoon" period. This phase of remission could be found in about 50% of children diagnosed with T1DM with recent evidence suggesting that the absence of diabetic ketoacidosis (DKA) at initial presentation, short duration of symptoms, older age at presentation, and strenuous exercise could be potential factors [2–5]. Previous studies have shown residual C-peptide secretion is associated with reduced risk of serious hypoglycemic episodes and long-term diabetic complications [6]. Therefore, prolonging the honeymoon period in newly diagnosed T1DM is a topic of intense interest and research in recent years [7].

During the honeymoon phase, exogenous insulin requirement is commonly reduced to below 50% of the initial insulin dose, but complete remission (insulin independence) remains rare. Most studies were done in pediatric subgroup patients, and the standard definition of partial clinical remission identified as the insulin dose-adjusted A1C was introduced in 2009 to allow for universal consensus [8]. The honeymoon period is a critical period for employing innovative treatments targeted at preserving residual beta-cell mass [9]. Recent data also suggest that obesity in individuals with T1DM could accelerate immune-mediated beta-cell destruction at the early stage following diagnosis [10, 11]. Studying the predictive and maintenance factors in this remission phase could improve our understanding in achieving immunotolerance and the potential to reduce, retard, or cure diabetes.

Adult-onset T1DM exhibits certain unique features when compared to childhood and adolescent-onset T1DM including higher beta-cell function at the onset, slower rate of beta-cell deterioration, and lower incidence of pancreatic autoantibodies [12]. Complete insulin withdrawal in new-onset T1DM has been reported in very few cases [13–15]. Herein, we report a case of a 24-year-old Thai patient with T1DM with sustained complete remission without antidiabetic medication for more than 5 years while maintaining low carbohydrate intake and regular exercise. Repeated mixed meal stimulation test (MMST) every 6–12 months showed preserved beta-cell functions. An informed written consent was obtained from the patient for publication of this case report which has been approved by the ethics committee of Theptarin Hospital, Bangkok, Thailand.

2. Case Presentation

A 24-year-old Thai male presented with a 6-month history of polyuria, polydipsia, and weight loss of 15 kilograms (baseline body weight 83 kilograms and BMI of 27.8 kg/m^2) in March 2016. The initial laboratory data showed plasma glucose of 398 mg/dL and glycated hemoglobin (A1C) of 9.3%. No ketonemia was observed. He was diagnosed with stage 3 of type 1 DM based on clinical presentation and positive autoantibodies of protein tyrosine phosphatase (anti-IA2). Antiglutamic acid decarboxylase (anti-GAD) was negative. He did not drink alcohol or smoke and denied using any drugs. He did not have a history of excessive soft drink or overintake of sugar-containing foods. No family history of diabetes was reported. Thyroid function tests and morning plasma cortisol level were normal. Lipid profiles were all in the normal range (total cholesterol, 168 mg/dL; plasma triglyceride, 73 mg/dL; plasma HDL, 68 mg/dL; and plasma LDL, 85 mg/dL). However, euthyroid Hashimoto's thyroiditis was also diagnosed based on his enlarged thyroid gland (30 grams) and positive thyroid autoantibodies. He was started on basal-bolus insulin regimen for only 2 months, and then A1C reversed to 5.9% within that time. Insulin was gradually withdrawn and completely stopped. Oral saxagliptin 5 mg and metformin 1,000 mg was initiated.

He came to Theptarin Hospital in May 2016 to seek second opinion. Next-generation sequencing (NGS) panel for monogenic diabetes including 34 monogenic diabetes-related genes (Table 1 in Supplementary Materials) and a mitochondrial mutation for maternally-inherited deafness and diabetes (MIDD, *mt A3243G*) (GemVCare, Shatin, Hong Kong) revealed negative results. The honeymoon period of T1DM was diagnosed, and he was advised to closely monitor his capillary plasma glucose. Oral antidiabetic medications were tapered within 2 months based on normal glycemic status. In the following months, the patient maintained low-carbohydrate diet (estimated at 90–120 gram per day) and strenuous aerobic exercise to keep his BMI at less than 23 kg/m^2. He denied any supplemental or herbal medicine usage. Results of retrospective 6-day continuous glucose monitoring (CGM) system (iPro™ 2 system, Medtronic MiniMed, Northridge, CA, USA) in the second year following diagnosis confirmed normoglycemia as shown in Figure 1. MMST was firstly evaluated at the second year after diagnosis to assess the reserved beta-cell function. This procedure was done by the ingestion of 6 mL/kg of Ensure® (Abbott, Illinois, USA) (1 calorie/mL; 65% carbohydrates, 21% protein, and 14% fat) after overnight fasting. Plasma C-peptide was measured by chemiluminescent immunoassay (IMMULITE®, Siemens) which had an interassay coefficient of variation of 3.3% at plasma C-peptide of 0.6 ng/mL. The result revealed preserved beta-cell function with stimulated C-peptide at 5.5 ng/dL. The patient maintains a healthy lifestyle with low-carbohydrate intake and regular exercise 5-6 times per week. His body weight was maintained at 60–63 kilograms (BMI: 20.3–21.3 kg/m^2) during the past 5-year period. A1C was maintained between 5.0 and 6.2% without any antidiabetic medication for more than 5 years as shown in Figure 2. Serial MMST in every 6–12 months still revealed preserved beta-cell functions.

Pancreatic autoantibodies had also been monitored during follow-up in order to understand ongoing autoimmune status in this unusual patient with T1DM. Interestingly, repeated anti-IA2 at 3 years after diagnosis showed lower titer at 549.4 IU/L and then turned negative in the fourth year after diagnosis. However, anti-IA2 converted to positive again (at the titer of 315.2 IU/L) at the latest follow-up as shown in Table 1. Anti-GAD also converted to positive at low-titer (28.9 IU/mL) in the fifth year after the onset of disease, while anti-ZnT8 was still positive at the latest follow-up. The patient was advised to maintain his bodyweight and healthy behavior together with closely regular OPD follow-ups. At the last follow-up (December 2020), he remained in remission without antidiabetic medication. No ketonuria was detected during follow-up.

3. Discussion

This case report highlights the potential for altering the natural history of T1DM in some patients by maintaining low-carbohydrate diet and a healthy lifestyle. To the best of our knowledge, our case represents the longest complete remission from any antidiabetic treatments in newly

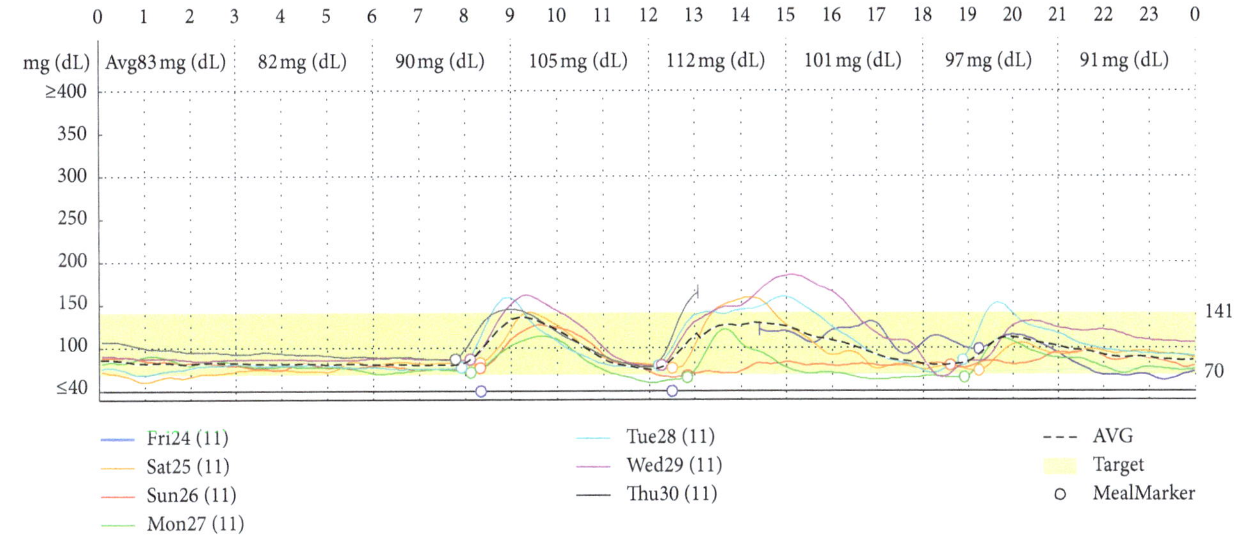

Figure 1: Results of retrospective 6-day continuous glucose monitoring (CGM) system (iPro™2 system, Medtronic MiniMed, Northridge, CA, USA) in the second year (November 2017) following diagnosis revealed normal glucose levels.

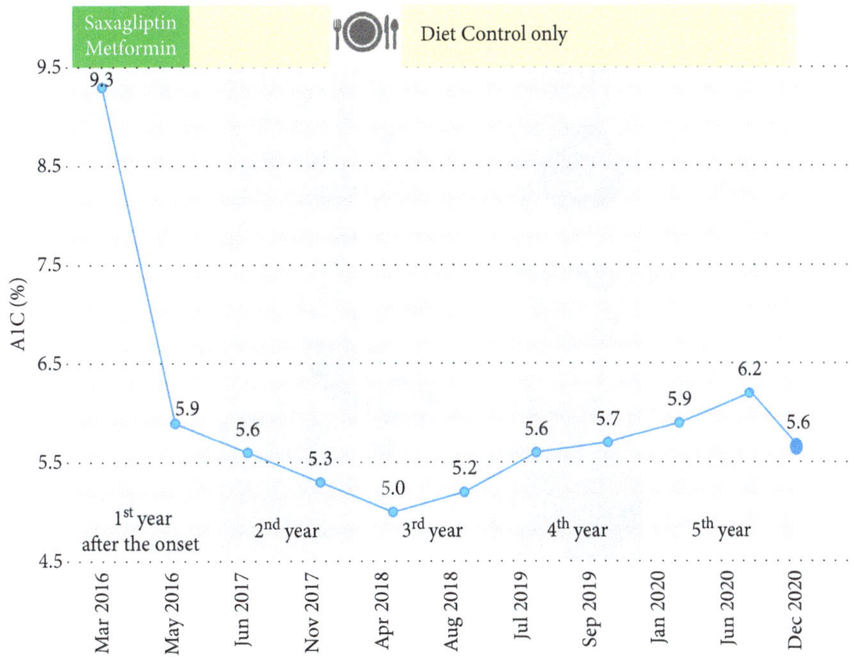

	Mar 2016	May 2016	Jun 2017	Nov 2017	Apr 2018	Aug 2018	Jul 2019	Sep 2019	Jan 2020	Jun 2020	Dec 2020
Stimulated plasma C-peptide (ng/mL)	N/A	N/A	N/A	5.5	6.3	5.5	4.8	N/A	N/A	5.2	4.9
Body Weight (kgs)	68.6	63.9	61.2	62.2	60.1	60.5	59.8	59.8	61.6	59.4	60.3

Figure 2: Clinical course and sequential laboratory data in this patient.

diagnosed people with T1DM. The honeymoon phase in this patient is sustained for more than 5 years, albeit with on-going positive pancreatic autoantibodies. The possibility of monogenic diabetes misdiagnosis was also excluded from genetic testing. This immunotolerance phenomenon is an example of metabolic flexibility and immune escape [16]. Currently, ongoing clinical trials attempt to prevent or slow disease progression by targeting immune system. However, progress and achievement remain limited.

Several other features present in this patient might also contribute to this exceptional clinical course as summarized in Figure 3. Age at the onset is a major determinant of beta-cell deterioration. Previous studies consistently confirmed that children with severe diabetic ketoacidosis at the time of diagnosis are less likely to enter a partial remission phase, reflecting more progressive and rapid destruction of beta-cell function [2–7]. During the honeymoon period, re-establishment of self-tolerance has also been shown to be

Table 1: Sequential pancreatic autoantibodies from the initial diagnosis to the fifth year of the development of T1DM.

	At the time of diagnosis (march 2016)	3rd year after the diagnosis (September 2018)	4th year after the diagnosis (January 2019)	5th year after the diagnosis (December 2020)
Anti-GAD (<5 IU/mL)	Negative	N/A	Negative	28.9
Anti-IA2 (<5 IU/mL)	>2,000	549.4	<7.5	315.2
Anti-ZnT8 (<15 IU/mL)	N/A	N/A	948	707.8

N/A: not available.

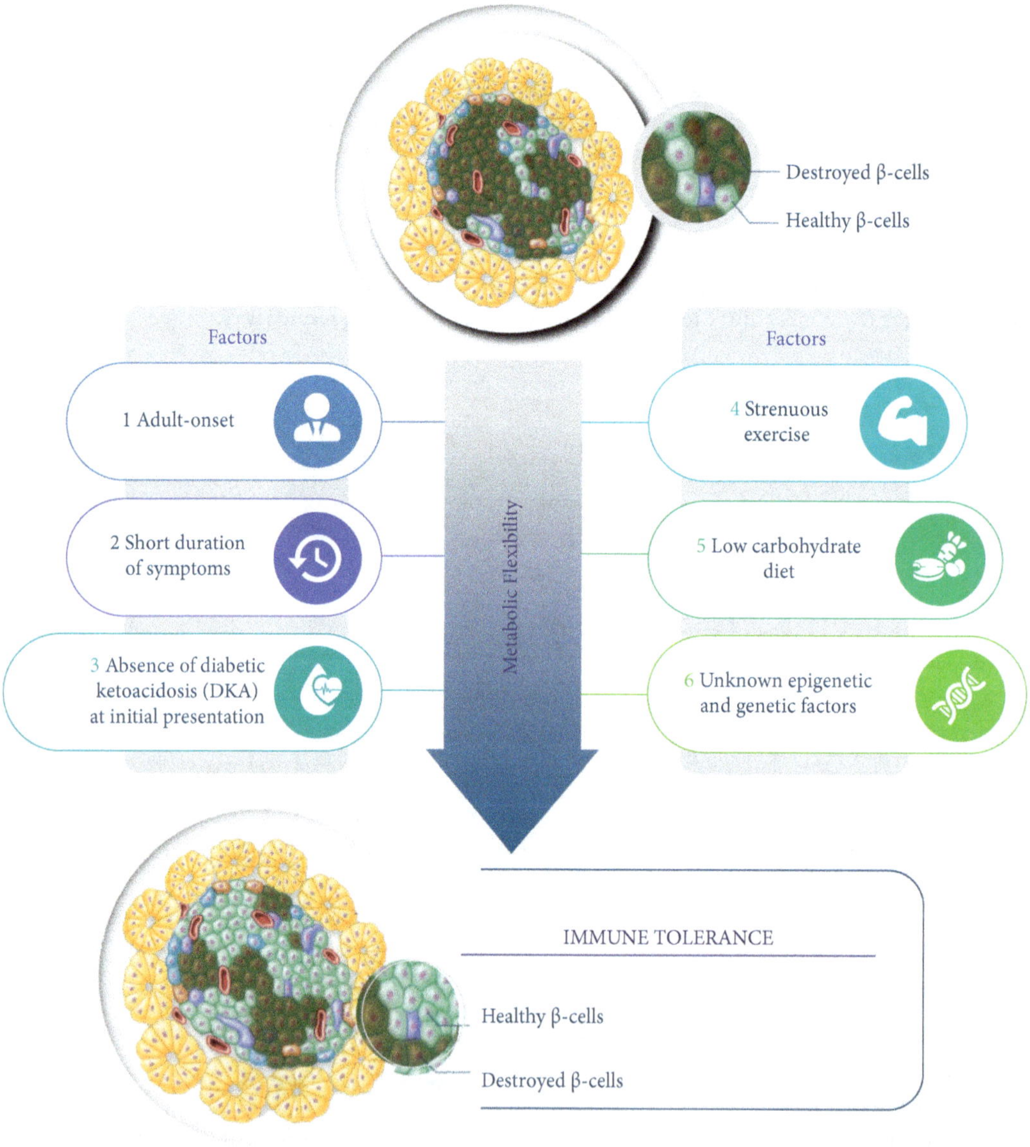

Figure 3: Postulated mechanisms of prolonged honeymoon period in this patient.

influenced by modifiable factors. Low-carbohydrate diet (less than 150 gram per day) and diet with low $n-6/n-3$ essential fatty acid ratio could prolong survival of experimental mice model with T1DM [17, 18]. Also, higher level of exercise in men with newly diagnosed T1DM showed the benefits in the extension of the honeymoon period and is five times longer when compared to sedentary men [19]. Therefore, the benefits of maintaining a healthy lifestyle following the diagnosis of T1DM should be investigated in more detail as a potential modifiable factor to delay beta-cell destruction. Nevertheless, it should be emphasized that carbohydrate should not be excessively restricted (less than 60 grams per day) in children and adolescents with T1DM given the increasing risk of eating disorders [20].

Although partial remission is well documented in T1DM, complete insulin withdrawal has been rarely reported. In reviewing literature, we found only four cases from 3 reports with complete remission of more than 1 year following the diagnosis of T1DM [13–15]. Three of the four cases were treated with oral sitagliptin as an off-label treatment. Our present case was also treated with dipeptidyl peptidase 4 (DPP-4) inhibitor (saxagliptin) for 2 months. Dietary factors and physical activity following the diagnosis of T1DM rather than initiating DPP4i in this patient might be a major factor to improve resilience toward autoimmunity. The potential immunoregulatory effects of this class of oral antidiabetic medication have been also reported in patients with latent autoimmune diabetes in adults (LADA) [21, 22]. Despite convincing clinical results using DPP-4 inhibitors to improve beta-cell function and attenuate autoimmunity in LADA, there are several differences between LADA and T1DM [23]. Further clinical studies are needed to understand the role of DPP-4 inhibitor as a disease-modifying medication in T1DM. Clinical studies on GLP-1 receptor agonists suggest possible benefit on the improvement of postprandial hyperglycemia and reduced insulin requirement in patients with T1DM. These effects were attributed to the effect of GLP-1 on gastric emptying and glucagon suppression, rather than a direct effect C-peptide release [24]. Other noninsulin adjunctive therapies for T1DM had also been extensively studied but yielded only small benefits [25].

The role of genetic and/or epigenetic factors that might influence the honeymoon phase remains poorly understood. Preclinical studies have shown changes in DNA methylation of beta-cell-specific CD8+ T cells related with the longevity of human autoreactive T-cell responses and the rate of T1DM progression [26], and this is consistent with recent studies showing immunological changes in peripheral T cells [27]. Manipulating epigenetic mechanisms in these autoreactive T cells might be one of the potential targets to reestablish self-tolerance.

4. Summary

We report an unusual case of T1DM with sustained remission of more than 5 years while a maintaining low-carbohydrate intake with regular exercise. Delaying autoimmune activity by reducing metabolic load in newly diagnosed T1DM might play a role in extending the honeymoon period together with unknown genetic and/or epigenetic factors. Longer duration of follow-up in this patient and further detailed studies in the mechanism of immune tolerance should provide an opportunity to develop innovative targets for curing or improving the prognosis of T1DM.

Disclosure

Parts of this manuscript had previously been presented as a poster at ENDO 2021, the Endocrine Society's annual meeting 2021, Virtual Meeting, and had been published as an abstract in Journal of the Endocrine Society 2021;5 (Suppl 1): A460.

Acknowledgments

The authors wish to thank the patient for allowing them to share his story with the medical community and to Dr. Tinapa Himathongkam for English language editing.

References

[1] J. T. Warshauer, J. A. Bluestone, and M. S. Anderson, "New frontiers in the treatment of type 1 diabetes," *Cell Metabolism*, vol. 31, no. 1, pp. 46–61, 2020.

[2] A. Schölin, C. Berne, E. Schvarcz, F. A. Karlsson, and E. Björk, "Factors predicting clinical remission in adult patients with type 1 diabetes," *Journal of Internal Medicine*, vol. 245, no. 2, pp. 155–162, 1999.

[3] M. Abdul-Rasoul, H. Habib, and M. Al-Khouly, "'The honeymoon phase' in children with type 1 diabetes mellitus: frequency, duration, and influential factors," *Pediatric Diabetes*, vol. 7, no. 2, pp. 101–107, 2006.

[4] P. Niedzwiecki, S. Pilacinski, A. Uruska, A. Adamska, D. Naskret, and D. Zozulinska-Ziolkiewicz, "Influence of remission and its duration on development of early microvascular complications in young adults with type 1 diabetes," *Journal of Diabetes and Its Complications*, vol. 29, no. 8, pp. 1105–1111, 2015.

[5] K. Nagl, J. M. Hermann, M. Plamper et al., "Factors contributing to partial remission in type 1 diabetes: analysis based on the insulin dose-adjusted HbA1c in 3657 children and adolescents from Germany and Austria," *Pediatric Diabetes*, vol. 18, no. 6, pp. 428–434, 2017.

[6] M. Fonolleda, M. Murillo, F. Vázquez, J. Bel, and M. Vives-Pi, "Remission phase in paediatric type 1 diabetes: new understanding and emerging biomarkers," *Hormone Research in Paediatrics*, vol. 88, no. 5, pp. 307–315, 2017.

[7] T. Zhong, R. Tang, S. Gong, J. Li, X. Li, and Z. Zhou, "The remission phase in type 1 diabetes: changing epidemiology, definitions, and emerging immuno-metabolic mechanisms," *Diabetes/metabolism research and reviews*, vol. 36, no. 2, p. e3207, 2020.

[8] H. B. Mortensen, P. Hougaard, P. Swift et al., "New definition for the partial remission period in children and adolescents with type 1 diabetes," *Diabetes Care*, vol. 32, no. 8, pp. 1384–1390, 2009.

[9] H. Aly and P. Gottlieb, "The honeymoon phase: intersection of metabolism and immunology," *Current Opinion in Endocrinology, Diabetes, and Obesity*, vol. 16, no. 4, pp. 286–92, 2009.

[10] A. Schölin, C. Törn, L. Nyström et al., "Normal weight promotes remission and low number of islet antibodies prolong the duration of remission in type 1 diabetes," *Diabetic Medicine*, vol. 21, no. 5, pp. 447–455, 2004.

[11] C. Ferrara-Cook, S. M. Geyer, C. Evans-Molina et al., "Excess BMI accelerates islet autoimmunity in older children and adolescents," *Diabetes Care*, vol. 43, no. 3, pp. 580–587, 2020.

[12] J. Karjalainen, P. Salmela, J. Ilonen, H.-M. Surcel, and M. Knip, "A comparison of childhood and adult type I diabetes mellitus," *New England Journal of Medicine*, vol. 320, no. 14, pp. 881–886, 1989.

[13] M. M. Lima-Martínez, E. Guerra-Alcalá, M. Contreras, J. Nastasi, J. A. Noble, and C. Polychronakos, "One year remission of type 1 diabetes mellitus in a patient treated with sitagliptin," *Endocrinology Diabetes and Metabolism Case*, vol. 2014, Article ID 140072, 2014.

[14] H. Moole, V. Moole, A. Mamidipalli et al., "Spontaneous complete remission of type 1 diabetes mellitus in an adult - review and case report," *Journal of Community Hospital Internal Medicine Perspectives*, vol. 5, no. 5, p. 28709, 2015.

[15] M. M. Pinheiro, F. M. Pinheiro, and M. A. Torres, "Four-year clinical remission of type 1 diabetes mellitus in two patients treated with sitagliptin and vitamin D3," *Endocrinology, Diabetes & Metabolism Case Reports*, vol. 2016, pp. 16–99, 2016.

[16] R. Tang, T. Zhong, C. Wu, Z. Zhou, and X. Li, "The remission phase in type 1 diabetes: role of hyperglycemia rectification in immune modulation," *Frontiers in Endocrinology*, vol. 10, p. 824, 2019.

[17] B. S. Lennerz, A. P. Koutnik, S. Azova, J. I. Wolfsdorf, and D. S. Ludwig, "Carbohydrate restriction for diabetes: rediscovering centuries-old wisdom," *Journal of Clinical Investigation*, vol. 131, no. 1, Article ID e142246, 2021.

[18] Y. Kagohashi and H. Otani, "Diet with a low $n-6/n-3$ essential fatty acid ratio when started immediately after the onset of overt diabetes prolongs survival of type 1 diabetes model NOD mice," *Congenital Anomalies*, vol. 50, no. 4, pp. 226–231, 2010.

[19] M. R. Chetan, M. H. Charlton, C. Thompson, R. P. Dias, R. C. Andrews, and P. Narendran, "The type 1 diabetes "honeymoon" period is five times longer in men who exercise: a case-control study," *Diabetic Medicine*, vol. 36, no. 1, pp. 127-128, 2019.

[20] C. E. Smart, F. Annan, L. A. Higgins, E. Jelleryd, M. Lopez, and C. L. Acerini, "ISPAD Clinical Practice Consensus Guidelines 2018: nutritional management in children and adolescents with diabetes," *Pediatric Diabetes*, vol. 19, no. 27, pp. 136–154, 2018.

[21] Y. Takeda, Y. Fujita, J. Honjo et al., "Reduction of both beta cell death and alpha cell proliferation by dipeptidyl peptidase-4 inhibition in a streptozotocin-induced model of diabetes in mice," *Diabetologia*, vol. 55, no. 2, pp. 404–412, 2012.

[22] Y. Zhao, L. Yang, Y. Xiang et al., "Dipeptidyl peptidase 4 inhibitor sitagliptin maintains β-cell function in patients with recent-onset latent autoimmune diabetes in adults: one year prospective study," *Journal of Clinical Endocrinology & Metabolism*, vol. 99, no. 5, pp. E876–E880, 2014.

[23] J. P. Palmer, C. S. Hampe, H. Chiu, A. Goel, and B. M. Brooks-Worrell, "Is latent autoimmune diabetes in adults distinct from type 1 diabetes or just type 1 diabetes at an older age?" *Diabetes*, vol. 54, no. 2, pp. S62–S67, 2005.

[24] M. A. Nauck and J. J. Meier, "GLP-1 receptor agonists in type 1 diabetes: a MAG1C bullet?" *The Lancet Diabetes & Endocrinology*, vol. 8, no. 4, pp. 262–264, 2020.

[25] C. S. Frandsen, T. F. Dejgaard, and S. Madsbad, "Non-insulin drugs to treat hyperglycaemia in type 1 diabetes mellitus," *The Lancet Diabetes & Endocrinology*, vol. 4, no. 9, pp. 766–780, 2016.

[26] A. E. Wiedeman, V. S. Muir, M. G. Rosasco et al., "Autoreactive CD8+ T cell exhaustion distinguishes subjects with slow type 1 diabetes progression," *Journal of Clinical Investigation*, vol. 130, no. 1, pp. 480–490, 2020.

[27] C. Bender, S. Rajendran, and M. G. von Herrath, "New insights into the role of autoreactive CD8 T cells and cytokines in human type 1 diabetes," *Frontiers in Endocrinology*, vol. 11, Article ID 606434, 2021.

4

A Dramatic Response of a Thyroid Lymphoma to R-CHOP Chemotherapy Reversing Mechanical Airway Obstruction and Respiratory Failure

Zeinab Alnahas[1] **and Mohamad H. Horani**[2]

[1]*Department of Internal Medicine, Cairo University, Giza, Egypt*
[2]*Chandler Regional Medical Center, AZ 1955 W Frye Rd, Chandler, AZ 85224, USA*

Correspondence should be addressed to Zeinab Alnahas; zeinab.elnahas@gmail.com

Academic Editor: Toshihiro Kita

Primary thyroid lymphoma is an extremely rare thyroid malignancy that usually occurs in patients with preexisting Hashimoto thyroiditis and commonly presents in older women. The most common type is non-Hodgkin's lymphoma of B-cell origin, particularly diffuse large B-cell lymphoma (DLBCL), which is primarily treated with chemotherapy and radiotherapy. We reported an 83-year-old woman with a past medical history of hypothyroidism who suffered dysphagia and dyspnea secondary to a large thyroid mass. Her CT neck scan showed an enlarged thyroid mass with pathological cervical lymphadenopathy and marked tracheal narrowing. The ultrasound-guided biopsy confirmed the diagnosis of DLBCL of the thyroid. A few days later, she experienced respiratory distress and failure that required endotracheal intubation and mechanical ventilation. She was not considered for tracheostomy or surgical interventions, and after discussion with her family, the decision was made to start R-CHOP therapy (rituximab, cyclophosphamide, doxorubicin, vincristine, and prednisone) which resulted in a marked reduction of the thyroid size and reversal of the mechanical airway obstruction, enabling her extubation. This case report demonstrated the dramatic response of a large thyroid lymphoma to R-CHOP therapy, reducing the thyroid size and its fatal obstructive complications, including mechanical airway obstruction, within a few days of the initiation of R-CHOP therapy.

1. Background

Primary thyroid lymphoma is extremely rare and accounts for <5% of all thyroid malignancies and <2% of extranodal lymphomas, with an estimated incidence of 2 per 1 million each year [1]. It usually occurs in patients with preexisting Hashimoto thyroiditis who are at 67% greater risk of developing thyroid lymphoma compared to those without thyroiditis. Primary thyroid lymphoma commonly affects women, typically between 60 and 70 years [2]. According to the 2008 World Health Organization's classification of lymphomas, almost all thyroid lymphomas are non-Hodgkin's lymphoma of B-cell origin, with diffuse large B-cell lymphoma (DLBCL) being the most common subtype accounting for 50–70%, followed by mucosa-associated lymphoid tissue (MALT) lymphoma, representing 25–30% of all thyroid lymphomas [3]. DLBCL tends to follow an aggressive course and usually presents with an enlarging anterior neck mass that might cause local obstructive symptoms in up to 30% of the patients, including dyspnea, dysphagia, hoarseness, and stridor [4]. However, B-symptoms such as fever, weight loss, and night sweats are uncommon and present in about 10% of the patients [5]. Thyroid lymphoma treatment and prognosis depend on the tumor's histology and staging. However, surgery has a limited role, and the standard treatment for thyroid lymphoma is chemotherapy and radiotherapy [6]. This case report shows a dramatic response to chemotherapy in a patient with mechanical airway obstruction due to large thyroid lymphoma, which facilitated her extubation.

2. Case Presentation

An 83-year-old woman with a past medical history significant for type 2 diabetes, coronary heart disease, and hypothyroidism controlled on L-thyroxine replacement therapy was presented with 3 months history of gradually progressive dysphagia. It was associated with left-sided neck pain with swallowing, choking on food, and shortness of breath. She denied fever, chills, or excessive sweats. Local examination of her neck revealed a large firm thyroid mass associated with left cervical lymphadenopathy. Her CT neck scan with intravenous contrast showed an enlarged, probably malignant thyroid gland with a marked amount of adjacent pathologic lymph nodes and marked transverse narrowing of the trachea to approximately 8.6 mm with no retrosternal extension (Figure 1). Also, her CT abdominal scan with intravenous contrast showed a 3.6 cm lesion of the medial right hepatic lobe (segment 8) concerning for metastases. The patient underwent an ultrasound-guided thyroid biopsy, and the results confirmed the diagnosis of DLBCL of the neck and thyroid. A few days later, the patient experienced respiratory distress and failure secondary to mechanical airway obstruction that required urgent intubation and mechanical ventilation. The discussion among different specialties, including general surgery, concluded that the patient was not a candidate for surgical intervention or tracheostomy, and recommendations were to proceed to palliative chemotherapy. She started R-CHOP chemotherapy (rituximab, cyclophosphamide, doxorubicin, vincristine, and prednisone), followed by a marked reduction in the thyroid size and relieving of the tracheal compression on the following CT neck scan (Figure 2). Her condition dramatically improved, and she was extubated after 5 days of receiving the first cycle of R-CHOP therapy.

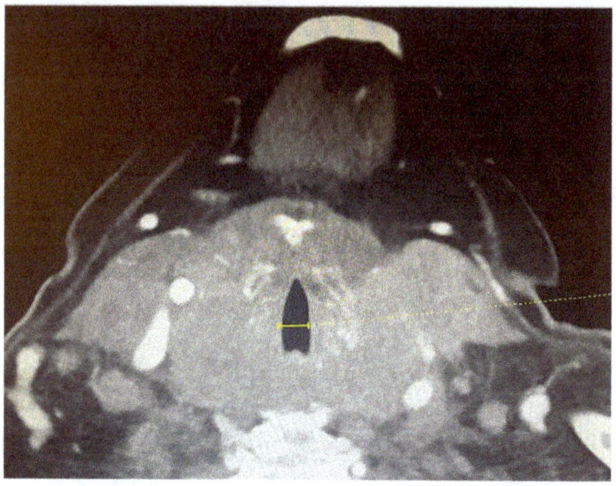

FIGURE 1: CT neck scan with contrast showed a markedly enlarged bilateral thyroid gland measured approximately 7.8 × 7.2 cm, with marked transverse narrowing of the trachea at the level of the thyroid gland to approximately 8.6 mm (solid yellow line).

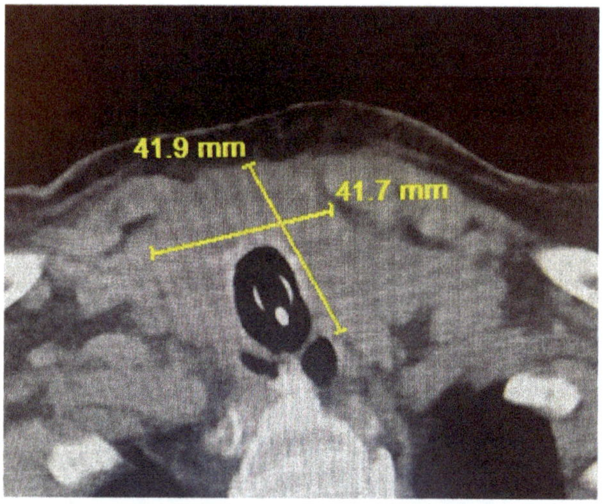

FIGURE 2: Following chemotherapy, the patient's CT neck scan with contrast showed a significant decrease in the thyroid size measured approximately 4.2 × 4.2 cm, with marked improvement in tracheal narrowing.

3. Discussion

Although the development of primary thyroid lymphoma on the top of preexisting thyroiditis is uncommon and usually occurs in 0.5% of cases, most lymphoma cases arise in a background of thyroiditis. Thyroid lymphoma should be suspected in patients with thyroiditis experiencing a rapidly enlarging neck mass [7]. Ultrasound-guided needle biopsy of the thyroid mass is the standard diagnostic testing, although in some cases, open biopsy is needed to confirm the diagnosis [1]. Pretreatment evaluation using comprehensive imaging of the chest, abdomen, and pelvis is crucial for determining the tumor staging, predicting prognosis, and establishing optimal therapeutic options [4]. Traditionally, the primary treatment for thyroid lymphomas was surgery and radiotherapy. However, due to significant relapse rate, poor survival rates, and the tumor sensitivity to chemotherapy and radiotherapy, the current standard practice, especially for DLBCL, is multimodality therapy with combination chemotherapy and loco-regional radiotherapy [8].

Multiagent chemotherapy generally includes cyclophosphamide, doxorubicin, vincristine, and prednisone (CHOP), and recently, the monoclonal anti-CD20 rituximab was added to the CHOP regimen (R-CHOP) [9]. Rituximab can act synergistically with chemotherapy and induce cell lysis of thyroid lymphoma through direct and indirect mechanisms, including induction of apoptosis, complement-mediated cytolysis, and antibody-dependent cell cytotoxicity [10]. Treatment of thyroid lymphoma with R-CHOP significantly improved the complete response rates and reduced treatment failure and relapse rates. Moreover, it increased the overall survival rates compared with CHOP alone without significant additional toxicity. In a small case series by Jonak et al. [11], who studied the effectiveness of R-CHOP therapy in elderly patients with DLBCL of the thyroid who were considered unfit for surgery or inoperable, treatment with R-CHOP resulted in complete remission of the lymphoma without evidence of disease recurrence for 2 years after initiation of the therapy [11]. In our case report, initiation of R-CHOP therapy in an elderly patient with a large thyroid lymphoma complicated by mechanical airway obstruction and respiratory failure was associated with a marked reduction in the thyroid size and reversal of the mechanical airway obstruction within a few days of receiving the first cycle of R-CHOP therapy.

4. Conclusion

Our case report demonstrates dramatic reversal of mechanical airway obstruction caused by a thyroid lymphoma within a few days of initiation of R-CHOP therapy. These cases are usually considered terminal and do not undergo aggressive surgical interventions. R-CHOP chemotherapy needs to be considered in these cases before considering hospice care.

References

[1] G. Sangalli, G. Serio, C. Zampatti, G. Lomuscio, and L. Colombo, "Fine needle aspiration cytology of primary lymphoma of the thyroid: a report of 17 cases," *Cytopathology*, vol. 12, no. 4, pp. 257–263, 2001.

[2] G. A. Derringer, L. D. R. Thompson, R. A. Frommelt, K. E. Bijwaard, C. S. Heffess, and S. L. Abbondanzo, "Malignant lymphoma of the thyroid gland," *The American Journal of Surgical Pathology*, vol. 24, no. 5, pp. 623–639, 2000.

[3] E. S. Jaffe, "The 2008 WHO classification of lymphomas: implications for clinical practice and translational research," *Hematology*, vol. 2009, no. 1, pp. 523–531, 2009.

[4] C. Onal, Y. X. Li, R. C. Miller et al., "Treatment results and prognostic factors in primary Thyroid lymphoma patients: a rare cancer network study," *Annals of Oncology*, vol. 22, no. 1, pp. 156–164, 2011.

[5] M. Alzouebi, J. R. Goepel, J. M. Horsman, and B. W. Hancock, "Primary thyroid lymphoma: the 40 year experience of a UK lymphoma treatment centre," *International Journal of Oncology*, vol. 40, no. 6, pp. 2075–2080, 2012.

[6] S. A. Stein and L. Wartofsky, "Primary thyroid lymphoma: a clinical review," *The Journal of Clinical Endocrinology & Metabolism*, vol. 98, no. 8, pp. 3131–3138, 2013.

[7] N. Watanabe, J. Y. Noh, H. Narimatsu et al., "Clinicopathological features of 171 cases of primary thyroid lymphoma: a long-term study involving 24,553 patients with Hashimoto's disease," *British Journal of Haematology*, vol. 153, no. 2, pp. 236–243, 2011.

[8] E. T. Pavlidis and T. E. Pavlidis, "A review of primary thyroid lymphoma: molecular factors, diagnosis and management," *Journal of Investigative Surgery*, vol. 32, no. 2, pp. 137–142, 2019.

[9] Y. J. Chai, J. H. Hong, D. H. Koo et al., "Clinicopathological characteristics and treatment outcomes of 38 cases of primary thyroid lymphoma: a multicenter study," *Annals of Surgical Treatment and Research*, vol. 89, no. 6, pp. 295–299, 2015.

[10] G. Cartron, H. Watier, J. Golay, and P. Solal-Celigny, "From the bench to the bedside: ways to improve rituximab efficacy," *Blood*, vol. 104, no. 9, pp. 2635–2642, 2004.

[11] C. Jonak, M. Troch, L. Müllauer, B. Niederle, M. Hoffmann, and M. Raderer, "Rituximab plus dose-reduced cyclophosphamide, mitoxantrone, vincristine, and prednisolone are effective in elderly patients with diffuse large B-cell lymphoma of the thyroid," *Thyroid*, vol. 20, no. 4, pp. 425–427, 2010.

5

Challenging Case of Ectopic ACTH Secretion from Prostate Adenocarcinoma

Wanling Zeng and Joan Khoo

Department of Endocrinology, Changi General Hospital, 2 Simei Street 3 529889, Singapore

Correspondence should be addressed to Wanling Zeng; zeng.wanling@singhealth.com.sg

Academic Editor: Toshihiro Kita

Cushing's syndrome (CS) secondary to ectopic adrenocorticotrophic hormone (ACTH)-producing prostate cancer is rare with less than 50 cases reported. The diagnosis can be challenging due to atypical and variable clinical presentations of this uncommon source of ectopic ACTH secretion. We report a case of Cushing's syndrome secondary to prostate adenocarcinoma who presented with symptoms of severe hypercortisolism with recurrent hypokalaemia, limb oedema, limb weakness, and sepsis. He presented with severe hypokalaemia and metabolic alkalosis (potassium 2.5 mmol/L and bicarbonate 36 mmol/L), with elevated 8 am cortisol 1229 nmol/L. ACTH-dependent Cushing's syndrome was diagnosed with inappropriately normal ACTH 57.4 ng/L, significantly elevated 24-hour urine free cortisol and unsuppressed cortisol after 1 mg low-dose, 2-day low-dose, and 8 mg high-dose dexamethasone suppression tests. ^{68}Ga-DOTANOC PET/CT showed an increase in DOTANOC avidity in the prostate gland, and his prostate biopsy specimen was stained positive for ACTH and markers for neuroendocrine differentiation. He was started on ketoconazole, which was switched to IV octreotide in view of liver dysfunction from hepatic metastases. He eventually succumbed to the disease after 3 months of his diagnosis. It is imperative to recognize prostate carcinoma as a source of ectopic ACTH secretion as it is associated with poor clinical outcomes, and the diagnosis can be missed due to atypical clinical presentations.

1. Introduction

Ectopic secretion of adrenocorticotropic hormone (ACTH) is responsible for approximately 10–20% of all causes of Cushing syndrome [1]. The classic sources of ectopic ACTH secretion include bronchial carcinoid tumours, small cell lung carcinoma, thymoma, medullary thyroid carcinoma (MTC), gastroenteropancreatic neuroendocrine tumours (NET), and phaeochromocytomas [2]. Ectopic adrenocorticotropic syndrome (EAS) is diagnostically challenging due to its variable clinical manifestations; however, prompt recognition and treatment is critical. Ectopic ACTH production from prostate carcinoma is rare, and there are less than 50 cases published to date. Here, we report a case of ectopic Cushing's syndrome secondary to prostate adenocarcinoma who did not present with the typical physical features of Cushing's syndrome, but instead with features of severe hypercortisolism such as hypokalaemia, oedema, and sepsis.

2. Case Presentation

A 61-year-old male presented to our institution with recurrent hypokalaemia, lower limb weakness, and oedema. He had a history of recently diagnosed metastatic prostate adenocarcinoma, for which he was started on leuprolide and finasteride. Other medical history includes poorly controlled diabetes mellitus and hypertension of 1-year duration. He presented with hypokalaemia of 2.7 mmol/L associated with bilateral lower limb oedema and weakness, initially attributed to the intake of complementary medicine, which resolved with potassium supplementation and cessation of the complementary medicine. One month later, he was readmitted for refractory hypokalaemia of 2.5 mmol/L and progression of the lower limb weakness and oedema. On examination, his blood pressure (BP) was 121/78 mmHg, and body mass index (BMI) was 24 kg/m^2. He had no Cushingoid features of rounded and plethoric facies, supraclavicular or dorsocervical fat pad, ecchymoses, and no purple striae on the abdominal examination. He had mild bilateral lower limb proximal weakness and oedema.

His initial laboratory findings of severe hypokalaemia with metabolic alkalosis (potassium 2.5 mmol/L and bicarbonate 36 mmol/L), raised 24-hour urine potassium (86 mmol/L), suppressed plasma renin activity and aldosterone, central hypothyroidism, and elevated morning serum cortisol (1229 nmol/L) (Table 1) raised the suspicion for endogenous hypercortisolism. Furthermore, hormonal evaluations confirmed ACTH-dependent Cushing's syndrome with inappropriately normal ACTH (56 ng/L) and failure of cortisol suppression after 1 mg low-dose, 2-day low-dose, and 8 mg high-dose dexamethasone suppression tests (Table 2). His 24-hour urine free cortisol (UFC) was significantly elevated at 20475 (59–413) nmol/day.

To identify the source of excessive cortisol secretion, magnetic resonance imaging (MRI) of the pituitary fossa and computed tomography (CT) of the thorax, abdomen, and pelvis were performed. Pituitary MRI was unremarkable, and CT scan showed the known prostate lesion with extensive liver, lymph nodes, and bone metastases (Figure 1). To confirm that the prostate cancer was the source of ectopic ACTH production, gallium-68 labelled somatostatin receptor positron emission tomography (PET)/CT (68Ga-DOTANOC) was done, which showed an increased DOTANOC avidity in the inferior aspect of the prostate gland (Figure 2). Immunohistochemical staining of his prostate biopsy specimen was requested, and it stained positive for ACTH and markers of neuroendocrine differentiation (synaptophysin and CD 56) (Figures 3 and 4), establishing the diagnosis of EAS secondary to prostate cancer.

The patient was started on potassium chloride 3.6 g 3 times daily and spironolactone 25 mg once daily with normalisation of serum potassium. His BP was controlled with the addition of lisinopril and terazosin to spironolactone and ketoconazole, and his blood glucose was well controlled with metformin and sitagliptin. To manage the hypercortisolism, he was treated with ketoconazole 400 mg twice daily with an initial improvement of serum cortisol from 2048 nmol/L to 849 nmol/L (Figure 5). Systemic platinum and etoposide-based chemotherapy was recommended for the treatment of his prostate cancer after a multidisciplinary discussion, but it was delayed due to severe bacterial and viral infection. With the development of liver dysfunction, ketoconazole was switched to intravenous octreotide 100 mcg three times daily as metyrapone was not readily available in our country. However, the efficacy was suboptimal with marginal reduction of serum cortisol from 3580 nmol/L to 3329 nmol/L (Figure 5). The patient continued to deteriorate and was deemed to be medically unfit for chemotherapy or bilateral adrenalectomy.

TABLE 1: Investigations done during his 2nd admission.

Renal panel	Value (normal range)
Urea	3.9 (2.7–6.9 mmol/L)
Sodium	143 (136–146 mmol/L)
Potassium	2.5 (3.6–5.0 mmol/L)
Chloride	94 (100–107 mmol/L)
Bicarbonate	36 (19.0–29.0 mmol/L)
Creatinine	41 (37–75 umol/L)
Estimated glomerular filtration rate	>90 (mL/min/1.73 m^2)
24-hour urine potassium	86 mmol/L
Hormonal workup	
Plasma renin activity	<0.6 (0.6–3.0 ng/mL/h)
Aldosterone	<4.0 (≤21 ng/dL)
8 am cortisol	1229 nmol/L
Free thyroxine	5.5 (10–20 pmol/L)
Thyroid stimulating hormone	0.378 (0.4–4.0 mIU/L)
Others	
Prostate-specific antigen	89 (0.0–4.0 ug/L)
HbA1c	9.0%

He was referred to palliative care services, and he eventually demised due to cancer progression within 3 months of his diagnosis.

3. Discussion

Ectopic ACTH secretion is an uncommon cause of Cushing's syndrome accounting for approximately 9–18% of the patients with Cushing's syndrome [3]. Clinical presentation is highly variable depending on the aggressiveness of the underlying malignancy, but patients typically present with symptoms of severe hypercortisolism such as hypokalaemiaa, oedema, and proximal weakness which were the presenting complaints of our patient [4]. The classical symptoms of Cushing's syndrome are frequently absent due to the rapid clinic onset resulting in diagnostic delay [5].

Prompt diagnosis and localisation of the source of ectopic ACTH secretion are crucial due to the urgent need for treatment initiation. The usual sources include small cell lung carcinoma, bronchial carcinoid, medullary thyroid carcinoma, thymic carcinoid, and pheochromocytoma. CT of the thorax, abdomen, and pelvis should be the first-line imaging modality, and its sensitivity varies with the type of tumour ranging from 77% to 85% [6]. Functional imaging such as 18-fluorodeoxyglucose-PET and gallium-68 labelled somatostatin receptor PET/CT can be useful in localising the source of occult EAS, determining the neuroendocrine nature of the tumour or staging the underlying malignancy [3, 6]. As prostate cancer is an unusual cause of EAS, we proceeded with 68Ga-DOTANOC PET/CT in our patient to localise the source of ectopic ACTH production.

The goals of management in EAS include treating the hormonal excess and the underlying neoplasm as well as managing the complications secondary to hypercortisolism [3]. Prompt management of the cortisol excess is paramount as complications such as hyperglycaemia, hypertension, hypokalaemia, pulmonary embolism, sepsis, and psychosis can develop especially when UFC is more than 5 times the upper limit of normal [3]. Ideally, surgical resection is the

Table 2: Diagnostic workup for hypercortisolism.

	Value (normal range)
8 am cortisol	1229 nmol/L
ACTH	56.0 (10–60 ng/L)
1 mg overnight dexamethasone suppression test	1327 nmol/L
2-day low-dose dexamethasone suppression test	1447 nmol/L
8 mg high-dose dexamethasone suppression test	1229 ≥ 1424 nmol/L
24-hour UFC	20475 (59–413 nmol/day)

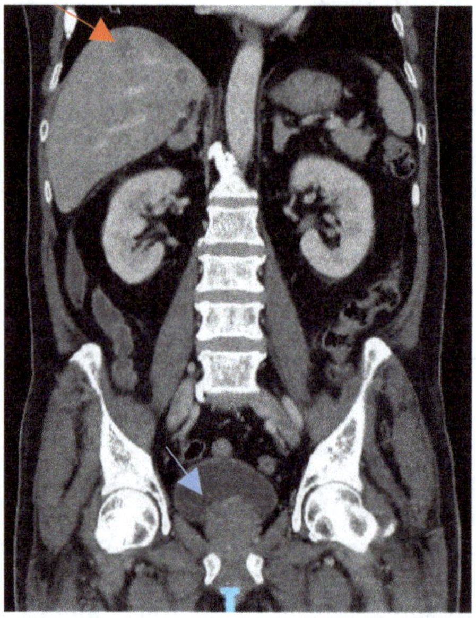

Figure 1: CT thorax abdomen and pelvis showing prostate cancer (blue arrow) with liver metastases (red arrow).

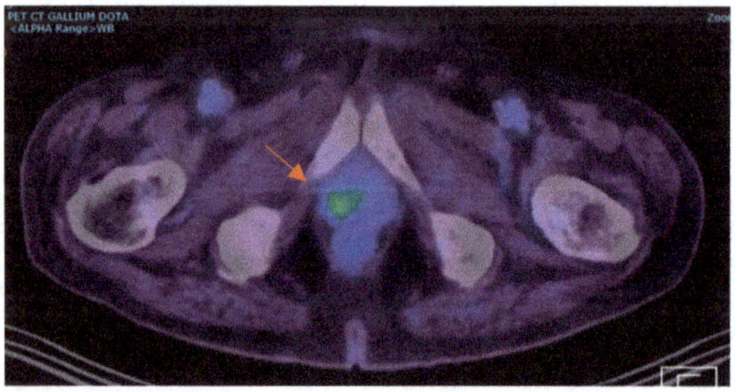

Figure 2: Ga68-DOTANOC PET/CT demonstrating increased DOTANOC avidity seen in the inferior aspect of the right side of the prostate gland (red arrow).

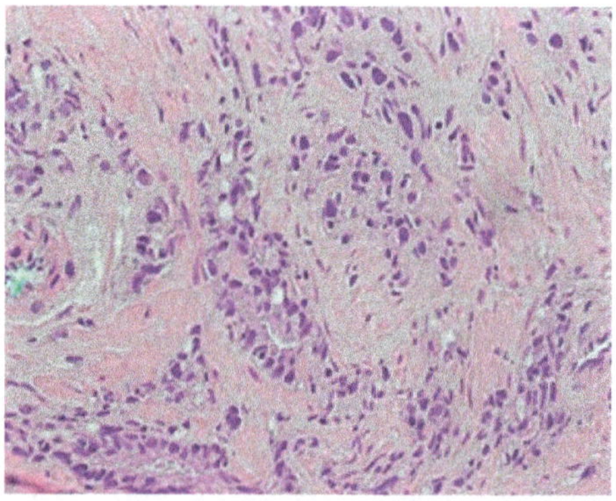

Figure 3: Hematoxylin and eosin staining showing acinar adenocarcinoma of the prostate featuring enlarged, pleomorphic cells infiltrating as solid nests and cords with poorly differentiated glands (Gleason score 5 + 4 = 9).

first-line management, but this may not be feasible in metastatic, advanced, or occult diseases.

Pharmacological agents are frequently required with steroidogenesis inhibitors such as ketoconazole and metyrapone, which reduce cortisol production effectively and rapidly [3, 6], the main drawback of ketoconazole being its hepatic toxicity. The efficacy of ketoconazole is reported to be 44%, metyrapone 50–75%, and ketoconazole-metyrapone combination therapy 73% [3, 7]. Mitotane, typically used in adrenocortical carcinoma, is effective in controlling cortisol excess but has a slow onset of action [3, 8]. Etomidate infusion can be used for short-term rapid control of severe symptomatic hypercortisolism and can serve as a bridge to definitive therapy [9]. Mifepristone, a glucocorticoid receptor antagonist, is indicated mainly in difficult to control hyperglycaemia secondary to hypercortisolism [8]. Somatostatin analogue has been proposed as a possible pharmacological therapy due to the expression of somatostatin receptors by ACTH secreting tumours [8, 10]. Bilateral adrenalectomy should be considered in patients with severe symptomatic hypercortisolism and life-threatening complications who cannot be optimally managed with medical therapies, especially in patients with occult EAS or

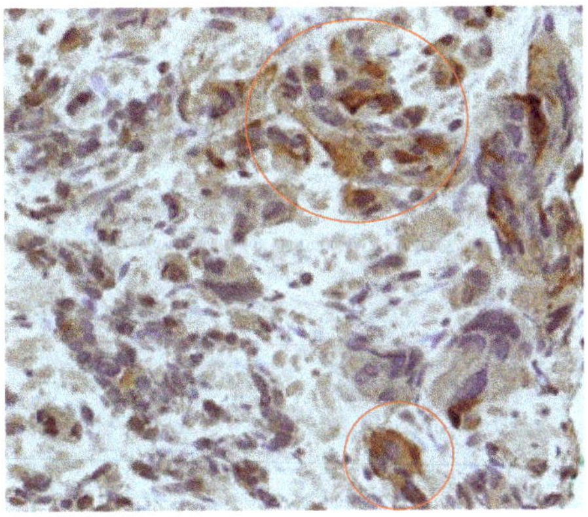

FIGURE 4: Positive ACTH immunohistochemical staining of prostate tumour (within the circle).

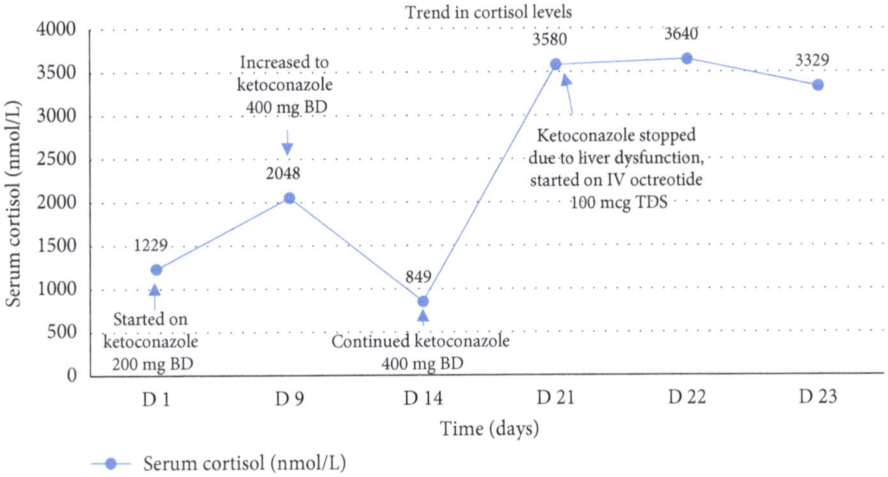

FIGURE 5: The trend in cortisol levels on pharmacological therapy.

metastatic disease [3, 8]. Bilateral adrenalectomy results in immediate improvement in cortisol levels and symptoms secondary to hypercortisolism [11]. However, surgical complications, morbidity, and mortality are high in patients with uncontrolled hypercortisolism [8], and our patient was deemed by his oncologist and surgeon to have too high a risk for bilateral adrenalectomy. For the treatment of prostate carcinoma, platinum and etoposide-based chemotherapies have been used, but their efficacy is limited with a median survival of 7.5 months [4, 12]. The side effects of chemotherapy can be severe with an enhanced risk of infection due to both cortisol and chemotherapy-mediated immunosuppression. Prompt control of hypercortisolism prior to chemotherapy and surgical procedure is strongly suggested to attenuate life-threatening complications such as infection, thrombosis, and bleeding with chemotherapy or surgery as well as to improve prognosis [3, 13].

There are rare reports of ectopic ACTH secretion from prostate carcinoma. These tumours were predominantly of small cell or mixed cell type, and pure adenocarcinoma with neuroendocrine differentiation are less common [4, 5]. There is a strong correlation between the prognosis and the types of malignancy in patients with EAS, and patients with prostate carcinoma have a poor prognosis [4]. These patients had metastatic disease at presentation, and the median survival was weeks to months despite medical treatment, chemotherapy, and even bilateral adrenalectomy [4], as seen with our patient who passed away within 3 months of his diagnosis.

In conclusion, adenocarcinoma of the prostate is a rare cause of EAS. The diagnosis and management are complex and challenging requiring specialised expertise with multidisciplinary involvement. The presentation can be atypical, and it is imperative to suspect and recognise prostate carcinoma as a source of ectopic ACTH secretion. Prompt initiation of treatment is important, as it is a rapidly progressive and aggressive disease associated with intense hypercortisolism resulting in high rates of mortality and morbidity.

Acknowledgments

The authors would like to thank the Pathology Department of Changi General Hospital for their contribution to this case.

Acknowledgments

The authors would like to thank the Pathology Department of Changi General Hospital for their contribution to this case.

References

[1] I. Ilias, D. J. Torpy, K. Pacak, N. Mullen, R. A. Wesley, and L. K. Nieman, "Cushing's syndrome due to ectopic corticotropin secretion: twenty years' experience at the national institutes of health," *Journal of Clinical Endocrinology & Metabolism*, vol. 90, no. 8, pp. 4955–4962, 2005.

[2] J. Newell-Price, P. Trainer, M. Besser, and A. Grossman, "The diagnosis and differential diagnosis of cushing's syndrome and pseudo-cushing's states," *Endocrine Reviews*, vol. 19, no. 5, pp. 647–672, 1998.

[3] J. Young, M. Haissaguerre, O. Viera-Pinto, O. Chabre, E. Baudin, and A. Tabarin, "Management of endocrine disease: cushing's syndrome due to ectopic ACTH secretion: an expert operational opinion," *European Journal of Endocrinology*, vol. 182, no. 4, pp. R29–R58, 2020.

[4] M. S. Elston, V. B. Crawford, M. Swarbrick, M. S. Dray, M. Head, and J. V. Conaglen, "Severe Cushing's syndrome due to small cell prostate carcinoma: a case and review of literature," *Endocrine Connections*, vol. 6, no. 5, pp. R80–R86, 2017.

[5] O. M. Alshaikh, A. A. Al-Mahfouz, H. Al-Hindi, A. B. Mahfouz, and A. S. Alzahrani, "Unusual cause of ectopic secretion of adrenocorticotropic hormone: cushing syndrome attributable to small cell prostate cancer," *Endocrine Practice*, vol. 16, no. 2, pp. 249–254, 2010.

[6] A. Sundin, R. Arnold, E. Baudin et al., "ENETS consensus guidelines for the standards of care in neuroendocrine tumors: radiological, nuclear medicine and hybrid imaging," *Neuroendocrinology*, vol. 105, no. 3, pp. 212–244, 2017.

[7] J.-B. Corcuff, J. Young, P. Masquefa-Giraud, P. Chanson, E. Baudin, and A. Tabarin, "Rapid control of severe neoplastic hypercortisolism with metyrapone and ketoconazole," *European Journal of Endocrinology*, vol. 172, no. 4, pp. 473–481, 2015.

[8] L. K. Nieman, B. M. K. Biller, J. W. Findling et al., "Treatment of cushing's syndrome: an endocrine society clinical practice guideline," *Journal of Clinical Endocrinology & Metabolism*, vol. 100, no. 8, pp. 2807–2831, 2015.

[9] T. B. Carroll, W. J. Peppard, D. J. Herrmann et al., "Continuous etomidate infusion for the management of severe cushing syndrome: validation of a standard protocol," *Journal of the Endocrine Society*, vol. 3, no. 1, pp. 1–12, 2019.

[10] K. Von Werder, O. A. Muller, and G. K. Stalla, "Somatostatin analogs in ectopic corticotropin production," *Metabolism*, vol. 45, pp. 129–131, 1996.

[11] N. Klomjit, D. J. Rowan, A. G. Kattah, I. Bancos, and S. J. Taler, "New-onset resistant hypertension in a newly diagnosed prostate cancer patient," *American Journal of Hypertension*, vol. 32, no. 12, pp. 1214–1217, 2019.

[12] R. Nadal, M. Schweizer, O. N. Kryvenko, J. I. Epstein, and M. A. Eisenberger, "Small cell carcinoma of the prostate," *Nature Reviews Urology*, vol. 11, no. 4, pp. 213–219, 2014.

[13] F. A. Collichio, P. D. Woolf, and M. Brower, "Management of patients with small cell carcinoma and the syndrome of ectopic corticotropin secretion," *Cancer*, vol. 73, no. 5, pp. 1361–1367, 1994.

6

Euglycemic Diabetic Ketoacidosis Secondary to Dapagliflozin in a Patient with Colon Malignancy

Eleni Papadokostaki[1] **and Evangelos Liberopoulos**[2]

[1]*Emergency Department, General Hospital of Heraklion "Venizeleio-Pananeio," Heraklion, 71409, Greece*
[2]*Department of Internal Medicine, Faculty of Medicine, University of Ioannina, Ioannina, 45110, Greece*

Correspondence should be addressed to Evangelos Liberopoulos; vaglimp@yahoo.com

Academic Editor: Mihail A. Boyanov

The use of sodium-glucose cotransporter 2 (SGLT2) inhibitors for the treatment of type 2 diabetes is steadily increasing. SGLT2 inhibitors are associated with weight loss, lowering of blood pressure, and low hypoglycemia risk along with beneficial cardiovascular and renoprotective effects. In view of the increasing use of SGLT2i, physicians must be aware of their adverse effects. Euglycemic diabetic ketoacidosis (euDKA) is a well-recognized adverse effect of SGLT2i. We present here a case of euglycemic diabetic ketoacidosis secondary to dapagliflozin use in a type 2 diabetic patient with colon cancer. To the best of our knowledge, this is first report of SGLT2 inhibitor-associated euDKA in a patient with underlying colon cancer.

1. Introduction

Diabetic ketoacidosis (DKA) is a serious acute metabolic complication of diabetes characterized by the triad of hyperglycemia (plasma glucose >250 mg/dL), metabolic acidosis (arterial pH <7.3 and serum bicarbonate <18 mEq/L), and ketosis. It usually affects people with type 1 diabetes, but type 2 diabetics are also at risk during acute illness, such as infection, trauma, or surgery [1]. Uncommonly, patients present with plasma glucose levels of less than 250 mg/dL, which is generally defined as euglycemic DKA (euDKA) [2]. Possible precipitating factors of euDKA include the recent use of insulin, decreased caloric intake, heavy alcohol consumption, chronic liver disease, and glycogen storage disorders [3]. Munro et al. first described euDKA in patients with type 1 diabetes in ketogenic stress who were vomiting or had reduced carbohydrate intake but continued to take insulin prior to presentation, as well as in pregnancy [2]. Of note, one study found no association between severity of hyperglycemia and metabolic acidosis in DKA [4].

euDKA is a well-recognized adverse effect of sodium-glucose cotransporter 2 (SGLT2) inhibitors, the newest drugs for the treatment of diabetes. Absence of hyperglycemia can delay diagnosis and treatment, thus requiring high clinical suspicion. Since their approval many cases of euDKA have been reported, prompting the FDA to issue a warning in May 2015 [5]. Here we report a type 2 diabetic patient who presented to the emergency department with euDKA secondary to dapagliflozin use.

2. Case Presentation

A 64-year-old-man presented to the Emergency Department of Venizeleio Hospital, Heraklion, Crete, with a 3 day history of nausea, vomiting, and abdominal pain. His medical history included type 2 diabetes and hypertension. He had had type 2 diabetes for 10 years and was being treated at the time with vildagliptin, metformin, and dapagliflozin. Dapagliflozin was added 8 months prior to admission. He reported a weight loss of 3 Kg following the commencing of dapagliflozin, but his weight appeared stable during the last 3 months. The A1C was 7.1% one month before admission. The patient noted that he suffered from recurrent episodes of abdominal pain the last 2 months.

At presentation the blood pressure was 130/80 mmHg, heart rate 95 beats/min, temperature 36.8°C, and oxygen saturation 98% on ambient air. The patient appeared mildly dehydrated with a BMI of 26.5 kg/m^2. The abdomen was soft with mild tenderness in the epigastrium and left upper quadrant. The remainder of the physical examination was normal.

An arterial blood gas analysis was performed and revealed metabolic acidosis pH 7.33, HCO_3^- 10.9 mEq/L, and PCO_2 21 mmHg with an increased anion gap at 29 mmol/L. Plasma glucose was mildly elevated at 203 mg/dL. Serum lactate was 1.1 mmol/L, i.e., within normal range. The rest of laboratory investigation was as follows: white blood cells 7860/μL, hemoglobin 14.8 g/dL, serum urea 84 mg/dL, serum creatinine 1.33 mg/dL, Na^+ 134 mmol/L, K^+ 4.6 mmol/L, and Cl^- 94 mmol/L. C-reactive protein level was moderately elevated at 8 mg/dL. Urinalysis showed glycosuria and ketonuria (glucose 4+, Oxone 4+). Measurement of serum ketones was not available.

The patient was diagnosed with euDKA possibly related to dapagliflozin use and was treated with intravenous fluids and insulin, with subsequent improvement of acid base disorders within the first 48 hours. He was also treated empirically with broad spectrum antibiotics. A computed tomography (CT) scan of the abdomen/pelvis with IV contrast was ordered to further evaluate the cause of the abdominal pain. The CT scan revealed ascending and transverse colonic dilatation proximal to a transition point in the splenic flexure and decompressed bowel distal to the obstruction, highly suspicious of colonic malignancy. Colonoscopy was then performed which showed splenic flexure cancer. The patient was transferred to the surgical clinic and underwent left hemicolectomy. He was discharged from the surgical clinic on the 9th postoperative day in good condition. Dapagliflozin was discontinued and basal-bolus insulin treatment was prescribed.

3. Discussion

SGLT2 inhibitors are the newest drugs for the treatment of type 2 diabetes. They act by preventing glucose reabsorption in the renal tubule, thus promoting glucosuria [6]. Their mechanism of action is independent of insulin, thus allowing their use in any stage of type 2 diabetes. Apart from their glucose-lowering action they exert some beneficial effects that make them very appealing in the treatment of diabetes. SGLT2 inhibitors are associated with a low incidence of hypoglycemia and have a favorable effect on body weight and blood pressure [7]. Moreover, cardiovascular outcomes trials (CVOTs) of empagliflozin, canagliflozin, and dapagliflozin demonstrated reduced atherosclerotic cardiovascular events in patients with established cardiovascular disease [8]. They have also showed benefits on reducing hospitalization for heart failure and progression of renal disease regardless of established atherosclerotic cardiovascular disease or history of heart failure [8]. Based on these findings American and European guidelines recommend SGLT2 inhibitors (or GLP-1 receptor agonists) with proven cardiovascular benefit for patients with type 2 diabetes and atherosclerotic cardiovascular disease (ASCVD) [9]. SGLT2 inhibitors are also recommended for patients with ASCVD in whom heart failure predominates as well as patients with chronic kidney disease [9]. SGLT2 inhibitors are also a preferable choice when weight loss is the main concern in diabetes treatment [9].

Adverse effects associated with SGLT2 inhibitors include mycotic genital infections (mostly vaginitis in women, balanitis in men) and euDKA [10]. SGLT2 inhibitors have also been associated with an increased risk of acute kidney injury, dehydration, and orthostatic hypotension [10]. Canagliflozin has been linked to lower-extremity amputations and bone fractures in some, but not all, studies [11, 12].

The mechanisms of SGLT2 inhibitor-associated euDKA are not fully elucidated. These agents decrease fasting and postprandial plasma glucose levels, which in turn decrease insulin secretion [13]. In contrast, glucagon secretion is increased as a result of diminished paracrine inhibition by insulin and the direct effect of SGLT2 inhibitors on pancreatic a-cells [14]. The lower insulin-to-glucagon ratio coupled with markedly elevated urinary glucose clearance favors ketogenesis [15]. Moreover, SGLT2 inhibitors are believed to reduce clearance of ketones by the kidneys [16]. Surprisingly, mild hyperketonemia has been proposed as one of the mechanisms responsible for the cardioprotection in the EMPA-REG OUTCOME trial [17].

Not all patients treated with SGLT2 inhibitors are susceptible to developing euDKA. Most patients with SGLT2 inhibitor-associated euDKA have type 1 diabetes or latent autoimmune diabetes in adults (LADA) or have long-standing insulin deficient type 2 diabetes and develop DKA in the presence of stress and illness [18]. In the case series from canagliflozin clinical trials, 6 of 12 patients had low C-peptide levels (≤0.51 ng/mL) and/or were positive for GAD65 antibodies [19]. Indeed, many cases of SGLT2 inhibitor-associated euDKA have occurred in individuals with presumed type 2 diabetes who were subsequently diagnosed with LADA and were positive for GAD65 antibodies [18]. Patients with type 1 diabetes have a higher risk of euDKA than those with type 2 diabetes and currently SGLT2 inhibitors are not approved for the treatment of type 1 diabetes. However, SGLT2 inhibitors have been investigated as an adjunctive therapy to insulin for patients with type 1 diabetes in clinical trials [20–22]. These trials have demonstrated increases in the absolute risk of DKA, which appear to be dose-dependent. In the EASE trials, empagliflozin improved glycemic control and weight in type 1 diabetes but increased the risk of ketoacidosis at the doses of 10 and 25 mg [22]. An international consensus on risk management of diabetic ketoacidosis in patients with type 1 diabetes treated with SGLT inhibitors has been recently published, providing data regarding the safety of SGLT inhibitors in type 1 diabetes [23].

Common precipitating factors for SGLT2 inhibitor-associated euDKA include abrupt insulin dose reduction, low caloric and fluid intake, acute illness (e.g., infection, gastroenteritis, myocardial infarction, and stroke), major surgical procedures, bariatric surgery, low carbohydrate diets, excessive alcohol intake, and prolonged starvation [24]. Under such stressful conditions, metabolism shifts from carbohydrate to fat oxidation, thereby predisposing patients treated with SGLT2 inhibitors to developing ketonemia and euDKA.

An analysis of case reports of SGLT2 inhibitor-related DKA from the FDA adverse event reporting system found an extremely wide range of age and body weight and a highly variable duration of SGLT2 inhibitor treatment before onset of DKA [25]. These data suggest that SGLT2 inhibitor-associated euDKA may not be limited to any particular demographic or comorbid subpopulation and can occur at any time of SGLT2 inhibitor use [25].

As already noted, euDKA also occurs in diabetic patients, both type 1 and type 2, who are not taking SGLT2 inhibitors. Therefore, when a patient taking an SGLT2 inhibitor presents with euDKA it cannot be known with certainty that the SGLT2 inhibitor caused euDKA in that individual. Although case reports are frequently cited to emphasize the euDKA risk with SGLT2 inhibitors, the baseline incidence of euDKA should be taken into account. Thus, true incidence in real clinical practice remains unknown.

The incidence of euDKA in randomized controlled trials of SGLT2 inhibitors with T2D is low. In the CANVAS trial a small number of events of diabetic ketoacidosis were observed with canagliflozin and placebo (0.6 vs. 0.3 participants with an event per 1000 patient years; hazard ratio, 2.33; 95% CI, 0.76 to 7.17) [11]. In EMPA-REG OUTCOME with approximately 7,000 patients, the frequency of reported events of DKA was less than 0.1% [26]. In DECLARE-TIMI 58, DKA was more common in the dapagliflozin than in placebo group (0.3% vs. 0.1%; hazard ratio, 2.18; 95% CI, 1.10 to 4.30) [27]. Data from 2 cohort studies indicate increased risk of DKA after initiation of SGLT2 inhibitors [10, 28]. A register-based cohort study from 2 countries, Sweden and Denmark, from July 2013 to December 2016, compared 17,213 new users of SGLT2 inhibitors with 17,213 new users of glucagon-like peptide 1 (GLP1) receptor agonists [10]. Use of SGLT2 inhibitors, as compared with GLP1 receptor agonists, was associated with a 2-fold increased risk of DKA [10]. A cohort study in the USA compared diabetic individuals who had newly started treatment with either an SGLT2 inhibitor or a dipeptidyl peptidase-4 (DPP4) inhibitor between April 1, 2013, and December 31, 2014. The unadjusted rate of DKA within 180 days after the initiation of an SGLT2 inhibitor was about twice the rate after the initiation of a DPP4 inhibitor before propensity-score matching to adjust for differences in individual characteristics (4.9 vs. 2.3 events per 1000 person years; HR, 2.1 (95% CI, 1.5, 2.9)). After propensity matching the hazard ratio was 2.2 (95% CI, 1.4, 3.6) [28].

The American Association of Clinical Endocrinologists and American College of Endocrinology in order to minimize the risk of SGLT2 inhibitor-associated DKA recommend stopping the SGLT2 inhibitor at least 24 hours prior to elective surgery, planned invasive procedures, or severe stressful physical activity; avoidance of abrupt insulin withdrawal or excessive dose decreases; and avoidance of excessive alcohol intake and/or very low carbohydrate or ketogenic diets [18]. Routine measurement of urine ketones is not recommended during use of SGLT2 inhibitors and can be confusing. This is because the nitroprusside reaction, which is a widely available method used to measure ketones in the urine, does not detect β-hydroxybutyrate, the predominant ketone product in ketoacidosis [1, 18]. Indeed, some investigators have recommended the use of serum β-hydroxybutyrate for diagnosis and monitoring of DKA [29]. Goldenberg et al. have also provided recommendations for prevention and diagnosis of SGLT2 inhibitor-related DKA. All patients should be educated on the signs and symptoms of DKA prior to starting an SGLT2 inhibitor. They should also be provided with clear instructions to seek medical help when they are experiencing symptoms suggestive of DKA, such as abdominal pain, nausea, vomiting, and fatigue [30].

In our patient euDKA probably developed due to acute illness because of the underlying colon malignancy and large bowel dilatation. The recurrent episodes of abdominal pain required further evaluation and led to colon malignancy diagnosis. To the best of our knowledge, this is first report of SGLT2 inhibitor-associated euDKA in a patient with underlying colon cancer. Further studies are needed to investigate whether malignancy increases the risk of euDKA when using an SGLT2 inhibitor.

4. Conclusion

SGLT2 inhibitors are generally well tolerated and make an appealing option because of their cardiovascular, renoprotective, and other benefits. euDKA is a possible adverse effect of SGLT2 inhibitors. It is important for clinicians to identify patients at risk of euDKA and provide relevant advice. A search for underlying malignancy may be warranted when no other risk factor is recognized.

References

[1] A. E. Kitabchi, G. E. Umpierrez, J. M. Miles, and J. N. Fisher, "Hyperglycemic crises in adult patients with diabetes," *Diabetes Care*, vol. 32, no. 7, pp. 1335–1343, 2009.

[2] J. F. Munro, I. W. Campbell, A. C. McCuish, and L. J. Duncan, "Euglycaemic diabetic ketoacidosis," *British Medical Journal*, vol. 2, no. 5866, pp. 578–580, 1973.

[3] A. Modi, A. Agrawal, and F. Morgan, "Euglycemic diabetic ketoacidosis: A review," *Current Diabetes Reviews*, vol. 13, no. 3, pp. 315–321, 2017.

[4] K. R. Brandt and J. M. Miles, "Relationship between severity of hyperglycemia and metabolic acidosis in diabetic ketoacidosis," *Mayo Clinic Proceedings*, vol. 63, no. 11, pp. 1071–1074, 1988.

[5] C. for D. E. and Research, "Drug Safety and Availability - FDA Drug Safety Communication: FDA revises labels of SGLT2 inhibitors for diabetes to include warnings about too much acid in the blood and serious urinary tract infections".

[6] A. A. Tahrani, A. H. Barnett, and C. J. Bailey, "SGLT inhibitors in management of diabetes," *The Lancet Diabetes & Endocrinology*, vol. 1, no. 2, pp. 140–151, 2013.

[7] B. C. Lupsa and S. E. Inzucchi, "Use of SGLT2 inhibitors in type 2 diabetes: weighing the risks and benefits," *Diabetologia*, vol. 61, no. 10, pp. 2118–2125, 2018.

[8] T. A. Zelniker, S. D. Wiviott, I. Raz et al., "SGLT2 inhibitors for primary and secondary prevention of cardiovascular and

renal outcomes in type 2 diabetes: a systematic review and meta-analysis of cardiovascular outcome trials," *The Lancet*, vol. 393, no. 10166, pp. 31–39, 2019.

[9] M. J. Davies, D. A. D'Alessio, J. Fradkin et al., "Management of hyperglycemia in type 2 diabetes, 2018. A consensus report by the american diabetes association (ADA) and the european association for the study of diabetes (EASD)," *Diabetes Care*, vol. 41, no. 12, pp. 2669–2701, 2018.

[10] P. Ueda, H. Svanström, M. Melbye et al., "Sodium glucose cotransporter 2 inhibitors and risk of serious adverse events: nationwide register based cohort study," *BMJ*, vol. 363, Article ID k4365, 2018.

[11] B. Neal, V. Perkovic, and K. W. Mahaffey, "Canagliflozin and cardiovascular and renal events in type 2 diabetes," *The New England Journal of Medicine*, 2017.

[12] M. Fralick, S. C. Kim, S. Schneeweiss, D. Kim, D. A. Redelmeier, and E. Patorno, "Fracture Risk After Initiation of Use of Canagliflozin," *Annals of Internal Medicine*, vol. 170, no. 3, p. 155, 2019.

[13] J. Rosenstock and E. Ferrannini, "Euglycemic diabetic ketoacidosis: a predictable, detectable, and preventable safety concern with SGLT2 inhibitors," *Diabetes Care*, vol. 38, no. 9, pp. 1638–1642, 2015.

[14] E. Ferrannini, E. Muscelli, S. Frascerra et al., "Metabolic response to sodium-glucose cotransporter 2 inhibition in type 2 diabetic patients," *The Journal of Clinical Investigation*, vol. 124, no. 2, pp. 499–508, 2014.

[15] E. Ferrannini, S. Baldi, S. Frascerra et al., "Shift to fatty substrate utilization in response to sodium–glucose cotransporter 2 inhibition in subjects without diabetes and patients with type 2 diabetes," *Diabetes*, vol. 65, no. 5, pp. 1190–1196, 2016.

[16] S. I. Taylor, J. E. Blau, and K. I. Rother, "SGLT2 inhibitors may predispose to ketoacidosis," *The Journal of Clinical Endocrinology & Metabolism*, vol. 100, no. 8, pp. 2849–2852, 2015.

[17] E. Ferrannini, M. Mark, and E. Mayoux, "CV protection in the EMPA-REG OUTCOME Trial: A thrifty substrate hypothesis," *Diabetes Care*, vol. 39, no. 7, pp. 1108–1114, 2016.

[18] Y. Handelsman, R. R. Henry, Z. T. Bloomgarden et al., "American association of clinical endocrinologists and American college of endocrinology position statement on the association of SGLT-2 inhibitors and diabetic ketoacidosis," *Endocrine Practice*, vol. 22, no. 6, pp. 753–762, 2016.

[19] N. Erondu, M. Desai, K. Ways, and G. Meininger, "Diabetic ketoacidosis and related events in the canagliflozin type 2 diabetes clinical program," *Diabetes Care*, vol. 38, no. 9, pp. 1680–1686, 2015.

[20] P. Dandona, C. Mathieu, M. Phillip et al., "Efficacy and safety of dapagliflozin in patients with inadequately controlled type 1 diabetes (DEPICT-1): 24 week results from a multicentre, double-blind, phase 3, randomised controlled trial," *Lancet Diabetes Endocrinol*, vol. 5, no. 11, pp. 864–876, 2017.

[21] C. Mathieu, P. Dandona, P. Gillard et al., "Efficacy and safety of dapagliflozin in patients with inadequately controlled type 1 diabetes (the depict-2 study): 24-week results from a randomized controlled trial," *Diabetes Care*, vol. 41, no. 9, pp. 1938–1946, 2018.

[22] J. Rosenstock, J. Marquard, L. M. Laffel et al., "Empagliflozin as adjunctive to insulin therapy in type 1 diabetes: the ease trials," *Diabetes Care*, vol. 41, no. 12, pp. 2560–2569, 2018.

[23] T. Danne, S. Garg, A. L. Peters et al., "International consensus on risk management of diabetic ketoacidosis in patients with type 1 diabetes treated with sodium-glucose cotransporter (SGLT) inhibitors," *Diabetes Care*, Article ID dc182316, 2019.

[24] B. M. Bonora, A. Avogaro, and G. P. Fadini, "Sodium-glucose co-transporter-2 inhibitors and diabetic ketoacidosis: A n updated review of the literature," *Diabetes, Obesity and Metabolism*, vol. 20, no. 1, pp. 25–33, 2018.

[25] G. P. Fadini, B. M. Bonora, and A. Avogaro, "SGLT2 inhibitors and diabetic ketoacidosis: data from the FDA Adverse Event Reporting System," *Diabetologia*, vol. 60, no. 8, pp. 1385–1389, 2017.

[26] B. Zinman, C. Wanner, J. M. Lachin et al., "Empagliflozin, cardiovascular outcomes, and mortality in type 2 diabetes," *The New England Journal of Medicine*, vol. 373, no. 22, pp. 2117–2128, 2015.

[27] S. D. Wiviott, I. Raz, M. P. Bonaca et al., "Dapagliflozin and cardiovascular outcomes in type 2 diabetes," *The New England Journal of Medicine*, vol. 380, no. 4, pp. 347–357, 2019.

[28] M. Fralick, S. Schneeweiss, and E. Patorno, "Risk of diabetic ketoacidosis after initiation of an SGLT2 inhibitor," *The New England Journal of Medicine*, vol. 376, no. 23, pp. 2300–2302, 2017.

[29] D. B. Sacks, M. Arnold, G. L. Bakris et al., "Guidelines and recommendations for laboratory analysis in the diagnosis and management of diabetes mellitus," *Diabetes Care*, vol. 34, no. 6, pp. e61–e99, 2011.

[30] R. M. Goldenberg, L. D. Berard, A. Y. Cheng et al., "SGLT2 inhibitor–associated diabetic ketoacidosis: clinical review and recommendations for prevention and diagnosis," *Clinical Therapeutics*, vol. 38, no. 12, pp. 2654–2664, 2016.

7

Occult Thyroid Carcinoma without Malignant Thyroid Gland Findings during Preoperative Examination: Report of Three Cases

Soji Toda,[1] Hiroyuki Iwasaki,[1] Nobuyasu Suganuma,[1] Yoichiro Okubo,[2] Hiroyuki Hayashi,[2] Katsuhiko Masudo,[3] Hirotaka Nakayama,[4] and Munetaka Masuda[4]

[1]*Department of Breast and Endocrine Surgery, Kanagawa Cancer Center, Yokohama, Japan*
[2]*Department of Pathology, Kanagawa Cancer Center, Yokohama, Japan*
[3]*Department of Breast and Thyroid Surgery, Yokohama City University Medical Center, Yokohama, Japan*
[4]*Department of Surgery, Yokohama City University School of Medicine, Yokohama, Japan*

Correspondence should be addressed to Soji Toda; s-toda@kcch.jp

Academic Editor: John Broom

Occult thyroid carcinoma preceded by clinical manifestations and findings from extrathyroidal tumors is rare. The lack of malignant findings in the thyroid during the preoperative examination makes diagnosis difficult. We encountered a 71-year-old man with a primary ectopic thyroid carcinoma causing superior vena cava syndrome. Although no malignant findings were found in the thyroid gland, biopsy of bone metastases led to the diagnosis of thyroid cancer. HE staining of bone metastases revealed nuclear features of papillary carcinoma, and immunostaining was positive for thyroglobulin and PAX-8. The second case involved an 84-year-old man with a mediastinal tumor and suspected thyroid cancer because of high thyroglobulin levels in blood. The pathological tumor finding was papillary thyroid cancer. The last case was that of a 56-year-old woman lacking preoperative thyroid examination malignant findings, but with cervical lymph node metastasis. The thyroglobulin level of the lymph node puncture fluid was useful for preoperative diagnosis. We performed total thyroidectomy plus bilateral modified neck dissection. Pathology revealed a 1 mm papillary carcinoma in the left lobe. All of these cases were difficult to diagnose. However, we combined the results of various tests such as radiographic imaging, blood tests, and immunohistological tests to diagnose our patients.

1. Introduction

Papillary thyroid cancer is the most common thyroid cancer and is likely to metastasize to the cervical lymph nodes often found in a thyroid mass. However, some thyroid cancers do not show malignant findings in the thyroid during preoperative examinations. These occult carcinomas are rare, and their diagnosis is difficult. In this paper, we report the cases of three patients with occult thyroid cancer preceded by clinical manifestations and findings from extrathyroidal tumors.

2. Case Presentation

Case 1 is a 71-year-old man who had facial edema for 9 months. He had jugular venous distention and eyelid edema. An enhanced computed tomography (CT) scan showed a 27 mm lump on the right side of the upper mediastinum, stenosis of the superior vena cava, and dilation of surrounding collateral vessels (Figure 1(a)). We diagnosed the patient as presenting superior vena cava syndrome due to superior mediastinal tumor.

Positron emission tomography-computed tomography (PET-CT) showed accumulation in the upper mediastinal tumor (SUVmax = 5.18), the left 1st and 4th ribs (SUVmax = 5.48), and lumbar vertebrae L1 and L2 (SUVmax = 7.64), but no hot spot in the thyroid (Figure 1(b)). A bone biopsy of the lumbar vertebrae revealed atypical epithelial cells with a follicular structure and nuclear groove on HE staining, and immunostaining was positive for thyroglobulin and PAX-8 (Figure 2), indicating the presence of a bone metastasis of papillary thyroid carcinoma.

Cervical ultrasonography showed no obvious malignancy in the thyroid. Tumor markers and thyroid function

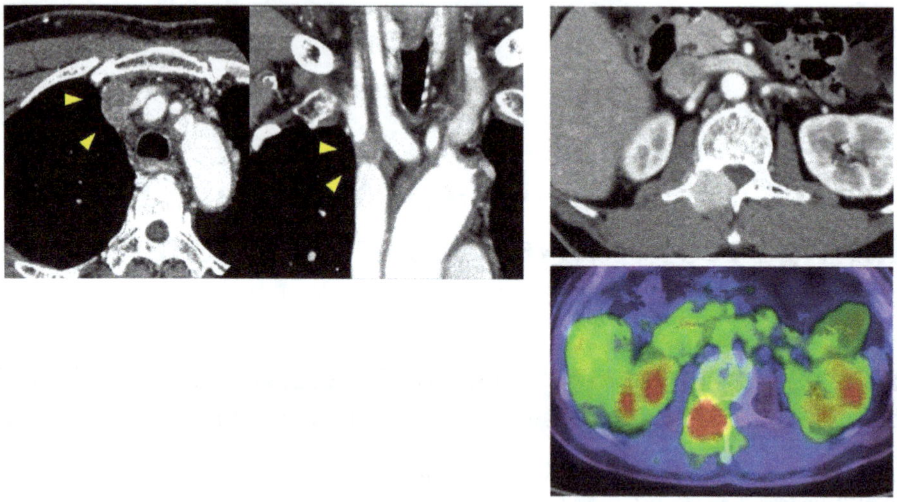

(a) (b)

FIGURE 1: CT and PET-CT findings. (a) Computed tomography showing a 27 mm lump on the right side of the upper mediastinum that is invading the superior vena cava. (b) PET-CT showing metastasis of the lumbar vertebrae.

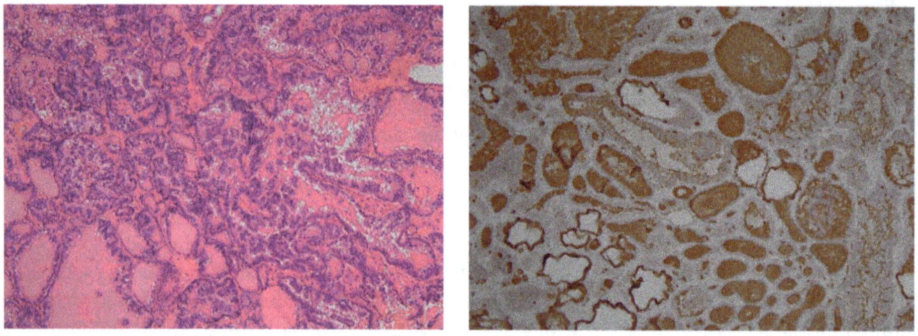

(a) (b)

FIGURE 2: Bone biopsy results of the lumbar vertebrae. HE staining showing a papillary structure and positive immunohistochemistry for thyroglobulin. (a) HE staining ×100. (b) Immunohistochemistry for thyroglobulin ×100.

tests were almost normal without thyroglobulin elevation (103 ng/mL).

We performed total thyroidectomy to administer radioiodine therapy and to reveal any primary tumor present in the thyroid. However, we found no papillary carcinoma in the gland.

The mediastinal tumor seemed to be firmly attached to the superior vena cava, and congestion was strong because of superior vena cava syndrome. Therefore, removing the superior mediastinal tumor or obtaining a biopsy was impossible. However, we suspected that the upper mediastinal tumor was the primary site because we found no other tumors. After surgery, we performed radioactive iodine (RAI) therapy as planned. A dosage of 100 mCi was administered to the patient. Although we observed uptake into the thyroid floor, we found no evidence of uptake into the mediastinum or bone. The thyroglobulin decreased to 26.1 ng/mL after RAI therapy. One year after surgery, there was no tumor growth and the superior vena cava syndrome was improving with the development of collateral circulation.

Case 2 is an 84-year-old man without remarkable medical history other than hyperlipidemia and prostatic hyperplasia. His chief complaint was cough, and an X-ray image showed an abnormal shadow on the upper mediastinum. A CT scan showed a 7.2 cm large mixed mass with a papillary solid component in the anterior mediastinum, and the trachea was compressed to the right and back. We could not confirm continuity with the thyroid; we found no lymph node metastases (Figure 3).

A PET-CT showed accumulation in the upper mediastinal tumor (SUVmax = 46.32) and pale nodules in the left

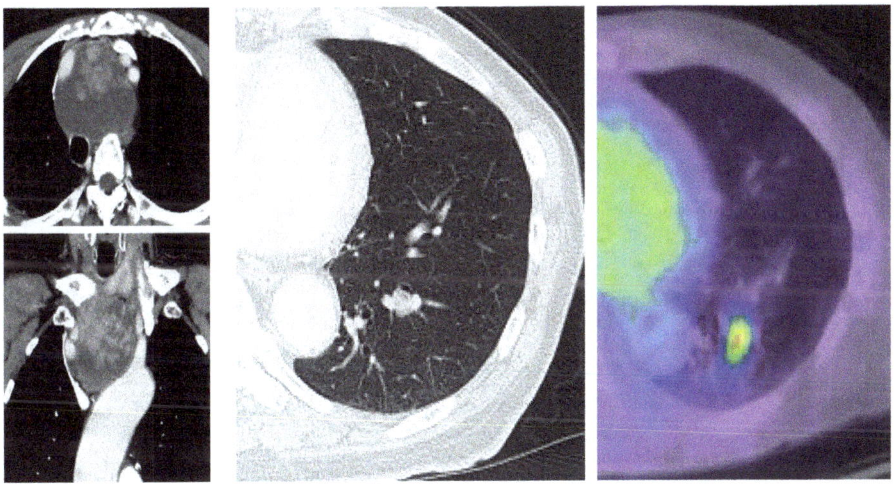

(a) (b)

FIGURE 3: CT images. (a) 7.2 cm mass in the anterior mediastinum. (b) Pulmonary metastasis.

lower lobe (SUVmax = 5.23; Figure 3). Neck ultrasonography revealed multiple nodules reminiscent of an adenomatous goiter in both lobes with no malignant appearance (the mediastinal tumors could not be visualized, and their continuity with the thyroid was unclear).

We performed endobronchial ultrasound-guided transbronchial needle aspiration (EBUS-TBNA) for diagnosis of the mediastinal tumor, but found no tumor cells, and the tumor's origin remained unknown.

In blood tests, the thyroid function was normal, but the thyroglobulin level rose to 2450 ng/mL. No other tumor markers were significant. We suspected that the mediastinal tumor originated from a thyroid cancer, and we decided to resect it.

The patient underwent total thyroidectomy, central neck dissection, and mediastinal tumor resection with sternal incision.

The mediastinal tumor adhered to the brachiocephalic artery and the right recurrent nerve on the right side, with the trachea and esophagus on the dorsal side and with the left recurrent laryngeal nerve on the left side. On the caudal side, a part of the thymus was resected together because the tumor also adhered to it.

Pathological findings included a fibrotic capsule and marked internal necrosis. The pathological report suggested a papillary carcinoma because of the preponderance of papillary growth and the presence of a papillary carcinoma nucleus (nuclear groove; Figure 4). We found no evidence of continuity between the mediastinal tumor and the thyroid. In addition, we noticed a 9 mm nodule in the isthmus of the thyroid and a nuclear finding of papillary carcinoma. We considered the nodule to represent a metastasis to the thyroid. We found no lymph node metastases. The thyroglobulin level decreased to 25.7 ng/mL after surgery. Administration of 131-iodine (100 mCi) resulted in strong accumulation in the thyroid bed and weak accumulation in lung metastasis. Therefore, we plan to follow-up the RAI therapy.

Case 3 is a 56-year-old woman without remarkable medical history. Her chief complaint was a neck mass. We found swelling of the lateral cervical lymph nodes upon examination. Neck ultrasonography showed no thyroid malignancies. Contrast-enhanced CT showed a hepatic hemangioma only, without findings suggesting a primary site (Figure 5). Upper gastrointestinal endoscopy and transvaginal ultrasonography were both normal.

Blood tests showed no tumor marker or thyroid function abnormalities, the thyroglobulin level was 37.9 ng/mL, and anti-thyroglobulin antibody was negative. Fine needle aspiration cytology of the lymph node revealed an adenocarcinoma without nuclear findings of papillary carcinoma. However, the thyroglobulin value of the puncture fluid was high (>500 ng/mL).

Since we suspected a cervical lymph node metastasis of thyroid cancer, we performed total thyroidectomy plus bilateral modified neck dissection to look for the primary tumor and for RAI therapy. A search through the excised thyroid with 4 mm slices revealed 1 mm of papillary carcinoma in the left lobe. We found metastases in 11 of 31 lymph nodes, with a maximum diameter of 23 mm. The metastatic lymph nodes had nuclear findings of papillary thyroid carcinoma (Figure 6).

The patient is considered to be at an ATA intermediate risk as she exhibited clinical N1 within all involved lymph nodes of <3 cm at their largest dimension [1]. She was recommended postoperative RAI, but she refused this procedure. TSH suppression therapy was performed, and TSH was suppressed under 0.1 μU/ml. Thyroglobulin levels decreased to <1 ng/mL following surgery. The patient did not experience recurrences up to 4 postoperative years.

3. Discussion

Occult thyroid carcinoma is a general term indicating clinically different situations that can be classified into five types as described below:

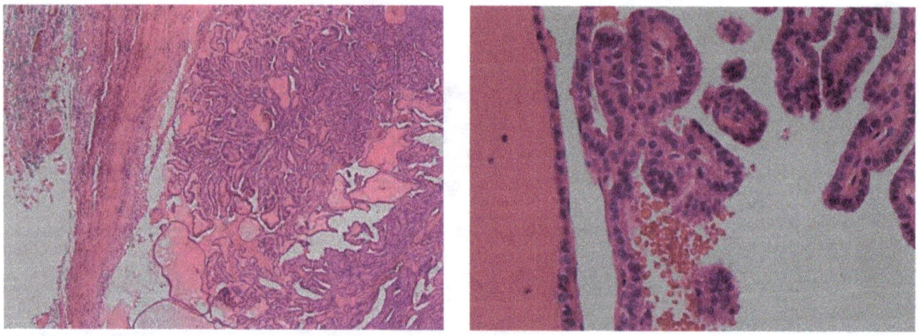

(a) (b)

Figure 4: Pathology results for a tumor. Mediastinal tumor growing in papillary shape with a fibrotic capsule. Tumor cells have nuclear groove and inclusion body (HE staining). (a) ×20. (b) ×400.

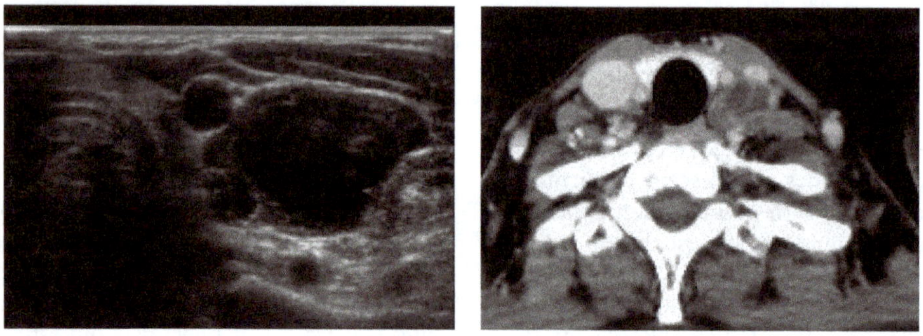

(a) (b)

Figure 5: Left lateral cervical lymph node imaging. Neck ultrasonography (a) and CT scan (b) images showing cervical lymph node swelling.

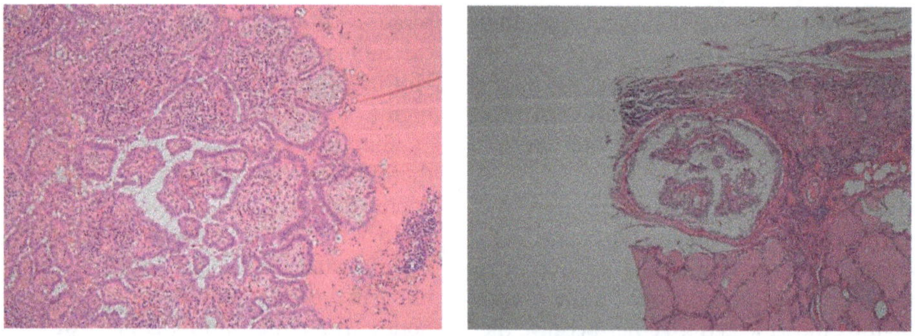

(a) (b)

Figure 6: Microscopic pathology slides of left cervical lymph nodes. (a) Left cervical lymph nodes had nuclear findings of papillary thyroid carcinoma. (b) 1 mm papillary carcinoma tumor in the left lobe (HE staining ×100).

Type 1 is sometimes found by autopsy or surgery for a benign lesion and is sometimes called latent cancer. Type 2 is a papillary thyroid microcarcinoma (PTMC) detected accidentally, mainly by ultrasonography. Type 3 is found with clinically apparent metastases of thyroid carcinoma, where the primary carcinoma is not detectable before surgery but is found in the final histological specimen. Type 4 originates from an ectopic thyroid gland. Type 5 has no carcinoma in the thyroid gland, only metastasis, also known as primary unknown cancer [2, 3].

The frequency of type 2 PTMC has increased because of improvements in diagnostic techniques such as ultrasonography [4], but the frequency of type 3 seems to have decreased. In addition, types 3, 4, and 5 are difficult to diagnose because no preoperative examination shows malignant thyroid findings. Therefore, these three types of occult cancer are clinically problematic. Of the three cases that we have encountered, patients with type 4 (cases 1 and 2) originated from ectopic thyroid gland tissue, and with type 3 (case 3) in an occult thyroid cancer. All of these are very rare cases.

Ultrasonography and fine needle aspiration cytology are useful and recommended for the diagnosis of thyroid cancers [1]. However, these diagnostic procedures are difficult in ectopic thyroid glands in the mediastinum because of anatomical complexity (presence of bones and lungs). We have encountered and reported two cases of patients with mediastinal tumors that were not thyroid cancers and were diagnosed after biopsy by bronchoscopy, immunohistological examination for PAX-8, thyroglobulin, and TTF-1 [5].

In case 1, we detected a papillary thyroid cancer from a bone metastasis biopsy. HE staining revealed an atypical epithelium and nuclear groove with follicular structure, and immunostaining was positive for thyroglobulin and PAX-8. Thus, we diagnosed the patient as having a metastasis of papillary thyroid cancer. The mediastinal tumor had displaced the superior vena cava, and the patient presented a superior vena cava syndrome. We thought that our patient presented a high bleeding risk because of the invasion of the superior vena cava and development of collateral circulation, and we decided not to resect the mediastinal tumor. We considered this ectopic thyroid as the primary tumor site because of the absence of another primary lesion (including in the thyroid gland).

In case 2, we performed EBUS-TBNA for a mediastinal tumor, but were not able to reach a diagnosis. We suspected a thyroid cancer because of the image findings and high blood thyroglobulin level. Thus, we performed both total thyroidectomy and mediastinal tumor resection by sternotomy. The mediastinal tumor pathological findings suggested a papillary thyroid cancer. A small papillary carcinoma was found in the thyroid gland, but the tumor volume was clearly smaller than the mediastinal tumor, and we think that the mediastinal tumor was the primary ectopic thyroid cancer.

Thus, we diagnosed the ectopic thyroid cancer by combining radiographic findings and immunostaining of specimens obtained by biopsy or surgery.

On the other hand, in case 3, we found no papillary thyroid cancer characteristics by cytology of the cervical lymph nodes. However, after measuring the thyroglobulin value of the puncture fluid, we found an adenocarcinoma derived from the thyroid gland. Uruno et al. reported that the measurements of thyroglobulin in the puncture fluid are useful for diagnosing cervical lymph node metastases in differentiated thyroid cancers [6]. Our results with case 3 support this idea. In addition, pathological examination of the thyroid gland after total thyroidectomy revealed a primary tumor in the thyroid gland, but its tumor size was so small that preoperative ultrasonography did not detect it.

Occult thyroid cancers in cervical lymph node metastases are intermediate to high risk, and RAI ablation should be considered [7]. If present in other metastases, RAI is recommended because distant metastases are considered an ATA high risk [1]. In cases where occult thyroid cancer is suspected, the metastasis site should be removed if possible for diagnostic and therapeutic purposes, and total thyroidectomy should be considered to allow for RAI, even if no thyroid gland findings are present.

Although few such cases have been reported, occult carcinoma exhibiting cervical cystic lymph node metastasis as the first manifestation has been reported. Verge et al. described seven papillary thyroid carcinomas that were discovered following a solitary lateral cervical cyst, and reported that ipsilateral modified neck dissection and total thyroidectomy followed by radioactive iodine therapy offered a favorable prognosis [8]. However, pathologic N1 with any metastatic lymph node >3 cm at its largest dimension is described as a high risk for ATA. When a tumor is discovered with cervical lymph node metastasis, the tumor size of lymph node metastasis is expected to be large. In high-risk cases, recurrence should be monitored, just as with regular PTC.

Occult papillary thyroid cancer is rare, and diagnosis is often impossible by ultrasonic examination or puncture aspiration cytology alone. Combining radiographic images, blood tests, immunohistological tests, and clinical signs is necessary. If occult thyroid cancer is suspected, total thyroidectomy should be considered even in the absence of malignant thyroid findings.

Acknowledgments

The authors would like to thank Enago (http://www.enago.jp) for editing a draft of this manuscript.

References

[1] B. R. Haugen, E. K. Alexander, K. C. Bible et al., "American thyroid association management guidelines for adult patients with thyroid nodules and differentiated thyroid cancer: the American thyroid association guidelines task force on thyroid nodules and differentiated thyroid cancer," *Thyroid*, vol. 26, no. 1, pp. 1–133, 2015.

[2] H. Liu, L. Lv, and K. Yang, "Occult thyroid carcinoma: a rare case report and review of literature," *International Journal of Clinical & Experimental Pathology*, vol. 7, no. 8, pp. 5210–5214, 2014.

[3] J. Boucek, J. Kastner, J. Skrivan et al., "Occult thyroid carcinoma," *Acta Otorhinolaryngologica Italica*, vol. 29, no. 6, pp. 296–304, 2009.

[4] L. Enewold, K. Zhu, E. Ron et al., "Rising thyroid cancer incidence in the United States by demographic and tumor characteristics, 1980–2005," *Cancer Epidemiology Biomarkers & Prevention*, vol. 18, no. 3, pp. 784–791, 2009.

[5] H. Yamazaki, H. Iwasaki, Y. Okubo et al., "Two cases of thyroid gland invasion by upper mediastinal carcinoma," *Endocrinology, Diabetes & Metabolism Case Reports*, vol. 2019, 2019.

[6] T. Uruno, A. Miyauchi, K. Shimizu et al., "Usefulness of thyroglobulin measurement in fine-needle aspiration biopsy specimens for diagnosing cervical lymph node metastasis in patients with papillary thyroid cancer," *World Journal of Surgery*, vol. 29, no. 4, pp. 483–485, 2005.

[7] Y. Ito, M. Hirokawa, M. Fukushima et al., "Occult papillary thyroid carcinoma: diagnostic and clinical implications in the era of routine ultrasonography," *World Journal of Surgery*, vol. 32, no. 9, pp. 1955–1960, 2008.

[8] J. Verge, J. Guixa, M. Alejo et al., "Cervical cystic lymph node metastasis as first manifestation of occult papillary thyroid carcinoma: report of seven cases," *Head & Neck*, vol. 21, no. 4, pp. 370–374, 1999.

8

A Unique Case of IGF-2 Induced Hypoglycemia Associated with Hepatocellular Carcinoma

Prachi Rana [1] **and Brian Kim** [2]

[1]*Department of Internal Medicine, Los Angeles County Hospital/University of Southern California, USA*
[2]*Department of Gastroenterology and Liver Diseases, Los Angeles County Hospital/University of Southern California, USA*

Correspondence should be addressed to Prachi Rana; prachirana02@gmail.com

Academic Editor: Lucy Mastrandrea

Tumor-induced hypoglycemia (TIH) associated with hepatocellular carcinoma (HCC) results from tumor production of insulin-like growth factor 2 (IGF-2), resulting in recurrent hypoglycemia. Serum levels of insulin-like growth factor 1 (IGF-1), insulin-like growth factor 2 (IGF-2), or pro-insulin-like growth factor 2 (pro-IGF-2) are required for the diagnosis. However, due to the limited availability of testing in many laboratories, this condition is often overlooked. As this condition is often overlooked, prompt recognition and implementation of tumor directed therapies and/or systemic therapies can help mitigate the consequences of hypoglycemia. We present a 38-year-old man with advanced multifocal HCC who presented with abdominal pain and was found to have recurrent symptomatic hypoglycemia. Evaluation revealed elevated levels of IGF-2, suggesting a diagnosis of HCC with production of IGF-2.

1. Introduction

Tumor-induced hypoglycemia (TIH) is a rare cause of hypoglycemia and is most commonly associated with tumor hyperinsulinism. However, TIH has been recently linked to nonislet-cell tumor hypoglycemia (NICTH) due to the production of insulin-like growth factor 1 (IGF-1), insulin-like growth factor 2 (IGF-2), autoantibodies to insulin, extrapancreatic insulinomas, or glucagon-like peptide (GLP1) [1]. We discuss a case of hepatocellular carcinoma (HCC) producing IGF-2. Although the exact incidence is unknown, it is generally associated with solid tumors of mesenchymal or epithelial origin with HCC being the most common cause of epithelial tumors [2]. Other malignant tumors associated with IGF-2 include leiomyosarcoma, fibrosarcoma, adrenal carcinoma, pheochromocytoma, and renal sarcoma [1]. This rare condition offers several diagnostic challenges due to the limited availability of testing for IGF-1, IGF-2, and pro-IGF-2. However, due to the rising incidence of chronic liver disease and HCC, this case highlights the importance of considering IGF-2 induced hypoglycemia in the differential for a patient presenting with recurrent hypoglycemia in the setting of known malignancy.

2. Case Presentation

We present a 38-year-old man with a history of alcoholic cirrhosis and newly diagnosed hepatocellular carcinoma who presented with sudden onset of abdominal pain. He presented with similar symptoms to another institution 2 months prior, and was diagnosed with HCC. Shortly thereafter, he underwent one round of chemoembolization though the specifics of his prior treatment were unknown. He remained asymptomatic until he presented to our emergency department with sudden onset of right upper quadrant abdominal pain. Past medical and social histories were significant for chronic alcohol use and alcoholic cirrhosis diagnosed several years prior. Upon arrival, a multiphase abdominal computed tomography (CT) scan demonstrated multifocal HCC with local invasion of the right hepatic vein and right portal vein (Figures 1 and 2). CT of the thorax showed no signs of distant metastatic disease. During his hospitalization, he experienced 40–50 episodes of symptomatic and asymptomatic hypoglycemia (38–67 mg/dL) requiring intravenous dextrose administration. There was initial concern for severe hypoglycemia due to prolonged food intolerance in the setting of poor appetite. However, after

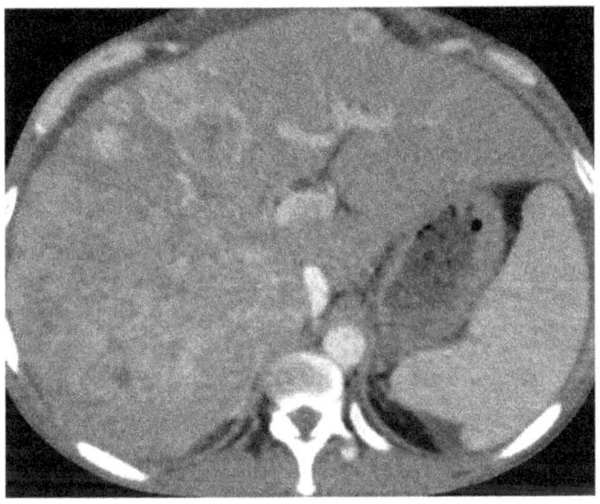

Figure 1: Multiphase abdominal computed tomography: Axial view through the liver showing extensive multifocal HCC.

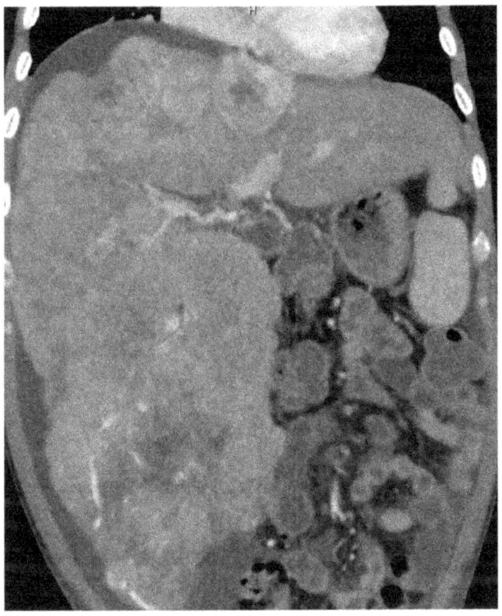

Figure 2: Multiphase abdominal computed tomography: Coronal view through the liver showing extensive multifocal HCC.

several episodes of hypoglycemia, further evaluation was pursued. Assessment revealed a normal morning cortisol level of 14.6 mcg/dL (normal 4.8–19.5 mcg/dL) and a mildly elevated thyroid stimulating hormone (TSH) level of 6.04 uIU/mL (normal 0.5–3.5 uIU/mL) with a normal free thyroxine level of 1.65 ng/dL (normal 0.93–1.7 ng/dL). Levels of insulin <0.4 uIU/mL (normal 2.6–24.9 uIU/mL) and C-peptide <0.1 ng/mL (normal 1.1–4.4 ng/mL) measured during an episode of hypoglycemia were low, indicating hypoinsulinemic hypoglycemia. The patient had no history of diabetes mellitus and was not on oral hypoglycemic agents. Two random levels of IGF-2 were elevated at 531 ng/mL and 535 ng/mL (normal 38–267 ng/mL) suggesting a diagnosis of HCC with production of IGF-2.

Hypoglycemia was initially treated with intravenous dextrose infusion. After work-up revealed elevated IGF-2 levels, nasogastric tube with enteral feeds and prednisone 40 mg/day were initiated, and he had no further episodes of hypoglycemia. Given his extensive tumor burden, he was started on immunotherapy with nivolumab. Shortly after completing his first treatment with nivolumab, he opted to pursue home hospice and passed away.

3. Discussion

The liver is the principal organ responsible for the production of IGF-1, IGF-2 and its regulating binding proteins, and insulin-like growth factor binding proteins (IGFBP). As demonstrated in murine models, TIH associated with IGF-2 is caused by the overexpression of the IGF-2 gene by the tumor, leading to an elevation of IGF-2 or its precursor pro- or big-IGF-2 [3]. The IGF-2 gene is structurally homologous to insulin and maintains insulin-like activity [1]. In a healthy individual, pro-IGF-2 accounts for 10–20% of the total IGF-2, while it accounts for 60–80% of the IGF-2 in a patient with NICTH [4]. Pro-IGF-2 and IGF-2 suppress both insulin and growth hormone (GH), which in turn decreases the production of IGF-1 and IGFBP-3, the principal binding protein for IGF-2. Furthermore, pro-IGF-2 inherently binds to IGFBP-3 poorly, thereby further increasing the availability of pro-IGF-2 to stimulate insulin receptors and glucose uptake. Continued stimulation of insulin receptors suppresses free fatty acid release and inhibits gluconeogenesis, glycogenolysis, and ketogenesis by the liver, further exacerbating hypoglycemia [1, 2, 4].

Evaluation of hypoglycemia will reveal low levels of insulin, pro-insulin, C-peptide, and β-hydroxybutyrate. Levels of GH and IGF-1 will also be low due to the suppressive effects of IGF-2. Total IGF-2 may be elevated or normal, while pro-IGF is elevated. The ratio of pro-IGF-2/IGF-2 and IGF-2/IGF-1 is usually elevated 3 : 1, and it may be helpful in cases where levels of IGF-2 are within the normal range (Figure 3). A ratio greater than 10 : 1 of IGF-2/IGF-1 is nearly diagnostic [2, 5, 6].

Initial management of hypoglycemia in NICTH is aimed at achieving and maintaining euglycemia. Supplementation with enteral and/or parenteral nutrition should be initiated promptly to prevent life threatening complications of severe hypoglycemia. Management of an IGF-2 producing tumor with surgical resection can potentially resolve hypoglycemia [2, 7, 8]. For patients with advanced disease, radiation, and/or chemotherapy have been shown to reduce hypoglycemia, although to a lesser degree [7]. When hypoglycemia persists after surgery, radiation, and/or chemotherapy, medical therapy with glucocorticoids or recombinant GH have been utilized. Glucocorticoids act by promoting hepatic gluconeogenesis, promoting lipolysis, and reducing peripheral glucose uptake. Glucocorticoids also help to decrease the levels of pro-IGF-2 either by decreased tumor production or increased clearance. Nevertheless, the effects of glucocorticoids are variable among patients, requiring close titration, and therapy is ineffective when it is discontinued. Recombinant GH functions similarly by increasing gluconeogenesis and glycogenolysis [2, 9].

Although NICTH is a rare cause of TIH, there is a well-established association between mesenchymal and epithelial tumors and production of IGF-2. Given the mortality associated with severe hypoglycemia, there should be a high clinical suspicion for hypoinsulinemic hypoglycemia in patients with recurrent hypoglycemia in the presence of known malignancy.

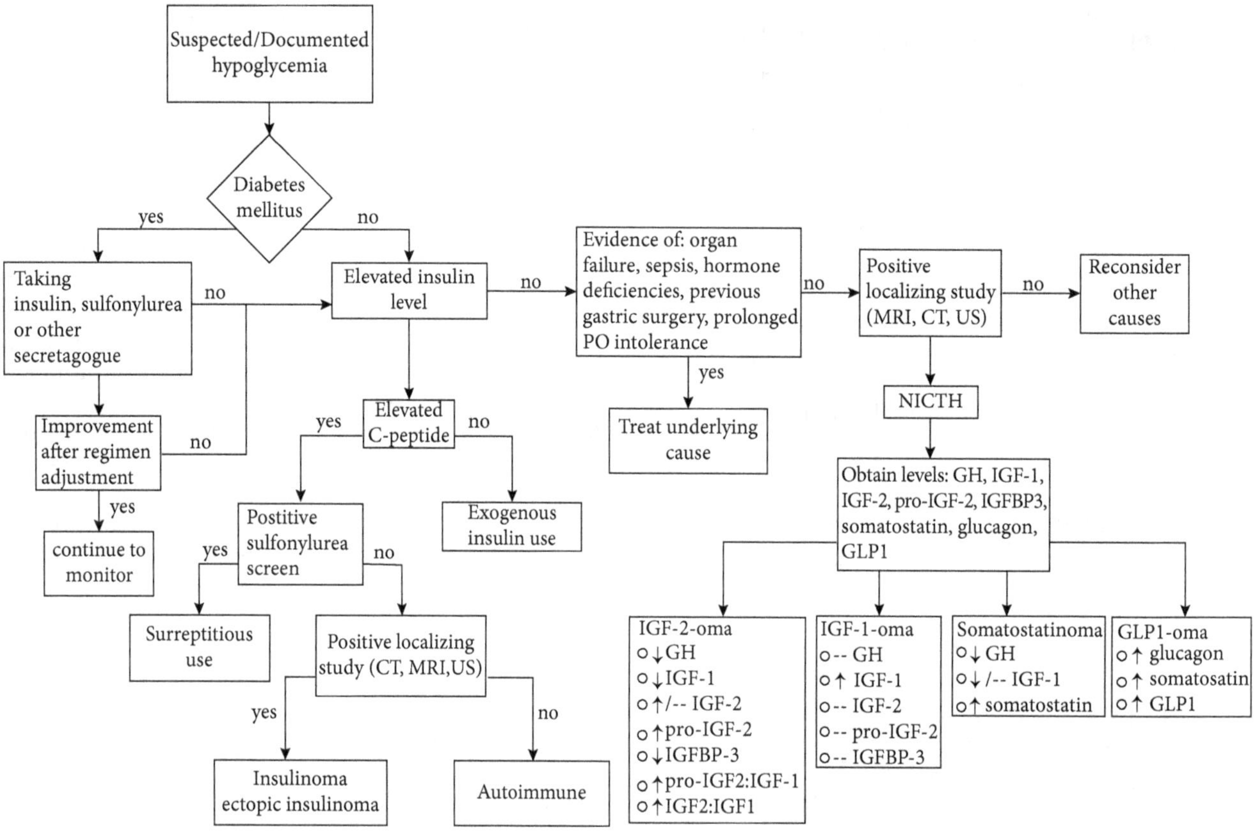

FIGURE 3: Diagnostic algorithm for patients with hypoglycemia. CT: computed tomography; MRI: magnetic resonance imaging; US: ultrasonography; GH: growth hormone; IGF: insulin-like growth factor; IGFBP: insulin-like growth factor binding protein; GLP: glucagon-like peptide; NICTH: non-islet cell tumor hypoglycemia; -- normal levels.

Ethical Approval

Our institution does not require ethical approval for reporting individual cases or case series.

Consent

Verbal informed consent was obtained from a legally authorized representative for anonymized patient information to be published in this article.

Authors' Contributions

Prachi R. contributed to the collection of the data and writing of the manuscript. Brian K. reviewed and edited the manuscript.

References

[1] P. Iglesias and J. J. Díez, "Management of endocrine disease: a clinical update on tumor-induced hypoglycemia," *European Journal of Endocrinology*, vol. 170, no. 4, pp. R147–R157, 2014.

[2] Y. Dynkevich, K. I. Rother, I. Whitford et al., "Tumors, IGF-2, and hypoglycemia: insights from the clinic, the laboratory, and the historical archive," *Endocrine Reviews*, vol. 34, no. 6, pp. 798–826, 2013.

[3] A. Adamek and A. Kasprzak, "Insulin-like growth factor (igf) system in liver diseases," *International Journal of Molecular Sciences*, vol. 19, no. 5, p. 1308, 2018.

[4] F. Miraki-Moud, A. B. Grossman, M. Besser, J. P. Monson, and C. Camacho-Hübner, "A rapid method for analyzing serum pro-insulin-like growth factor-ii in patients with non-islet cell tumor hypoglycemia," *The Journal of Clinical Endocrinology & Metabolism*, vol. 90, no. 7, pp. 3819–3823, 2005.

[5] P. Dutta, A. Aggarwal, Y. Gogate et al., "Non-islet cell tumor-induced hypoglycemia: a report of five cases and brief review of the literature," *Endocrinology, Diabetes & Metabolism Case Reports*, vol. 2013, 2013.

[6] C. Livingstone, "IGF2 and cancer," *Endocrine-Related Cancer*, vol. 20, no. 6, pp. R321–R339, 2013.

[7] J.-S. Huang and P.-H. Chang, "Refractory hypoglycemia controlled by systemic chemotherapy with advanced hepatocellular carcinoma: A case report," *Oncology Letters*, vol. 11, no. 1, pp. 898–900, 2016.

[8] W. H. Daughaday, M. A. Emanuele, M. H. Brooks, A. L. Barbato, M. Kapadia, and P. Rotwein, "Synthesis and secretion of insulin-like growth factor II by a leiomyosarcoma with associated hypoglycemia," *New England Journal of Medicine*, vol. 319, no. 22, pp. 1434–1440, 1988.

[9] J. D. Teale and V. Marks, "Glucocorticoid therapy suppresses abnormal secretion of big IGF-II by non-islet cell tumours inducing hypoglycaemia (NICTH)," *Clinical Endocrinology*, vol. 49, no. 4, pp. 491–498, 1998.

9

Adrenal Adenoma Anarchy: A Case of an ACTH-Secreting Pheochromocytoma

Michelle N. Lee,[1] WingYee Wan,[1] Dianna C. Chormanski,[2] and Maria I. Kravchenko[1]

[1]*Department of Medicine, Department of Endocrinology, San Antonio Military Medical Center, 3551 Roger Brooke Drive, JBSA Fort Sam Houston, San Antonio, TX 78234, USA*
[2]*Department of Pathology, San Antonio Military Medical Center, 3551 Roger Brooke Drive, JBSA Fort Sam Houston, San Antonio, TX 78234, USA*

Correspondence should be addressed to WingYee Wan; wingyee.wan.mil@mail.mil

Academic Editor: Lucy Mastrandrea

Introduction. Pheochromocytomas are rare neuroendocrine tumors that arise from sympathetic adrenomedullary chromaffin tissue. Depending on the amount of catecholamines they secrete, they have variable presentations. There have been reported cases of adrenocorticotrophic (ACTH) secreting pheochromocytomas that present with severe Cushing syndrome. Here, we present a pheochromocytoma with adrenocorticotrophic hormone (ACTH) cosecretion, which due to its rarity and variable presentation, may be a diagnostic challenge. *Presentation.* A 64-year-old woman with history of colon cancer presented with new-onset diabetes, worsening hot flashes, and hypertension. On CT imaging she had an enlarging right adrenal nodule (1.7 cm) with 60 Hounsfield units of attenuation and no PET avidity. Biochemical evaluation showed elevated urinary and plasma metanephrines, elevated plasma cortisol levels despite dexamethasone suppression, elevated late-night salivary cortisol, and high-normal adrenocorticotrophic hormone. The patient underwent laproscopic right adrenalectomy, and pathology confirmed pheochromocytoma. Her lab abnormalities and symptoms of hot flashes and hypertension improved postoperatively. *Conclusion.* This case demonstrates an unusual ACTH-secreting pheochromocytoma with subtle presentation and highlights the importance of obtaining a complete biochemical evaluation of incidental adrenal adenomas.

1. Introduction

Pheochromocytomas are rare neuroendocrine tumors that arise from sympathetic adrenomedullary chromaffin tissue. Presentations are variable depending on the amount of catecholamine secretion. Classically, patients present with the nonspecific triad of palpitations, headaches, and/or sweating, although recent studies have found only 17% of patients diagnosed with pheochromocytoma to present classically [1]. Another study by Gruber et al. reported 61% of pheochromocytomas to be asymptomatic and diagnosed on incidental imaging. Due to its nonspecific presentation, a high level of suspicion is needed for the diagnosis of a pheochromocytoma and rare ACTH-producing pheochromocytomas may be a diagnostic challenge. Patients can present with severe Cushing Syndrome (CS), resistant hypertension, diabetes mellitus, and hypokalemia. Due to the high prevalence of obesity, metabolic syndrome, diabetes mellitus, and hypertension, and the potentially subtle physical findings associated with cortisol excess, the diagnosis of CS alone can be challenging. Here, we report how an ACTH-secreting pheochromocytoma, being a rarity, can cause a delay in diagnosis and treatment.

2. Case Presentation

A 64-year-old woman with a history of hypertension, obesity, diabetes mellitus, and ileocecal carcinoma status post right hemicolectomy with ileal resection was evaluated in 2018 for hot flashes, worsening hypertension, and new-onset diabetes in association with an enlarging adrenal nodule. Physical exam was notable for an elevated blood pressure to 165/93 but did not reveal abdominal striae, central obesity, or hirsutism. She had a history of a 1.3 cm right adrenal nodule on CT abdomen/pelvis as early as 2012, found incidentally on evaluation for her colorectal cancer. It was not further evaluated until 2013, at which time it was stable in size (Figure 1). Her hormonal workup in 2013 was remarkable for elevated urine metanephrines to less than twice the upper limit of normal, an appropriately suppressed cortisol level on her overnight dexamethasone suppression test (DST), and normal renin and aldosterone levels (Table 1). The patient was again lost to follow-up for several years and continued to have poorly controlled hypertension and worsening diabetes mellitus. On surveillance CT in October 2018, the adrenal nodule was noted to have grown to 1.7 cm in size with 60 Hounsfield units of attenuation and no PET avidity (Figure 2). Repeat laboratory evaluation revealed elevated urinary metanephrines and elevated serum metanephrines, now three to four times the upper limit of normal (free metanephrines 403 pg/mL (0–62), free normetanephrine 482 mcg/mL (0–145)). She now had a nonsuppressed cortisol on DST (cortisol 11.4mcg/dL (0–3), dexamethasone 226 ng/dL), two elevated late night salivary cortisol readings (0.173 mcg/dL, 0.097 mcg/dL (0–0.090)), and a high-normal ACTH level of 45.62 pg/mL (6–50) (Table 1). The patient's serum potassium was consistently normal.

The patient was diagnosed with an ACTH-producing pheochromocytoma, and due to the lack of PET avidity, there was less concern for colon cancer metastasis. Doxazosin and a high salt diet were initiated prior to undergoing an uncomplicated laparoscopic right adrenalectomy in May 2019. Pathology confirmed pheochromocytoma with low mitotic index and positive for synaptophysin and chromogranin. Immunohistochemical staining confirmed ectopic hypersecretion of ACTH (Figures 3(a) and 3(b)).

Her hot flashes, hypertension, and diabetes significantly improved following surgery, and she no longer required doxazosin or insulin. Repeat laboratory testing showed normalization of her cortisol on DST (cortisol 0.4 mcg/dL, dexamethasone 240 ng/dL), normal ACTH (42 pg/mL), normal metanephrine levels (35 pg/mL), and only slightly elevated normetanephrine levels (189 pg/mL), deemed normal for her age and history of essential hypertension.

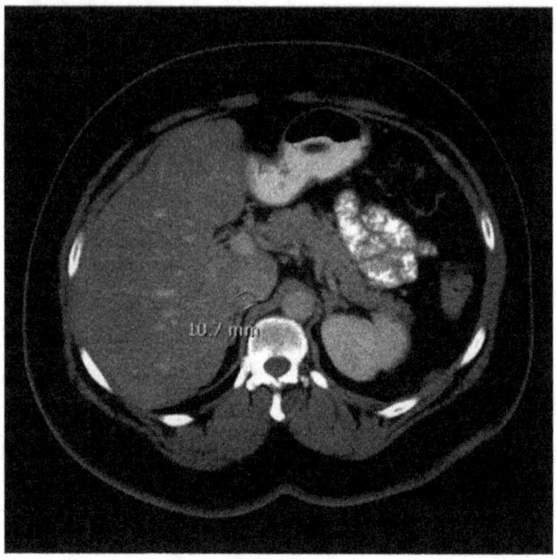

Figure 1: Initial CT imaging of incidental right adrenal nodule measuring 1.1 cm.

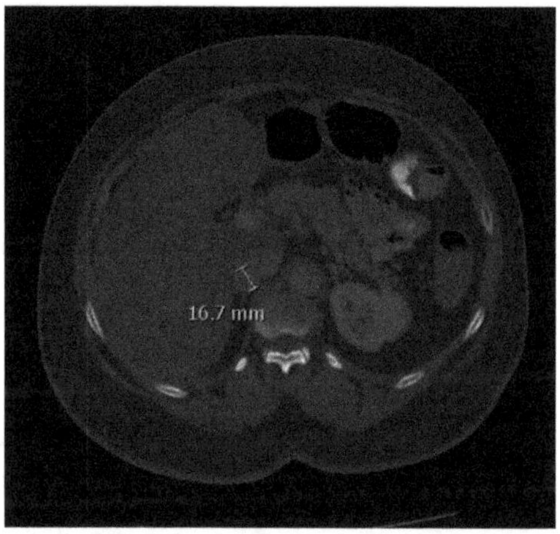

Figure 2: Follow-up CT noting an increase in size of the right adrenal nodule (1.7 cm) with 60 Hounsfield units of attenuation (right).

3. Discussion

Pheochromocytomas, although rare, are becoming more common due to incidental detection on CT. Gruber et al. identified that incidental pheochromocytomas were typically found in older patients, with fewer symptoms and with a smaller degree in elevation of urine and serum metanephrines compared to those diagnosed based on symptoms. Incidentally discovered pheochromocytomas were also found to require less cumulative phenoxybenzamine compared to those with symptoms [2].

This patient's pheochromocytoma was initially identified as an incidentaloma on multiple CT scans for surveillance of her colon cancer. Her symptoms of worsening hypertension and night sweats were not the classic triad presentation for a pheochromocytoma, which may be due to having only moderate catecholamine secretion. There was also a concern for subclinical Cushing's syndrome based on her nonsuppressed cortisol on DST and elevated late night salivary cortisol levels.

ACTH-producing pheochromocytomas are rarely diagnosed, comprising approximately 5% of cases of ectopic ACTH syndrome, with less than 100 reported cases [3]. It more commonly presents in women and unilaterally. Patients will typically present with severe CS with diabetes mellitus and significant hypokalemia and will less likely present with catecholamine excess [4]. The diagnosis can sometimes be challenging as symptoms are nonspecific, although they typically present less insidiously than classic Cushing's syndrome. Our patient's presentation was more insidious, without clinical symptoms or signs of Cushing's syndrome or hypokalemia that would suggest a secondary cause of her hypertension and diabetes mellitus. Hypertension and intermittent sweating or hot flashes were her only symptoms of catecholamine excess.

TABLE 1: Hormonal evaluation.

	Initial screening Jul 2013	Repeat screening Nov 2018	Jan 2019	Jun 2019 (1 month postoperative)
AM cortisol with 1 mg overnight DST	1.2 mcg/dL	7.3 mcg/dL	11.4 mcg/dL	0.4 mcg/dL
Late-night salivary cortisol at 0300 (0–0.090 mcg/dL)			0.175 mcg/dL, 0.173 mcg/dL, 0.097 mcg/dL	
24 hr urinary cortisol (36–137 mcg/24 hr)			89.0 mcg/24 hr	
Adrenocorticotrophic hormone (ACTH) (6.00–50 pg/mL)			45.62 pg/mL	
24 hr urinary metanephrines (74–297 mcg/24 hr)	505 mcg/24 hr	864 mcg/24 hr		
24 hr urinary normetanephrine (105–354 mcg/24 hr)	434 mcg/24 hr	690 mcg/24 hr		
24 hr urinary metanephrines, total (179–651 mcg/24 hr)	939 mcg/24 hr	1554 mcg/24 hr		
Plasma-free metanephrine (0–62 pg/mL)	—	403 pg/mL	199 pg/mL	35 pg/mL
Plasma-free normetanephrine (0–145 pg/mL)	—	482 pg/mL	176 pg/mL	189 pg/mL
Plasma renin (0.25–5.82 ng/mL/h)	1.77 ng/mL/h	1.121 ng/mL/h	—	—
Plasma aldosterone (0–30 ng/dL)	13 ng/dL	10.6 ng/dL	—	—

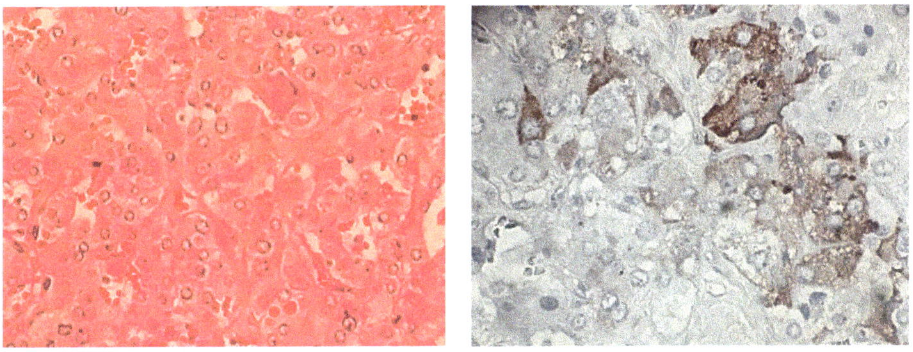

(a) (b)

FIGURE 3: (a) Hematoxylin and eosin stain demonstrating polygonal tumor cells with vesicular nuclei and some prominent nucleoli growing in a nested pattern. (b) Immunohistochemical stain for adrenocorticotrophic hormone demonstrating tumor cells with patchy positive staining (brown).

Patients with ectopic ACTH syndrome can present with variable ACTH as well, ranging from normal levels, as seen in our patient, to over 200 pg/ml [3, 5]. Although her preoperative ACTH was within normal limits, this was inappropriate in the setting of her hypercortisolism. Repeat ACTH postoperatively was slightly improved and appropriate for a preserved hypothalamus-pituitary-adrenal axis. Due to already having a diagnosis of a right pheochromocytoma, the decision to undergo an adrenalectomy was made prior to any further workup for hypercortisolism. The normal postoperative suppression of cortisol and positive ACTH staining of the tumor confirmed that her pheochromocytoma was the ectopic source. If further workup was necessary, for example, if ACTH staining was negative, the tumor could have been stained for CRH to assess for ectopic secretion. Additionally, a high dose DST or CRH stimulation test could assist in differentiating a pituitary from an ectopic source. High-dose DST is noted to have only 76.5% accuracy, as 20–30% of ectopic ACTH-producing tumors have functioning glucocorticoid receptors that can still suppress ACTH production [4].

It is important to treat the excess catecholamines and cortisol prior to surgery in ACTH-producing pheochromocytomas. Patients are typically treated with an alpha blocker in addition to other antihypertensives to control their hypertension. In the case of the hypercortisolism, treatment is dependent on the severity and may include metyrapone and/or ketoconazole to directly prevent further production of cortisol, potassium supplementation to correct hypokalemia, and insulin to control hyperglycemia. Medical therapies are usually tapered and discontinued following adrenalectomy. Patients with a unilateral adrenalectomy will typically still require a short course of steroids [3]. As our patient did not present with overt Cushing's syndrome, preoperative ketoconazole was not deemed necessary.

Unlike other ectopic ACTH-producing tumors, pheochromocytomas are usually benign and cured following unilateral adrenalectomy. Many other tumors that have been associated with ectopic ACTH production are usually metastatic at the time of diagnosis and may require palliative bilateral adrenalectomy [5, 6].

Abbreviations

ACTH: Adrenocorticotrophic hormone
CS: Cushing syndrome
DST: Dexamethasone suppression test
CRH: Corticotropin-releasing hormone.

Disclosure

The view(s) expressed herein are those of the authors and do not reflect the official policy or position of Brooke Army Medical Center, the U.S. Army Medical Department, the U.S. Army Office of the Surgeon General, the Department of the Army, the Department of the Air Force, or the Department of Defense or the U.S. Government.

References

[1] H. Falhammar, M. Kjellman, and J. Calissendorff, "Initial clinical presentation and spectrum of pheochromocytoma: a study of 94 cases from a single center," *Endocrine Connections*, vol. 7, no. 1, pp. 186–192, 2018.

[2] L. M. Gruber, R. P. Hartman, G. B. Thompson et al., "Pheochromocytoma characteristics and behavior differ depending on method of discovery," *The Journal of Clinical Endocrinology & Metabolism*, vol. 104, no. 5, pp. 1386–1393, 2019.

[3] J. N. Gabi, M. M. Milhem, Y. E. Tovar, E. S. Karem, A. Y. Gabi, and R. A. Khthir, "Severe cushing syndrome due to an ACTH-producing pheochromocytoma: a case presentation and review of the literature," *Journal of the Endocrine Society*, vol. 2, no. 7, pp. 621–630, 2018.

[4] M. F. Nijhoff, O. M. Dekkers, L. J. Vleming, J. W. A. Smit, J. A. Romijn, and A. M. Pereira, "ACTH-producing pheochromocytoma: clinical considerations and concise review of the literature," *European Journal of Internal Medicine*, vol. 20, no. 7, pp. 682–685, 2009.

[5] L. R. Salgado, M. C. B. V. Fragoso, M. Knoepfelmacher et al., "Ectopic ACTH syndrome: our experience with 25 cases," *European Journal of Endocrinology*, vol. 155, no. 5, pp. 725–733, 2006.

[6] H. Chen, J. L. Doppman, G. P. Chrousos, J. A. Norton, L. K. Nieman, and R. Udelsman, "Adrenocorticotropic hormone-secreting pheochromocytomas: the exception to the rule," *Surgery*, vol. 118, no. 6, pp. 988–995, 1995.

10

Bilateral Lipoadenoma of the Adrenal Glands and Humeral Brown Tumor: An Unusual Association

N. Messaoudi,[1] N. Bouichrat,[1] M. Karrou,[1] I. Assarrar,[1] S. Malki,[2] S. Elmahjoubi,[3] S. Rouf,[1] N. Karich,[2] A. Lachkar,[3] S. Sefiani,[4] M. Bouziane,[5] I. Kamaoui,[6] and H. Latrech[1]

[1]*Department of Endocrinology-Diabetology and Nutrition, Mohammed VI University Hospital Center, Faculty of Medicine and Pharmacy, University of Mohammed 1st, Oujda, Morocco*
[2]*Department of Anatomical Pathology, Mohammed VI University Hospital Center, Faculty of Medicine and Pharmacy, University of Mohammed 1st, Oujda, Morocco*
[3]*Department of Orthopedic Surgery B, Mohammed VI University Hospital Center, Faculty of Medicine and Pharmacy, University of Mohammed 1st, Oujda, Morocco*
[4]*AGDAL Anatomical Pathology Center, Rabat, Morocco*
[5]*Department of General Surgery, Mohammed VI University Hospital Center, Faculty of Medicine and Pharmacy, University of Mohammed 1st, Oujda, Morocco*
[6]*Department of Radiology, Mohammed VI University Hospital Center, Faculty of Medicine and Pharmacy, University of Mohammed 1st, Oujda, Morocco*

Correspondence should be addressed to H. Latrech; hlatrech@hotmail.fr

Academic Editor: Toshihiro Kita

Adrenal adenolipomas are rare lipomatous adrenal tumors that can be either functional or not. Only 7 cases have been reported in the English literature so far. However, brown tumors are benign, rare, historical lesions, with histological similarity to giant tumors that can be encountered in 1% of all primary hyperparathyroidism cases. We report the case of an unusual association of bilateral lipoadenoma of the adrenal glands and humeral brown tumor in a 35-year-old patient. He presented to the emergency department with a pathological fracture of the left humerus secondary to a brown tumor. The medical investigations have concluded to primary hyperparathyroidism. The screening for multiple endocrine neoplasia type 1 revealed the presence of bilateral nonsecreting adrenal masses whose anatomopathological study concluded adenolipomas. Adrenal tumors may constitute a part of multiple endocrine neoplasia type 1 in 20 to 40% of cases. In this view, it is necessary to check for the presence of other endocrine gland tumor locations such as primary hyperparathyroidism, neuroendocrine tumors of the duodenum and pancreas, or pituitary adenomas.

1. Introduction

Lipomatous tumors of the adrenal gland are a group of tumors that have in common a significant component of adipose tissue. They are usually benign and nonfunctional. Myelolipomas are the most frequently described entity in the literature; other tumors have also been described, such as teratomas, lipomas, angiomyolipomas, and exceptionally adrenal adenolipomas [1].

Adrenal adenolipomas are extremely rare lipomatous adrenal tumors that can be functional or not. They have been described for the first time in 1995 [2]. To our knowledge, only 7 cases have been reported in the English literature to date [1].

The association of adrenal adenolipoma and brown tumors has never been reported in the literature. This association may be part of a multiple endocrine neoplasia type 1 (MEN1). In this paper, we report the case of an unusual association of bilateral lipoadenoma of the adrenal glands and a humeral brown tumor in a 35-year-old patient.

2. Case Report

A 35-year-old patient with a medical history of gout under dietary regimen and an undocumented dysthyroidism in the mother was admitted to the emergency room for the management of a fracture of the left humerus without prior trauma (Figure 1).

Considering the suspicious osteolytic image of the fracture site on the standard X-ray (Figure 1), a magnetic resonance imaging (MRI) scan of the left arm was performed to confirm the presence of a centromedullary osteolytic tumor process of the left humeral diaphysis, responsible for a pathologic fracture.

Malignant hypercalcemia at 4.72 mmol/l and then 4.49 mmol/l (normal range: 2.1 mmol/l–2.6 mmol/l using the colorimetric spectrophotometric method) was discovered on the preoperative biological assessment, requiring intravenous rehydration (500 ml of 0.9% saline solution every 4 hours, i.e., 3 l per day) and 3 hemodialysis sessions followed by an infusion of zoledronic acid 4 mg. The blood calcium level decreased at 2.61 mmol/l.

The patient then underwent centromedullary nailing with bone biopsy. The anatomopathologic results showed a connective tissue and bone with thinned and rarefied trabeculae surrounded by osteoblasts (Figure 2(a)), associated with numerous multinucleated giant cells and siderophages (Figure 2(b)) compatible with a brown tumor.

The patient was then hospitalized in our endocrinology department for etiological assessment of his hypercalcemia.

The anamnesis found no functional signs, including the absence of previous bone pain or dental problems. The blood tests revealed a primary hyperparathyroidism made of hypercalcemia, a low phosphoremia at 17 mg/l (normal range: 24 mg/l–45 mg/l), a high biointact parathyroid hormone (iPTH) 1–84 at 795 pg/ml (normal range: 14.9 pg/ml–56.9 pg/ml), an elevated 24 h calciuria at 550 mg/24 h, and a low vitamin D at 7.8 ng/ml.

Cervical ultrasonography showed the presence of an oval nodule at the lower left parathyroid lodge that was bilobed, frankly hypoechoic with hypervascular Doppler signal, measuring 33 ∗ 32 ∗ 18 mm (Figure 3). The same parathyroid adenoma was located on the cervicothoracic computed tomography scan (Figure 4).

The evaluation of hypercalcemia impacts did not find any cardiac repercussions; however, the X-rays of the long bones showed multiple brown tumours in the ischiopubic ramus (Figure 5(a)), in the distal extremity of the femur and the upper end of the tibia (Figure 5(b)), and the pancreatic CT scan found small calcification of the head of the pancreas.

In view of the young age of the patient, the search for forms that fit into the context of multiple endocrine neoplasia has been initiated. CT scan of the adrenal glands and pancreas revealed the presence of bilateral adrenal masses, with embossed, multilocular contours, and a predominantly fat density, measuring 64 ∗ 59 ∗ 42 mm on the right gland and 102 ∗ 93 ∗ 69 mm on the left one (Figure 6). Acute adrenal insufficiency was eliminated on the blood serum ionogram (potassium was at 3.3 meq/l, and sodium was at 134 meq/l). Biochemical screening for adrenal hypersecretion

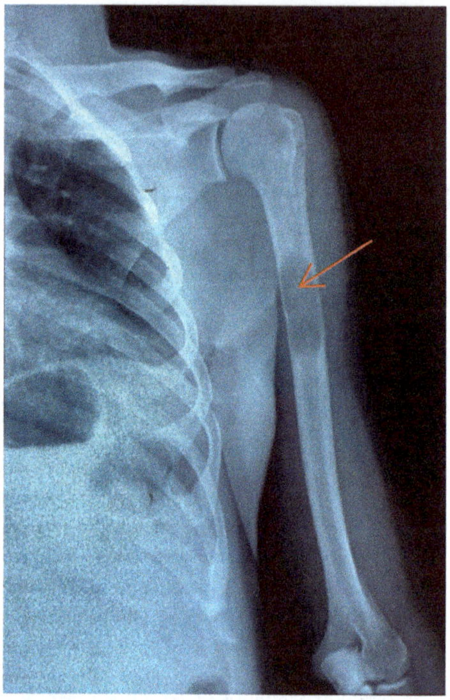

Figure 1: Standard X-ray showing a lytic lesion with cortical thinning and pathologic fracture in the left proximal humerus (red arrow).

found normal plasma catecolamines, with neither hypercorticism nor hyperaldosteronism.

Brain imaging did not find any pituitary mass. The blood test revealed normal gonadotropin and prolactin levels.

Furthermore, a hyperthyroidism was noted in the thyroid assessment with negative TSH-receptor-antibodies and calcitonin. Cervical ultrasound showed an enlarged thyroid gland measuring 63 cc with multiple Thyroid Imaging Reporting and Data System (TI-RADS) 3 nodules in the right thyroid lobe and a TI-RADS 4 nodule with a long-axis diameter of 5 cm in the left thyroid lobe.

The rest of the evaluation did not find any bronchial or thymic tumors or additional pancreatic abnormalities.

The case was discussed over a multidisciplinary meeting. The decision was to initially perform a bilateral adrenal tumorectomy, followed by a lower-left parathyroidectomy and a total thyroidectomy. The pathological analysis of the adrenal specimen was in favor of adrenal adenomyolipomas without signs of malignancy. A 250 μg Synacthen® test was performed. The cortisol level within 60 minutes reached 147 ng/ml.

Hypercalcemia was controlled by regular injections of zoledronic acid. Once normocalcemia was achieved, the patient underwent lower left parathyroidectomy with total thyroidectomy. The anatomopathological results confirmed the diagnosis of parathyroid adenoma without signs of malignancy (Figure 7). As for the thyroidectomy specimen, the histological study showed a vesicular carcinoma with capsular effraction and vascular emboli, classified pT3aNxMx (Figure 8), and a lymph node dissection with a radioiodine-131 therapy (RIT) will be scheduled.

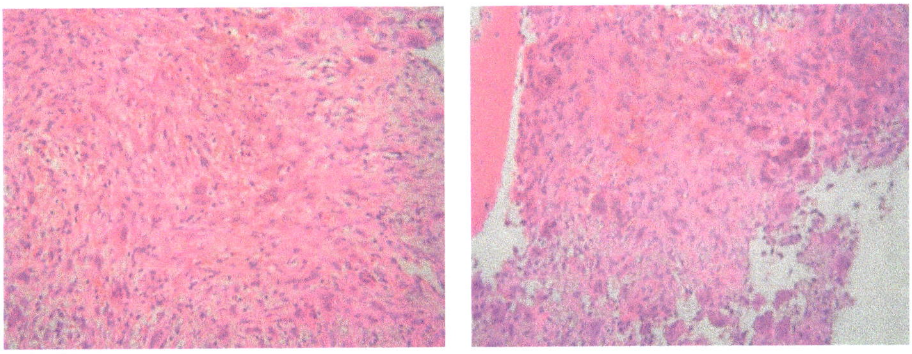

(a) (b)

Figure 2: (a) Proliferation of fibroblasts mixed with giant cells (magnification: 100x). (b) Bone infiltration by a brown tumor (magnification: 100x).

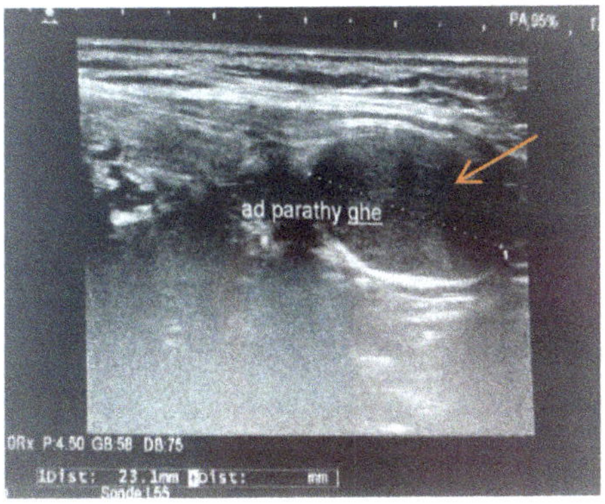

Figure 3: Cervical ultrasound showing an oval, well-defined, hypoechoic nodule, with regular contours, measuring 33 ∗ 32 ∗ 18 mm (red arrow).

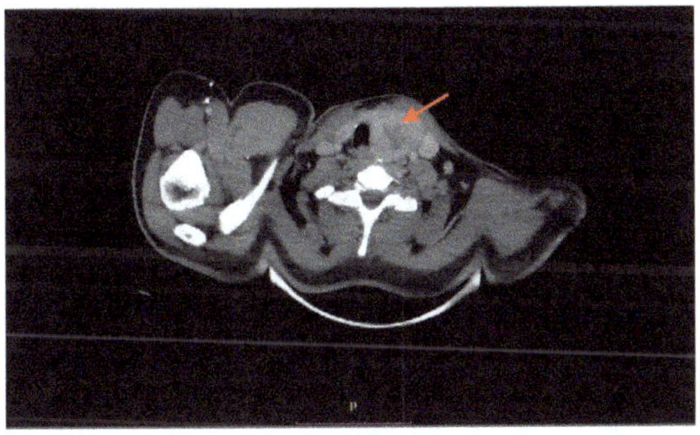

Figure 4: Cervicothoracic CT scan revealing a hypodense nodule in the posteroinferior pole of the left thyroid lobe (red arrow).

The postoperative evolution noted a normalization of phosphocalcic markers. The calcemia reached 2.3 mmol/l, and iPTH reached 11 pg/ml (normal range: 9,2 pg/ml–44,6 pg/ml). The genetic testing is still ongoing.

3. Discussion

Primary adrenal tumors are rare, with a poorly elucidated prevalence, most often discovered incidentally. Some studies estimate that the frequency of adrenal tumors increases with age and may reach 10% of the elderly population [3]. Adrenal tumors are classified according to their location, the uni- or bilateral localisation, functional or unfunctional character, and their evolutive profile. The most frequently encountered etiologies are nonfunctional benign adrenocortical adenomas in first rank followed by adrenal myelolipomas.

Adrenal myelolipoma is the most frequent and most described lipomatous adrenal tumor in the literature. It represents 3% of all adrenal tumors. Much rarer, other lipomatous tumors of the adrenal cortex can be found, such as teratomas, angiomyolipomas, lipomas, and more rarely adenolipomas.

Adrenal adenolipomas are extremely rare lipomatous adrenal tumors, first described in 1995 [2]. They have had several names: adrenal cortical adenomas with fat component in 1995 [2], adenomas with lipomatous metaplasia [4], and lipoadenomas [5, 6]. To date, only 7 cases of unilateral adenolipomas have been described in the English literature including 5 cases of secreting adenolipomas (Table 1). In our patient, the adrenal tumors are bilateral, nonsecreting and of fortuitous discovery even with their large size.

Despite the small sample size reported in the literature, the average age of the patients was 47.8 years with a female predominance (sex ratio M/F: 2/5). The size of the mass varied from 20 mm to 100 mm with an average of 60 mm, and a higher frequency on the right side (57%).

Adrenal adenolipomas are the main differential diagnosis with adrenal myelolipomas. They have the same clinical and radiological characteristics: the only difference resides in the histological pattern, as adrenal adenolipomas do not comprise hematopoietic tissues or calcifications [6]. Adrenal tumors, especially those of the adrenal cortex, whether functional or not, could be a part of a MEN1 in 20 to 40% of cases, which is why it is mandatory to screen for other endocrine gland tumor locations. Our case presents the unique association of adrenal adenolipoma and primary hyperparathyroidism complicated by a brown tumor. All can be integrated into MEN1.

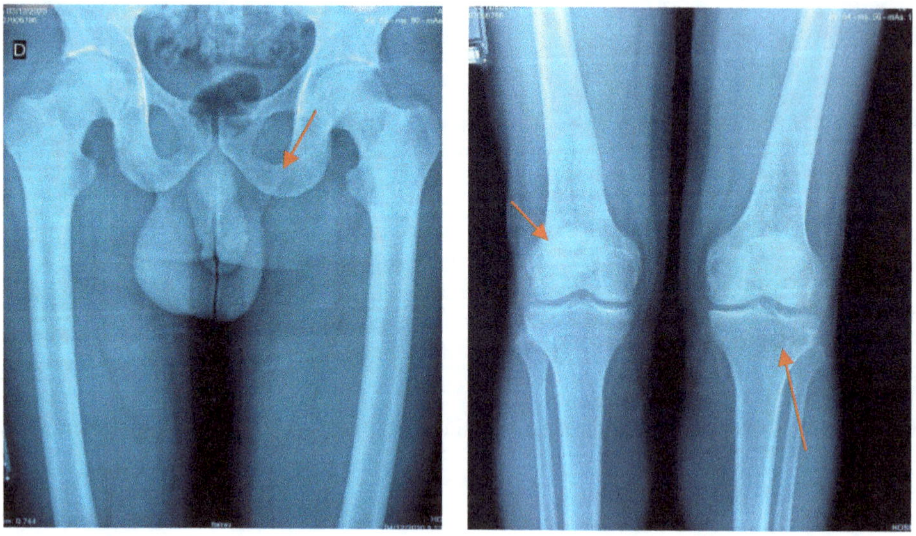

(a) (b)

FIGURE 5: Radiographs showing multiple well-limited osseous lytic lesions with sclerotic margins (red arrows). (a) Ischiopubic ramus. (b) The distal extremity of the femur and the upper end of the tibia.

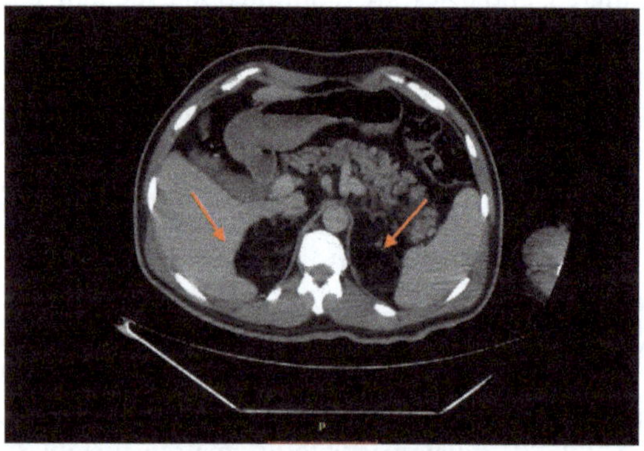

FIGURE 6: Abdominal CT scan showing bilateral multilocular adrenal masses, with a predominantly fat density (−75 UH), measuring 64 ∗ 59 ∗ 42 mm on the right gland and 102 ∗ 93 ∗ 69 mm on the left gland (red arrows).

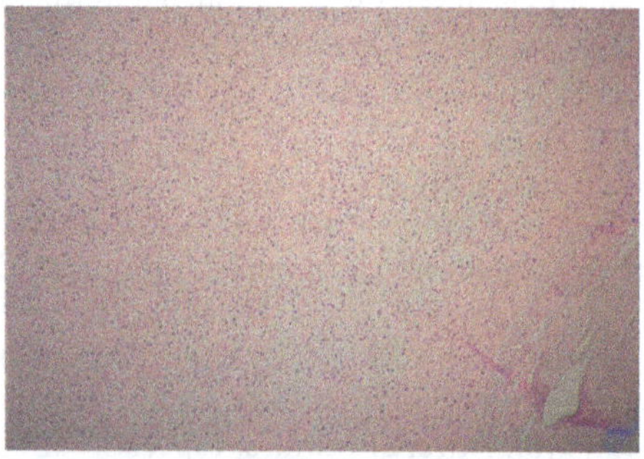

FIGURE 7: Magnification 100x, showing well-circumscribed tumor proliferation with thin fibrous capsule. Tumor cells are monotonous not atypical (HE: 100x).

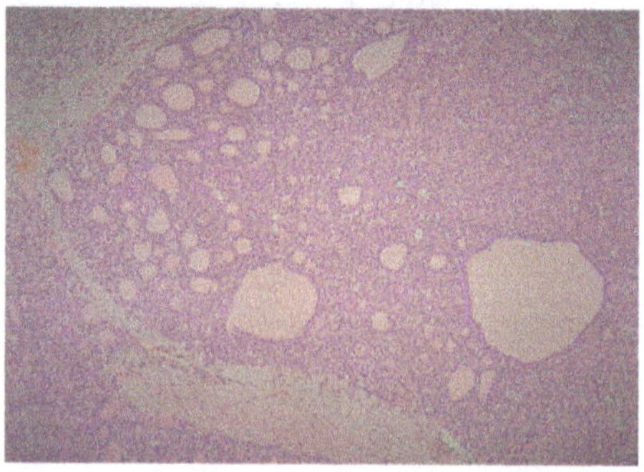

FIGURE 8: Magnification 100x, showing tumor proliferation of vesicular pattern with capsular invasion (HE: 100x).

MEN1 is a rare genetic syndrome, first described in 1954 [9], also known as Wermen's syndrome [10], and is listed in the McKusik classification "OMIM 131100" [11]. It is defined by the association, in the same individual or in related persons belonging to the same family, of hyperparathyroidism, pancreatic or duodenal neuroendocrine tumors, pituitary adenoma, adrenal cortical tumors, and bronchial, thymic, or gastric neuroendocrine tumors. Other tumor proliferations of nonendocrine tissues can also be encountered, such as angiofibromas, lipomas, and collagenomas. Its prevalence is poorly known and is estimated at 25/100,000, affecting all age ranges from 5 to 82 years. The clinical (Table 2) and biological onset symptoms appear around the fifth decade in 94% of cases [10]. It can be sporadic in 10 to 14% of cases.

Hyperparathyroidism is the most common condition in MEN1 [9]. It is found predominantly in females and is fortuitously discovered in 75% to 80% of cases through a systematic measurement of blood calcium levels. The clinical signs are secondary to hypercalcemia: renal colic, bone pain, and pathologic fractures.

The bone manifestations are various, including fibrocystic osteitis, brown tumors, and pathological fracture.

Table 1: Characteristics of adenolipomas described in the literature.

Reference	Age	Sex	Discovery circumstances	Localization	Size (mm)	Secretion
Sato et al. [2]	47	M	Abdominal pain	Left	35	Absent
Papotti et al. [4]	79	F	Abdominal pain	Left	60	Present
Papotti et al. [4]	46	F	Fortuitous	Right	110	Present
Uriev et al. [5]	51	F	Cushing's syndrome	Left	40	Present
Mylarappa et al. [7]	12	F	Hirsutism	Right	100*80	Present
Martins et al. [8]	53	F	Cushing's syndrome	Right	28	Present
Luo et al. [6]	46	M	Abdominal pain	Right	20*15*13	Absent
Our case	35	M	Fortuitous	Bilateral	Right: 64*59*42 Left: 102*93*69	Absent

Table 2: Clinical manifestations of MEN1 syndrome.

Clinical manifestations	Prevalence (%)
Hyperparathyroidism	90
Neuroendocrine tumors of the duodenum and pancreas	Nonfunctioning: 55 Gastrinoma: 40 Insulinoma 10 Glucagonoma <1 VIPoma <1
Pituitary adenomas	40
Adrenocortical tumors	20–40
Pheochromocytomas	<1
Neuroendocrine thymic tumors	2
Bronchopulmonary neuroendocrine tumors	5
Angiofibromas	85
Collagenomas	70
Lipomas	30
Other tumors	
Meningioma	8
Ependymoma, melanoma, thyroid	0–25

Brown tumors are benign, rare, historical lesions, with histological similarity to giant tumors. They result directly from the action of parathormone on the bone structure. The brown color is secondary to hemosiderin deposits. They are encountered in 1% of primary hyperparathyroidism cases [12]. Their radiological aspects include lytic lesions, with well-limited contours, without sclerosis, being either eccentric or cortical, with thinning, blowing, or rupture of the cortex [13]. In most cases, the brown tumors secondary to primary hyperparathyroidism are unique and are most often located in the facial bones, more rarely in the long bones, pelvis, spine, and base of the skull [14]. Only a few cases of multiple brown tumors have been reported in the literature [15]. In our case, the patient presented with multiple lytic lesions with cortical thinning and a pathologic fracture in the left proximal humerus.

The first step in the treatment of brown tumors is the management of primary hyperparathyroidism. Some authors report spontaneous resorption of these tumors after parathyroidectomy [16].

Our patient has 3 conditions that are part of MEN1: primary hyperparathyroidism, an adrenocortical tumor, and a vesicular carcinoma of the thyroid. The genetic study for the MEN1 mutation is currently ongoing. Due to the strong clinical presumption, the patient requires regular and strict surveillance given the risk of the appearance of other tumor conditions.

4. Conclusion

Adrenal adenolipomas are very rare tumors. Their diagnosis is based on histopathology. The current progress of imaging, the development of new strategies of hormonal evaluation, and histological analysis allow a better understanding and studying of their characteristics. In view of the frequency of associations that often take part of MEN1, the screening for other endocrine disorders is necessary when an adrenal mass is diagnosed, whatever its particularities. In order of frequency, a systematic dosage of the calcemia is needed in order to make an early diagnosis of hyperparathyroidism and to avoid the development of complications such as the brown tumors reported in our patient. To our knowledge, this particular association has never been described before in the existing literature.

Consent

A written and signed consent was provided by the patients to publish the findings of this case report.

Disclosure

N. Messaoudi and N. Bouichrat are co-first authors.

References

[1] A. K.-Y. Lam, "Lipomatous tumours in adrenal gland: WHO updates and clinical implications," *Endocrine-Related Cancer*, vol. 24, no. 3, pp. R65–R79, 2017.

[2] N. Sato, Y. Watanabe, T. Saga, K. Mitsudo, M. Dohke, and K. Minami, "Adrenocortical adenoma containing a fat component: CT and MR image evaluation," *Abdominal Imaging*, vol. 20, no. 5, pp. 489-490, 1995.

[3] E. P. M. Corssmit and O. M. Dekkers, "Screening in adrenal tumors," *Current Opinion in Oncology*, vol. 31, no. 3, pp. 243–246, 2019.

[4] M. Papotti, A. Sapino, E. Mazza, S. Sandrucci, M. Volante, and G. Bussolati, "Lipomatous changes in adrenocortical adenomas: report of two cases," *Endocrine Pathology*, vol. 7, no. 3, pp. 223–228, 1996.

[5] L. Uriev, I. Maslovsky, D. Ben-Dor, and F. Barak, "Adrenal lipoadenoma," *Pathology Discovery*, vol. 2, no. 1, 2014.

[6] J. Luo, L. Chen, Q. Wen et al., "Case report lipoadenoma of the adrenal gland: report of a rare entity and review of literature," *International Journal of Clinical and Experimental Pathology*, vol. 8, 2015.

[7] P. Mylarappa, A. Pathade, D. Ramesh, and T. Javali, "Virilizing lipoadenoma of the adrenal gland in a pre-pubertal girl: a rare case," *Indian Journal of Urology*, vol. 30, no. 2, p. 219, 2014.

[8] R. G. Martins, R. Agrawal, D. M. Berney et al., "Differential diagnosis of adrenocorticotropic hormone-independent cushing syndrome: role of adrenal venous sampling," *Endocrine Practice*, vol. 18, no. 6, pp. e153–e157, 2012.

[9] A. Al-Salameh, C. Baudry, and R. Cohen, "Update on multiple endocrine neoplasia type 1 and 2," *La Presse Médicale*, vol. 9, no. September, pp. 722–731, 2018.

[10] G. Singh, N. J. Mulji, and I. Jialal, *Multiple Endocrine Neoplasia Type 1*, StatPearls, Treasure Island, FL, USA, 2021, https://www.ncbi.nlm.nih.gov/books/NBK536980/.

[11] V. A. McKusick, *Mendelian Inheritance in Man: A Catalog of Human Genes and Genetic Disorders*, Johns Hopkins University Press, Baltimore, MD, USA, 1994.

[12] Q. X. Ngo, D. Q. Ngo, T. D. Tran, D. T. Le, G. N. Hoang, and Q. V. Le, "Multiple brown tumors with primary hyperparathyroidism mimicking bone metastases [ ]," *International Journal of Surgery Case Reports*, vol. 79, no. February, pp. 375–378, 2021.

[13] A. Slama, Z. Mziou, L. Walha, B. Sriha, and H. Kochtali, "Les tumeurs brunes des maxillaires," *Actualités Odonto-Stomatologiques*, vol. 238, pp. 169–176, 2007.

[14] A. kumar Yadav, E. Pawar, A. Harsoor, P. kumar G S, and H. Rohra, "Primary hyperparathyroidism with extensive brown tumours and distal humerus fracture-A case report," *International Journal of Surgery Case Reports*, vol. 66, no. January, pp. 421–424, 2020.

[15] E. Ullah, M. Ahmad, S. A. Ali, and N. Redhu, "Primary hyperparathyroidism having multiple Brown tumors mimicking malignancy," *Indian Journal of Endocrinology and Metabolism*, vol. 16, no. 6, pp. 1040–1042, 2012.

[16] F. Malika, L. Taali, A. Mohamed et al., "Tumeur brune du maxillaire révélatrice d'hyperparathyroidie primaire: a propos d'un cas et revue de la littérature," *Pan African Medical Journal-ISSN*, vol. 14, no. 21, pp. 1937–8688, 2013.

11

Aggressive Papillary Thyroid Carcinoma Presenting with Metastasis to the Pancreas

Firas Warda[1,2] **Sam Ho**[3] **Enoch Kuo**[3] **Dinesh Rao**[4] **and Marilu Jurado-Flores**[1,2]

[1]*Division of Endocrinology, Diabetes, and Metabolism, University of Florida College of Medicine-Jacksonville, Jacksonville, FL 32209, USA*
[2]*Department of Medicine, University of Florida College of Medicine-Jacksonville, Jacksonville, FL 32209, USA*
[3]*Department of Pathology, Immunology and Laboratory Medicine, University of Florida College of Medicine-Gainesville, Gainesville, FL 32610, USA*
[4]*Department of Radiology, University of Florida College of Medicine-Jacksonville, Jacksonville, FL 32209, USA*

Correspondence should be addressed to Firas Warda; firas.warda@jax.ufl.edu

Academic Editor: Mihail A. Boyanov

Papillary thyroid cancer is the most common type of thyroid cancer. Aggressive forms tend to metastasize to the lungs and bones, but the abdomen is a rare site of metastasis. We present a 46-year-old male patient who presented with a neck mass associated with shortness of breath and hemoptysis. He was found to have a large thyroid mass on imaging. He underwent a total thyroidectomy with bilateral neck dissection, with pathology showing a multifocal tall cell variant of papillary thyroid carcinoma with lymphovascular invasion in both thyroid lobes. Due to recurrent findings of residual thyroid tissue on whole-body scan imaging, the patient underwent radioactive iodine ablation therapy twice, with poor response to therapy, suggested by persistently elevated thyroglobulin levels. However, the residual tissue responded to external beam radiation. After the initial response to radiation, thyroglobulin was noted to have increased again, prompting a PET-CT after administration of recombinant TSH. PET showed a focal area of increased uptake in the head of the pancreas. The patient underwent the Whipple procedure for resection of the metastasis. Pathology showed papillary thyroid carcinoma with strong and diffuse staining for TTF-1 and thyroglobulin. The patient was started on lenvatinib in the postoperative period and is currently tolerating treatment well with evidence of decreasing thyroglobulin levels. Intra-abdominal metastasis from a thyroid malignancy source is quite rare and can be challenging as far as diagnosis and treatment. Surgical resection can be curative and can be followed by radioactive iodine ablation therapy if cancer cells show avidity. Tyrosine kinase inhibitors can be used in refractory disease. New research is being conducted on new agents that can reverse the resistance to radioactive iodine therapy.

1. Introduction

Papillary thyroid cancer (PTC) continues to be the most common thyroid cancer with the incidence being on the rise likely due to increased use of imaging modalities and ease of detection [1]. Since 1975, the incidence of thyroid cancer has tripled, and the entire increase has essentially been attributed to PTC [2]. Unfortunately, up to 10% of patients with papillary and follicular thyroid carcinomas present with distant metastasis [3]. A study done by Durante et al. showed that the 10-year survival in patients with well-differentiated thyroid carcinoma is reduced from 80–95% to 14% in patients older than 40 years of age with macronodular lung metastases or multiple bone metastasis [4]. Thyroid cancer metastasis to the gastrointestinal tract is unusual and only accounts for 0.5–1% of all distant metastases [5]. PTC metastasis to the pancreas is extremely rare [6], with only a dozen of cases reported in the literature to the best of our knowledge. Here, we present a patient with an initial diagnosis of mpT4a, N1b papillary thyroid cancer with pancreatic metastasis detected on positron emission tomography-computed tomography (PET-CT) and confirmed after undergoing radical pancreaticoduodenectomy, close to three years after initial diagnosis.

2. Case Presentation

The patient is a 46-year-old male who complained of a neck mass that he noticed 4 months prior to presentation, associated with hoarseness, shortness of breath, and occasional hemoptysis. Physical exam showed a 5 cm mass in the anterior neck fixed to the trachea with extension to the left thyroid lobe and hoarseness of voice. Subsequent pharyngoscopy showed tracheal narrowing and paralysis of the left vocal cord. Computed tomography (CT) scan of the neck soft tissue showed a large thyroid mass arising from the left thyroid gland (Figure 1) with extension into the posterior upper mediastinum (Figure 2), paravertebral space, and left tracheoesophageal region with severe narrowing of the trachea (Figure 3), and right tracheoesophageal lymphadenopathy. He underwent total thyroidectomy, along with central, left-sided, and right tracheoesophageal lymph node dissection. Intraoperatively, left recurrent laryngeal nerve invasion of the tumor was noted in addition to circumferential encasement of the trachea. The postoperative period was complicated by severe and persistent hypocalcemia, requiring IV and oral calcium loading and initiation of calcitriol. Pathology showed a multifocal bilateral tall cell variant of papillary thyroid carcinoma, 6.5 cm in the greatest dimension, with perineural and lymphovascular invasion, and metastasis to one left-sided lymph node. The posterior resection margin of the left thyroid lobe and isthmus was involved by the papillary carcinoma.

Following thyroid hormone withdrawal, a whole-body scan along with single-photon emission computed tomography (SPECT) showed a focal area of increased radiotracer activity within the right thyroid bed representing residual thyroid tissue. There was a subtle area of increased uptake in the left thyroid bed representing residual malignancy. No evidence of distant metastatic disease was found. The patient was treated with 200 μCi of ^{131}I radioactive iodine, followed by a postablative whole-body scan, which showed a focal area of increased radiotracer uptake at the left thyroid bed and prominent soft tissue indentation on the left posterolateral trachea, likely representing residual neoplasm. Four months later, the patient presented with hemoptysis and shortness of breath, for which CT of the chest was done and showed a large thyroid mass causing significant tracheal and esophageal luminal narrowing as well as esophageal leftward displacement. Postwithdrawal whole-body scan showed only minimal increase in radiotracer activity within the thyroid bed. Following a second treatment with 200 μCi of ^{131}I radioactive iodine, postablative whole-body scan showed relatively minimal uptake within the tumor, suggesting a poor response to therapy. Unfortunately, a tracheostomy tube and percutaneous endoscopic gastrostomy (PEG) tube had to be placed for airway protection and feeding, respectively. The patient underwent 35 treatments of external beam radiation (EBR), after which thyroglobulin levels decreased to 1.3 ng/mL from 270 ng/mL, and the tumor size partially decreased. The patient was monitored with neck ultrasonography every 3–6 months, which repeatedly showed no residual thyroid tissue or suspicious lymphadenopathy. Approximately 3 years after diagnosis, the thyroglobulin level increased to 4.1 ng/mL. PET-CT scan showed a focus of intense activity corresponding to the area of the pancreatic head without a clear anatomical correlate (Figure 4). Magnetic resonance imaging (MRI) with contrast could not be done at the time as the patient was suffering from a contrast-induced acute kidney injury. Due to esophageal stenosis, endoscopic ultrasound could not be performed. After

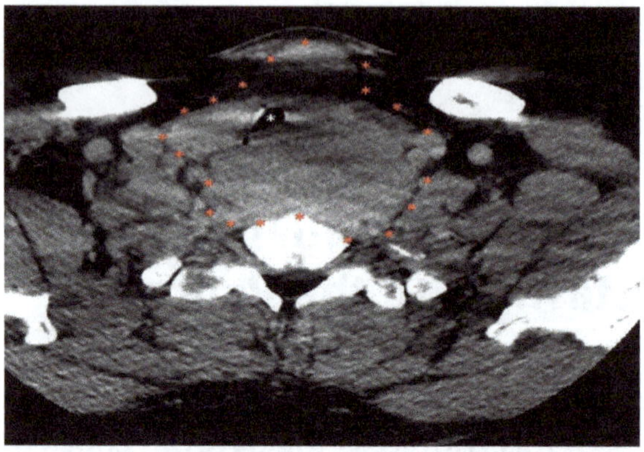

FIGURE 1: Enhanced axial computed tomography image at the level of the upper trachea demonstrating a large thyroid mass (red asterisks) resulting in compression and right lateral displacement of the trachea (white asterisk).

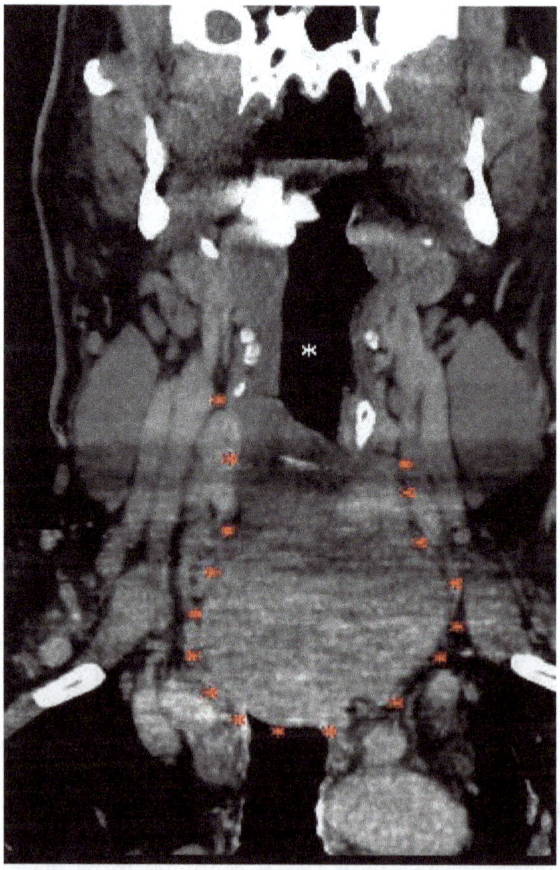

FIGURE 2: Enhanced coronal computed tomography image demonstrating a large thyroid mass (red asterisk) with invasion of the superior mediastinum. The airway (white asterisk) is displaced outside the field of view of this image.

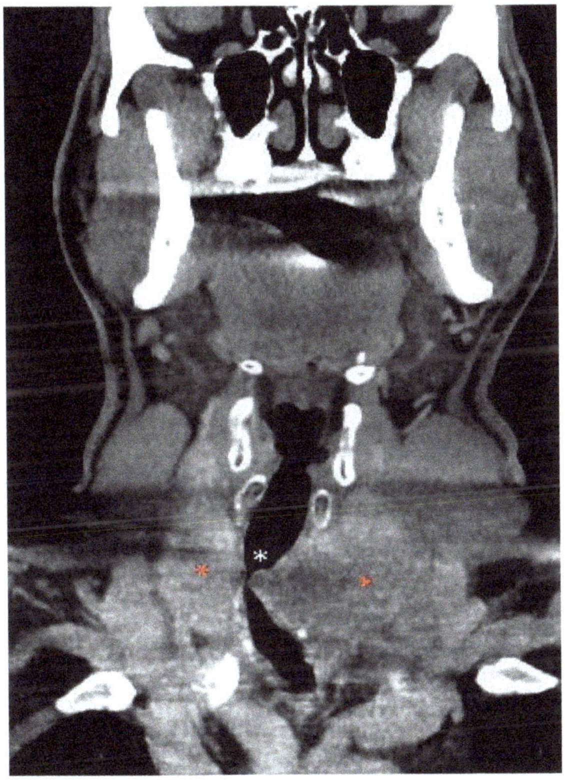

Figure 3: Enhanced coronal computed tomography image demonstrating severe narrowing of the trachea (white asterisk) by bilateral thyroid lobe tumor (red asterisks).

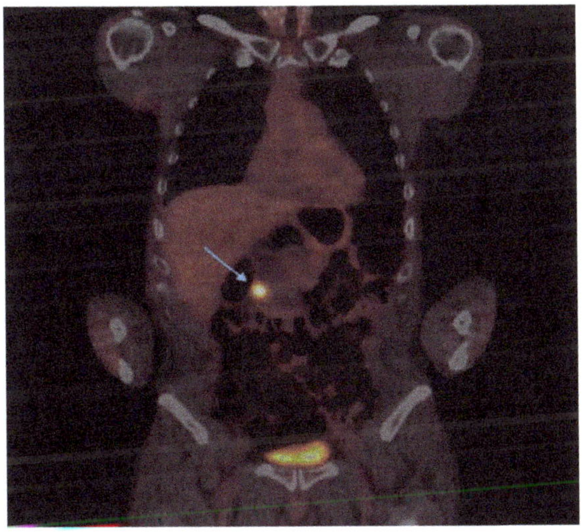

Figure 4: Positron emission tomography-computed tomography scan showing a focus of intense activity corresponding to the area of the pancreatic head (blue arrow) without a clear anatomical correlate.

discussion with the surgical oncology team and patient, he underwent radical pancreaticoduodenectomy and placement of a gastrostomy-jejunostomy tube. Pathology showed metastatic papillary thyroid carcinoma involving the pancreas (Figure 5), 3.0 cm in the greatest dimension, with the tumor showing strong and diffuse nuclear staining for TTF-1 and cytoplasmic

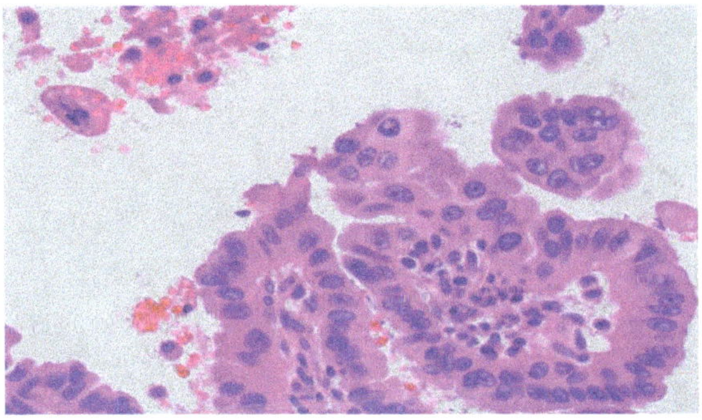

Figure 5: Hematoxylin and eosin stain. The tumor consisted of papillae lined by cells with the hallmark nuclear features of papillary thyroid cancer, such as nuclear grooves and pseudoinclusions. No psammoma bodies were seen. Overall, the histologic appearance was consistent with metastatic papillary thyroid carcinoma.

staining for thyroglobulin (Figure 6). Sixteen peripancreatic lymph nodes and one pericystic lymph node were removed during the operation and found to be negative for carcinoma. Genetic analysis was performed on the pancreatic lesion using Guardant 360 assay (Guardant Health Inc., Redwood City, CA). Gene amplification was detected in BRAF, KRAS, EGFR, and PIK3CA genes. Alteration in the promoter region of the TERT gene was also reported. Finally, fusion events involving RET, NTRK1, NTRK2, NTRK3, BRAF, and EGFR genes were reported as well. The patient was assessed by a medical oncologist, who started the patient on lenvatinib. The latest thyroglobulin level was 2.9 ng/mL. Unfortunately, lenvatinib treatment caused TSH to increase drastically, for which thyroid hormone dose was increased. The patient suffered from debilitating depression secondary to his medical condition, with notable and significant weight loss, prompting palliative care team involvement for goals of care discussion.

3. Discussion

While primary pancreatic tumors make up most pancreatic masses, metastatic lesions can be found in the pancreas, mainly from lung and renal primary malignancies [7]. Metastasis from PTC occurs in up to 34% of patients on follow-up after diagnosis and initial treatment, but it is usually local and rarely distant, with the liver being the most common site of metastasis in the gastrointestinal tract [8]. Aside from our case, there are only 15 reports of PTC metastasis to the pancreas in the literature [9]. Mean age at presentation was roughly 56.5 years. Like our patient, all reported cases had aggressive PTC on initial diagnosis, and mutations in the BRAFV600E gene were commonly found [8, 10–12]. Tall cell variant of PTC, which is known to be more aggressive in nature, was reported in only 3 patients in addition to our patient [6, 10, 13]. However, many cases showed nonavidity to radioactive iodine, which is known to be a poor prognostic factor as the loss of the sodium-iodine symporter is a sign of dedifferentiation [6, 8, 11–14]. It is well known that differentiated thyroid cancer has a female predominance, but strikingly, 11 of the reported cases including our patient were males. Most patients with

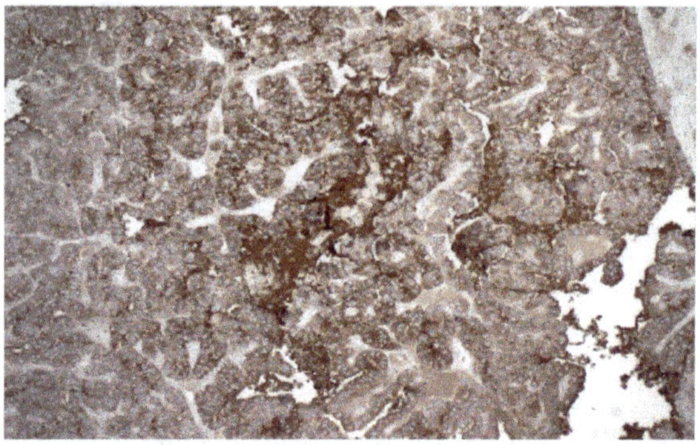

FIGURE 6: Immunohistochemistry for thyroglobulin was diffusely positive in tumor cells. This pattern confirms the tumor's thyroid origin.

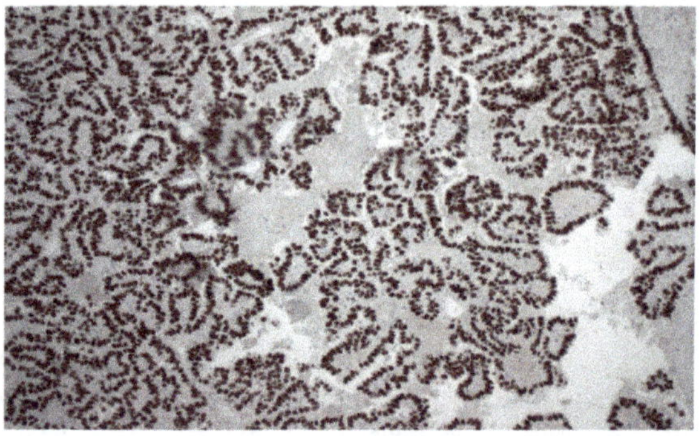

FIGURE 7: Immunohistochemistry for thyroid transcription factor-1 (TTF-1) was diffusely positive in tumor cells. This supports the tumor's thyroid origin.

pancreatic metastasis have undergone surgical resection, followed by tyrosine kinase inhibitor (TKI) therapy in only 3 cases [8, 9, 12]. Histologically, almost all cases reported positive staining for TTF-1 and thyroglobulin, except for one case [9]. Unique to two cases was the positive staining for Ki67 [9, 15]. In terms of location, the head of the pancreas was the most common location of metastasis, although 3 cases report multifocal disease in the tail and the body [15–17]. Lastly, the timing of presentation after primary tumor diagnosis varied widely between cases, starting as early as one month and as late as thirteen years. Only one case reported the metastatic disease at the same time as the primary cancer diagnosis [16].

The emergence of multiple targeted therapies has provided more hope in targeting metastatic thyroid cancer based on gene mutations that it may have. Some of the important gene mutations to screen for in thyroid cancer include BRAFV600E, RAS, RET, telomerase reverse transcriptase (TERT), and neurotrophic tyrosine kinase (NTRK) [18]. Depending on the gene mutation present, therapy can be specific for each patient.

Gene expression classifier (GEC) advancements have made it easier to detect such mutations at the time of fine-needle aspiration performance, which has been helpful in further stratifying patients with indeterminant nodules. This has reduced the number of patients that undergo surgery for such nodules given the high sensitivity of such tests [19].

As some aggressive forms of thyroid cancer become refractory to radioactive iodine, some agents were studied to determine whether they can resensitize thyroid cancer to radioactive iodine. Of interest, selumetinib (AZD6244), which is a mitogen-activated protein kinase (MAPK) inhibitor, was studied by Ho et al. in 2013 and found to produce a clinically significant increase in iodine uptake in a subgroup of patients with iodine-refractory thyroid cancer with RAS and BRAF gene mutations [18]. Dabrafenib (GSK2118436) was also studied by Rothenberg et al. in 2015 and showed benefit in redifferentiation of thyroid cancer in patients with BRAF gene mutation [20].

In our patient, metastasis developed despite TSH suppression, and surgical resection of the pancreatic metastasis was thought to be of benefit given it was the only site detected on the PET scan. Extensive discussion needs to be held with patients regarding future targeted therapy if any of the gene mutations return positive as such therapy is expected to cause a lengthy list of side effects.

4. Conclusion

We present an unfortunate case of aggressive primary thyroid cancer that has metastasized to the pancreas, a rare site of abdominal metastasis. Few points can be learnt from this case and previous similar cases:

(i) Despite the rarity of abdominal metastasis from primary thyroid cancer, it should always be considered as a possibility in a patient with rising thyroglobulin levels, especially with a history of high-risk features.

(ii) Developing ultrasensitive thyroglobulin assays that can detect even minimal serum levels can aid in early detection and prompt evaluation [21].

(iii) Discussion should be held with the patient regarding treatment options, including surgical interventions, medical therapy, radiation therapy, or combination of more than one.

(iv) Further studies (and possibly updated guidelines) should look further at the appropriate frequency of biochemical and radiological monitoring of patients with aggressive disease.

(v) Tyrosine kinase inhibitors continue to be the mainstay of medical treatment of aggressive papillary thyroid cancer that is refractory to radioactive iodine treatment. However, the long list of side effects must be discussed with patients, particularly the need for a higher dose of the thyroid hormone.

(vi) Multidisciplinary team including endocrinology, medical oncology, radiation oncology, general surgery, and palliative care must be involved in the care of such patients.

(vii) More studies need to be conducted regarding the psychosocial burdens of thyroid cancer recurrence and active persistent disease on patients.

References

[1] C. La Vecchia, M. Malvezzi, C. Bosetti et al., "Thyroid cancer mortality and incidence: a global overview," *International Journal of Cancer*, vol. 136, no. 9, pp. 2187–2195, 2015.

[2] L. Davies and H. G. Welch, "Current thyroid cancer trends in the United States," *JAMA Otolaryngology-Head & Neck Surgery*, vol. 140, no. 4, pp. 317–322, 2014.

[3] E. L. Mazzaferri, "Long-term outcome of patients with differentiated thyroid carcinoma: effect of therapy," *Endocrine Practice*, vol. 6, no. 6, pp. 469–476, 2000.

[4] C. Durante, N. Haddy, and E. Baudin, S. Leboulleux and D. Hartl, J. P. Travagli, B. Caillou, S. Leboulleux, D. Hartl et al., Long-term outcome of 444 patients with distant metastases from papillary and follicular thyroid carcinoma: benefits and limits of radioiodine therapy," *Journal of Clinical Endocrinology & Metabolism*, vol. 91, no. 8, pp. 2892–2899, 2006.

[5] J. Klubo-Gwiezdzinska, D. Morowitz, D. Van Nostrand et al., "Metastases of well-differentiated thyroid cancer to the gastrointestinal system," *Thyroid*, vol. 20, no. 4, pp. 381–387, 2010.

[6] R. Jobran, Z. W. Baloch, and V. Aviles, E. F. R., S. Schwartz, E. F. Rosato, S. Schwartz, and V. A. LiVolsi, Tall cell papillary carcinoma of the thyroid: metastatic to the pancreas," *Thyroid*, vol. 10, no. 2, pp. 185–187, 2000.

[7] L. J. Layfield and E. A. Jarboe, "Cytopathology of the pancreas: neoplastic and nonneoplastic entities," *Annals of Diagnostic Pathology*, vol. 14, no. 2, pp. 140–151, 2010.

[8] A. S. Alzahrani, A. AlQaraawi, F. Al Sohaibani, H. Almanea, and H. Abalkhail, "Pancreatic metastasis arising from a BRAFV600E-positive papillary thyroid cancer: the role of endoscopic ultrasound-guided biopsy and response to sorafenib therapy," *Thyroid*, vol. 22, no. 5, pp. 536–541, 2012.

[9] A. A. Machado, R. B. Luciano Lenz, I. R. Josino, and Martin Ac Cordero, A. V. Safatle-Ribeiro, G. A. D. Paulo, E. R. Baba, R. S. Uemura, and F. M. Filho, Pancreatic metastasis from papillary thyroid carcinoma: a case report," *JOP. Journal of Pancreas (Online)*, vol. 21, no. 6, pp. 151–155, 2020.

[10] M. Davidson, R. J. Olsen, A. A. Ewton, and R. J. Robbins, "Pancreas metastases from papillary thyroid carcinoma: a review of the literature," *Endocrine Practice*, vol. 23, no. 12, pp. 1425–1429, 2017.

[11] T. Borschitz, W. Eichhorn, C. Fottner et al., "Diagnosis and treatment of pancreatic metastases of a papillary thyroid carcinoma," *Thyroid*, vol. 20, no. 1, pp. 93–98, 2010.

[12] M. A. Tunio, K. R. Mushabbab AlAsiri, and W. AlShakweer, "Pancreas as delayed site of metastasis from papillary thyroid carcinoma," *Case Reports in Gastrointestinal Medicine 2013*, vol. 2013, Article ID 386263, 6 pages, 2013.

[13] A. A. Siddiqui, L. Olansky, R. N. Sawh, and W. M. Tierney, "Pancreatic metastasis of tall cell variant of papillary thyroid carcinoma: diagnosis by endoscopic ultrasound-guided fine needle aspiration," *JOP: Journal of the Pancreas*, vol. 7, no. 4, pp. 417–422, 2006.

[14] A. Meyer and M. Behrend, "Is pancreatic resection justified for metastasis of papillary thyroid cancer?" *Anticancer Research*, vol. 26, no. 3B, pp. 2269–2273, 2006.

[15] X. O. Li, Z. P. Li, P. Wang et al., "Pancreatic metastasis of papillary thyroid carcinoma: a case report with review of the literature," *International Journal of Clinical and Experimental Pathology*, vol. 7, no. 2, pp. 819–22, 2014.

[16] H. Ren, N. Ke, C. Tan, X. Wang, W. Cao, and X. Liu, "Unusual metastasis of papillary thyroid cancer to the pancreas, liver, and diaphragm: a case report with review of literature," *BMC Surgery*, vol. 20, no. 1, pp. 82–84, 2020.

[17] A. Angeles-Angeles, F. Chable-Montero, B. Martinez-Benitez, and J. Albores-Saavedra, "Unusual metastases of papillary thyroid carcinoma: report of 2 cases," *Annals of Diagnostic Pathology*, vol. 13, no. 3, pp. 189–196, 2009.

[18] A. L. Ho, R. K. Grewal, R. Leboeuf et al., "Selumetinib-enhanced radioiodine uptake in advanced thyroid cancer," *New England Journal of Medicine*, vol. 368, no. 7, pp. 623–632, 2013.

[19] R. T. Kloos, "Molecular profiling of thyroid nodules: current role for the Afirma gene expression classifier on clinical decision making," *Molecular Imaging and Radionuclide Therapy*, vol. 26, no. Suppl 1, pp. 36–49, 2017.

[20] S. M. Rothenberg, D. G. McFadden, E. L. Palmer, G. H. Daniels, and L. J. Wirth, "Redifferentiation of iodine-refractory BRAF V600E-mutant metastatic papillary thyroid cancer with dabrafenib," *Clinical Cancer Research*, vol. 21, no. 5, pp. 1028–1035, 2015.

[21] A. Flores-Rebollar, I. Pérez-Díaz, S. Lagunas-bárcenas, B. García-martínez, R. Rivera-Moscoso, and R. Fagundo-Sierra, "Clinical utility of an ultrasensitive thyroglobulin assay in the follow-up of patients with differentiated thyroid cancer: can the stimulation test be avoided in patients with an intermediate recurrence risk?" *Acta Otorhinolaryngologica Italica*, vol. 38, no. 3, pp. 188–193, 2018.

12

Three Successful Pregnancies in a Patient with Recurrent Cushing's Disease

W. Benothman, G. Saad, M. Kacem, and K. Ach

Endocrinology Unit, Department of Endocrinology, Farhat Hached University Hospital, Avenue Ibn El Jazzar, Sousse 4000, Tunisia

Correspondence should be addressed to W. Benothman; benothmanwafaa@gmail.com

Academic Editor: Suat Simsek

The association of pregnancy and Cushing's disease (CD) is rare. A 28-year-old woman was admitted for clinical suspicion of Cushing's syndrome. The investigations confirmed the diagnosis of CD with secondary hypogonadotropic hypogonadism due to an invasive pituitary macroadenoma. The patient underwent transsphenoidal adenomectomy, and histopathology showed an adrenocorticotropic hormone pituitary adenoma. Initial remission of CD ensued, and fertility was restored as the patient had 2 uncomplicated pregnancies. Five years and 10 months after surgery, a third spontaneous pregnancy was confirmed with underlying recurrent CD. Having mild hypercortisolism, CD was managed expectantly. The outcome was a healthy full-term neonate with no maternal complications during pregnancy or labor. Our case highlights the challenge faced by physicians of choosing the optimal approach to active CD in pregnancy. In cases where maternal and fetal complications are mild, conservative approach may be used and specific treatment can be postponed until after delivery.

1. Introduction

Cushing's disease (CD) is a severe endocrinopathy caused by a pituitary corticotroph adenoma that primarily affects females of childbearing age [1]. However, pregnancy rarely occurs during the course of CD due to the influence of hypercortisolism on the reproductive axis [2]. The best approach to women with active CD who become pregnant is still controversial [3]. Cushing's syndrome (CS) in pregnancy is deemed an obstetric high-risk condition associated with significant morbidity. Therefore, it requires careful surveillance and early effective treatment [4].

We report a case of a patient operated for an invasive pituitary corticotroph macroadenoma with initial remission. She had three successful uneventful pregnancies, the last one being in the setting of CD recurrence.

2. Case Report

A 28-year-old woman was referred to our endocrinology department by her urologist for clinical suspicion of CS and recently diagnosed diabetes mellitus (DM). She was admitted in the urology department for an acute kidney failure and a urinary tract infection secondary to bilateral ureteral calculi. She had a five-month history of headaches, menstrual irregularity, hirsutism, and depressive symptoms. On physical examination, she had facial plethora, purple abdominal striae, and normal blood pressure. Her body mass index was 22 kg/m^2. Her laboratory results showed serum potassium concentration at 2 mmol/L, blood glucose level of 17 mmol/L, and both high levels of cholesterol and low-density lipoprotein cholesterol at 6.88 and 4.92 mmol/L, respectively. The patient also had hypercalciuria. Dual X-ray absorptiometry (DXA) confirmed osteoporosis (T-score at −3.2). NPH insulin, psychotropics, and bisphosphonate treatment was started. Her endocrinological workup revealed a plasma adrenocorticotropic hormone (ACTH) level of 152.4 pg/ml (normal <50 pg/ml), morning serum cortisol (MC) of 760 μg/L, 24 h urine-free cortisol (UFC) of 975 μg (normal <45 μg), and unsuppressed cortisol after 1 mg overnight dexamethasone suppression test. Low-dose dexamethasone suppression testing (LDST) showed a plasma cortisol level of 660 μg/L and 24 h UFC of 1500 μg. High-dose dexamethasone suppression testing (HDST) was performed with a postsuppression cortisol level of 280 μg/L (>50% suppression from baseline serum cortisol). The patient showed both normal prolactin level and thyroid function; however, low gonadotropin levels were detected. These results were compatible with a pituitary-dependent CS. Pituitary magnetic resonance imaging (MRI) showed a right 17 mm adenoma with right cavernous sinus invasion and sellar floor erosion. Visual fields were normal (Figure 1).

These investigations confirmed the diagnosis of CD and a secondary hypogonadotropic hypogonadism due to an invasive pituitary macroadenoma. We could not find any sign of an accompanying multiple endocrine neoplasia type 1. Following a three-month pretreatment with ketoconazole (600 mg/day) and cabergoline (2 mg/week), the patient underwent transsphenoidal adenomectomy. Resection was deemed complete by the neurosurgeon. Adenoma cells stained positive for ACTH and were negative for prolactin, luteinizing hormone, follicle-stimulating hormone, growth hormone, and thyroid-stimulating hormone.

Clinical remission of CD ensued, accompanied by a resolution of DM and dyslipidemia and a normalization of both serum potassium and calcium excretion levels. Hormonal tests confirmed the remission with no hypoadrenalism. ACTH, MC, and 24 h UFC levels, at 3 months after surgery, were 15 pg/ml, 110 μg/L, and 60 μg (<4 times the upper limit of normal), respectively. Pituitary MRI showed no persistent mass. The preoperative hypogonadism was functional as gonadotropin levels were normal.

Five and seventeen months after the surgery, she had two spontaneous uneventful pregnancies with successful maternal-fetal outcomes and with no intrapartum or postpartum complications, such as pregnancy-induced hypertension or gestational diabetes. DXA showed improvement of bone density, as T-score was at −1.7. At follow-up, the patient was still at remission, confirmed by a two-year and a half postsurgery hormonal workup. She had regular menstrual cycles. The bone density went back to normal.

Three years and a half after the transsphenoidal surgery, pituitary MRI showed tumor remnant invading the right cavernous sinus. The patient had no clinical signs of CS. However, the endocrine laboratory assessment revealed high ACTH concentration exceeding 100 pg/ml. Plasma cortisol level was not suppressed with LDST (>18 μg/L). In light of these findings, recurrent CD was diagnosed. Shortly after, the patient had an extrauterine pregnancy with an intrauterine device *in situ*. Afterwards, she was lost to follow-up.

Five years and 8 months after her surgery, she returned for reexamination. She still had no clinical features of hypercortisolemia. Her menstrual cycles were regular. Biochemical workup was as follows: 24 h UFC 150 μg, ACTH 156 pg/ml, and cortisol after 1 mg overnight dexamethasone suppression 20 μg/L. Two months later, on her next visit, the patient reported a confirmed pregnancy at 5 weeks of amenorrhea. The pituitary MRI, performed at 3 weeks of amenorrhea, visualized a macroadenoma remnant measuring 8 × 10 mm invading the right cavernous sinus (grade 4 of Knosp) (Figure 2). All investigations confirmed again the diagnosis of recurrent CD with mild hypercorticism. Due to the risk of maternal complications and the possibility of unpredictable fetal anomalies, therapeutic abortion was discussed as an option, but the patient refused. CD was then managed expectantly.

Throughout her pregnancy, she had no specific treatment, in particular, no dopamine agonists. She had normal blood pressure and manifested no signs of pituitary apoplexy. Laboratory tests were in normal range. Both the oral glucose (75 gr) tolerance test at the 26th week of amenorrhea and the thyroid function were normal. Ultrasound imaging showed normal fetal growth and anatomy with no signs of macrosomia, hydramnios, or intrauterine growth retardation. Monitored closely by her obstetrician and us and at full term, the patient delivered a healthy male infant, weighing 3250 grams, by vaginal delivery.

Three months postpartum, the patient still had clinical "eucorticism," and she reported that she was breastfeeding. MC was 156 μg/L. Plasma cortisol levels were not suppressed with LDST. The pituitary MRI showed that the adenoma remained stable after pregnancy (Figure 3). A multidisciplinary collaboration between us, neurosurgeons, and radiation oncologists is being arranged for the management of the recurrent CD. Decision will be made after discussion with the patient.

3. Discussion

One of the unique aspects of our case is that CD was caused by a pituitary corticotroph macroadenoma. ACTH-secreting macroadenomas account for only about 6% of all CD cases [5]. Initial remission was achieved with a transsphenoidal surgery. Shortly after, fertility was restored and the patient had 2 uncomplicated pregnancies. As the diagnosis of CD recurrence was established, a third pregnancy was confirmed. Adding another unusual aspect to our case, pregnancy is exceptionally rare in CS. The first case was reported in 1953 by Hunt and McConahey [6]. More than 200 cases have been reported in the literature since then [7]. The most frequent etiology of CS diagnosed during pregnancy is adrenal adenoma (40 to 60% of the cases), whilst in nonpregnant women, it is pituitary lesions (CD in 70% of the cases). Such difference is still poorly understood [8, 9]. It has been suggested that hypersecretion of both cortisol and androgens in CD is associated with impaired fertility, in contrast to an almost exclusive hypersecretion of cortisol with minimal androgen production in peripheral CS [10].

It is normal to observe changes in the pituitary gland and endocrine function during pregnancy. Often extending into the suprasellar space towards the optic chiasm, the pituitary gland increases nearly 1.5 times in size [11]. The increased sensitivity of pituitary corticotrophs to CRH, their decreased sensitivity to cortisol's negative feedback inhibition, and a placental CRH production are responsible of the rise of maternal plasma ACTH and cortisol. Plasma concentrations of both hormones typically reach levels comparable to those observed in patients with CD and increase during labor [12, 13]. This transient, but physiologic, relative

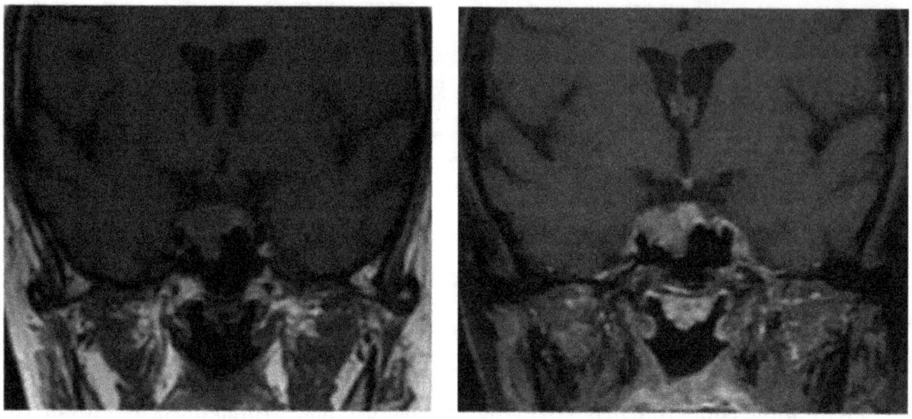

(a) (b)

Figure 1: Pregadolinium (a) and postgadolinium (b) T1-weighted coronal images of pituitary MRI showing 17 mm adenoma with right cavernous sinus invasion and sellar floor erosion.

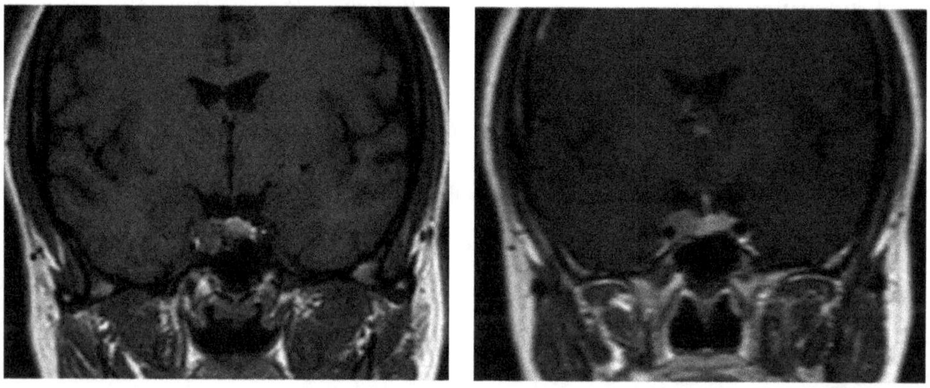

(a) (b)

Figure 2: Pregadolinium (a) and postgadolinium (b) T1-weighted coronal images of pituitary MRI showing 10 mm adenoma with right cavernous sinus invasion.

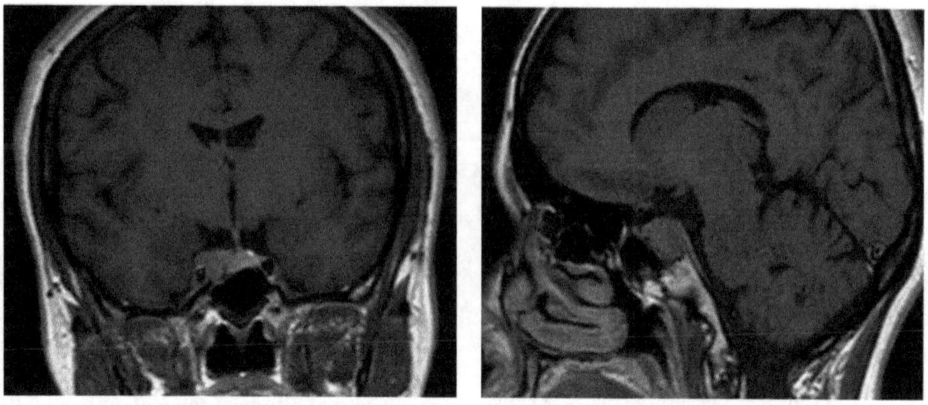

(a) (b)

Figure 3: Coronal (a) and sagittal (b) images of pituitary MRI showing 10 mm hypoenhancing adenoma with invasion of the right cavernous sinus.

hypercortisolism during gestation and the immediate postpartum period may somehow promote tumorigenesis resulting in a higher risk of ACTH-secreting pituitary adenomas and CD following pregnancy [13]. In an exploratory study by Palejwala et al. [14], over one-fourth of all women of reproductive age with CD appeared to have symptomatic disease onset within 1 year of childbirth. The median number of pregnancies in the pregnancy-associated CD cohort was 2 suggesting that repeated "exposure" to the stress of pregnancy may also be a significant factor. Two thirds of women of reproductive age and nonpregnancy-associated CD had no pregnancies prior to their diagnosis of CD. This fact, and that CD affects both sexes, strongly advocates that the gestational changes may be just one possible factor among many others that ultimately leads to a clinically significant corticotroph adenoma.

In light of these findings, the factors in our case of a recurrent CD are the repeated exposure to pituitary corticotroph hyperactivity during 2 peripartum periods and essentially the likely incomplete surgical resection. Even though exeresis was deemed complete by the neurosurgeon and early postsurgery imaging, it is greatly difficult to obtain such result for macroadenomas. The subsequent growth of remnant tumor cells was responsible for the relapse of the hypercortisolism. Extensive experience on nonpregnant patients with CD has noted that, following transsphenoidal surgery, a considerable proportion of individuals has normal plasma and urinary levels of cortisol without developing adrenal insufficiency, just as our case. The clinical symptoms improved but, in most cases, hypercortisolism reappeared during follow-up [15]. Actuarial recurrence rates of CD after initial successful transsphenoidal surgery at 1, 2, 3, and 5 years were 0.5, 6.7, 10.8, and 25.5%, respectively [16]. The diagnosis of recurrence was confirmed three years and a half after the surgery for our patient, roughly 2 years after her last pregnancy. It is quite possible that the gestational hypercortisolemia was responsible of an earlier recurrence, as the adenoma remnant was stimulated by the hormonal milieu during the two pregnancies.

Approximately 40% of patients with CD during pregnancy received treatment during gestation. Of these, 11.3% women only received medical treatment [8]. Surgery is the first-line treatment for CD in pregnant and nonpregnant patients, with reported live birth rates up to 87% following transsphenoidal adenomectomy or adrenalectomy [4]. Due to their potential harmful or teratogenic effects and their delayed results, other options to treat hypercortisolism, such as radiotherapy and mitotane, are contraindicated during gestation [17]. In all cases of successfully treated CD with transsphenoidal surgery, the procedure was performed between the end of the first trimester and the early second trimester, an optimum period with lower maternal and fetal complications. Medical therapy is a second treatment option, generally initiated during the second or third trimesters. The most common steroidogenesis inhibitors were metyrapone followed by ketoconazole and cyproheptadine used in 61%, 15%, and 11% of cases, respectively [4]. Dopamine agonists, the only available molecules in Tunisia, have been successfully used for CD in minority of pregnant patients with no major adverse effects noted [8]. Testing more than 6,000 pregnancies, the safety of bromocriptine in pregnancy, both for the mother and the fetus, was demonstrated. The few studies regarding the safety of cabergoline in pregnancy showed no higher rate of maternal-fetal complications and it is currently an FDA pregnancy category B drug [18]. The stage of pregnancy, etiology, severity of hypercortisolism, and potential benefit of treatment, all contribute to treatment decision-making [2]. Pregnant women with mild hypercortisolism, as our patient, and/or diagnosed late in gestation may be managed expectantly, and causal treatment deferred until after delivery. Potential risks of surgical or medical treatment might exceed the benefits. Pregnancy during CD presents great maternal-fetal risks. Metabolic and cardiovascular parameters should be monitored closely, and hyperglycemia or hypertension should be treated appropriately upon diagnosis [19, 20]. However, some authors suggested that treatment of mild hypercortisolism prevents adverse outcomes, as it increases live birth rate, avoids disease worsening, and reduces the risk of preeclampsia [12]. The most frequently stated maternal complications in CS are hypertension (68%), diabetes (25%), preeclampsia (14%), osteoporosis and fractures (5%), heart failure (3%), and maternal death (2%) [21, 22]. Due to placental enzymes such as 11β-hydroxysteroid dehydrogenase type 2, the fetus is normally protected from maternal hypercortisolism. The enzyme converts glucocorticoids to inactive metabolites [23]. However, complications can occur, and the most common ones include prematurity (43%), intrauterine growth restriction (21%), stillbirth (6%), spontaneous abortion or intrauterine death (5%), and hypoadrenalism (2%) [21].

It has been stated that maternal and fetal outcomes are better in patients with CD than in those with peripheral CS [24]. Furthermore, just like in our case, uncomplicated pregnancies ending with vaginal delivery have been reported in women with CS, especially in those treated with no complete remission. It appears that morbidity is rather related to the severity of underlying hypercortisolism [19]. As hypercortisolism was mild in our case, no such complications had been noted.

The pituitary gland rapidly returns to its normal size after the immediate postpartum period, regardless of breastfeeding status [25]. The pituitary MRI showed that the adenoma remained stable after pregnancy for our patient. The choice of treatment method for the recurrent CD will be discussed in a multidisciplinary concertation meeting.

4. Conclusion

Pregnancy with preexisting CD poses a challenge to physicians because of its association with maternal and fetal morbidities. The decision on treating CD during pregnancy and choice of treatment method must be approached on a case-by-case basis. A multidisciplinary approach consisting of endocrinology, obstetrics, endocrine surgery, and anesthesiology is highly recommended. A conservative approach may be used and a specific treatment can be postponed until after delivery in cases with mild maternal-fetal complications.

References

[1] K. Tang, L. Lu, M. Feng et al., "The incidence of pregnancy-associated Cushing's disease and its relation to pregnancy; a retrospective study," *Front Endocrinol (Lausanne)*, vol. 11, p. 305, 2020.

[2] S. P. Ildefonso-Najarro, E. A. Plasencia-Dueñas, C. J. Benites-Moya, J. Carrion-Rojas, and M. J. Concepción-Zavaleta, "Pregnancy during the course of Cushing's syndrome: a case report and literature review," *Endocrinology, Diabetes & Metabolism Case Reports*, vol. 2020, no. 1, pp. 20–0022, 2020.

[3] M. Almalki, "Cabergoline use for Cushing's disease during pregnancy: mini review," *Clinical Research and Trials*, vol. 3, no. 2, pp. 1-2, 2017.

[4] K. Jolly, A. Darr, W. Arlt, S. Ahmed, and N. Karavitaki, "Surgery for Cushing 's disease in pregnancy: our experience and a literature review," *Annals of the Royal College of Surgeons of England*, vol. 101, no. 1, pp. e26–e31, 2019.

[5] Y. S. Woo, A. M. Isidori, W. Z. Wat et al., "Clinical and biochemical characteristics of adrenocorticotropin-secreting macroadenomas," *The Journal of Clinical Endocrinology & Metabolism*, vol. 90, no. 8, pp. 4963–4969, 2005.

[6] A. B. Hunt and W. M. McConahey, "Pregnancy associated with diseases of the adrenal glands*," *American Journal of Obstetrics and Gynecology*, vol. 66, no. 5, pp. 970–987, 1953.

[7] X. Zhang, H. Liao, X. Zhu, D. Shi, and X. Chen, "A successful pregnancy in a patient with secondary hypertension caused by adrenal adenoma: a case report," *BMC Pregnancy and Childbirth*, vol. 19, no. 1, pp. 1–8, 2019.

[8] F. Caimari, E. Valassi, P. Garbayo et al., "Cushing's syndrome and pregnancy outcomes: a systematic review of published cases," *Endocrine*, vol. 55, no. 2, pp. 555–563, 2017.

[9] T. Brue, V. Amodru, and F. Castinetti, "Management of endocrine disease: management of Cushing's syndrome during pregnancy: solved and unsolved questions," *European Journal of Endocrinology*, vol. 178, no. 6, pp. R259–R266, 2018.

[10] M. A. Buescher, H. D. McClamrock, and E. Y. Adashi, "Cushing syndrome in pregnancy," *Obstetrics & Gynecology*, vol. 79, no. 1, pp. 130–137, 1992.

[11] H. Dinç, F. Esen, A. Demirci, A. Sari, and H. R. Gümele, "Pituitary dimensions and volume measurements in pregnancy and post partum," *Acta Radiologica*, vol. 39, no. 1, pp. 64–69, 1998.

[12] J. R. Lindsay and L. K. Nieman, "The hypothalamic-pituitary-adrenal axis in pregnancy: challenges in disease detection and treatment," *Endocrine Reviews*, vol. 26, no. 6, pp. 775–799, 2005.

[13] G. Mastorakos, "Maternal and fetal hypothalamic-pituitary-adrenal axes during pregnancy and postpartum," *Annals of the New York Academy of Sciences*, vol. 997, no. 1, pp. 136–149, 2003.

[14] S. K. Palejwala, A. R. Conger, A. A. Eisenberg et al., "Pregnancy-associated Cushing's disease? An exploratory retrospective study," *Pituitary*, vol. 21, no. 6, pp. 584–592, 2018.

[15] J. Estrada, J. García-Uría, C. Lamas et al., "The complete normalization of the adrenocortical function as the criterion of cure after transsphenoidal surgery for Cushing's disease," *Journal of Clinical Endocrinology & Metabolism*, vol. 86, no. 12, pp. 5695–5699, 2001.

[16] C. G. Patil, D. M. Prevedello, S. P. Lad et al., "Late recurrences of Cushing's disease after initial successful transsphenoidal surgery," *The Journal of Clinical Endocrinology & Metabolism*, vol. 93, no. 2, pp. 358–362, 2008.

[17] S. Leiba, R. Weinstein, B. Shindel et al., "The protracted effect of o,p'-DDD in Cushing's disease and its impact on adrenal morphogenesis of young human embryo," *Annales d'Endocrinologie*, vol. 50, no. 1, pp. 49–53, 1989.

[18] A. Nakhleh, L. Saiegh, M. Reut, M. S. Ahmad, I. W. Pearl, and C. Shechner, "Cabergoline treatment for recurrent Cushing's disease during pregnancy," *Hormones (Athens)*, vol. 15, no. 3, pp. 453–458, 2016.

[19] N. Polli, F. P. Giraldi, and F. Cavagnini, "Cushing's disease and pregnancy," *Pituitary*, vol. 7, no. 4, pp. 237–241, 2004.

[20] M. Ragonese, O. R. Cotta, F. Ferraù, F. Trimarchi, and S. Cannavò, "How to diagnose and manage Cushing's disease during pregnancy, when hypercortisolism is mild?" *Gynecological Endocrinology*, vol. 28, no. 8, pp. 637–639, 2012.

[21] J. R. Lindsay, J. Jonklaas, E. H. Oldfield, and L. K. Nieman, "Cushing's syndrome during pregnancy: personal experience and review of the literature," *The Journal of Clinical Endocrinology & Metabolism*, vol. 90, no. 5, pp. 3077–3083, 2005.

[22] O. Lekarev and M. I. New, "Adrenal disease in pregnancy," *Best Practice & Research Clinical Endocrinology & Metabolism*, vol. 25, no. 6, pp. 959–973, 2011.

[23] C. E. Andreescu, R. A. Alwani, J. Hofland et al., "Adrenal Cushing's syndrome during pregnancy," *European Journal of Endocrinology*, vol. 177, no. 5, pp. K13–K20, 2017.

[24] A. Yawar, L. M. Zuberi, and N. Haque, "Cushing's disease and pregnancy: case report and literature review," *Case Report*, vol. 13, no. 3, pp. 296–299, 2007.

[25] A. D. Elster, T. G. Sanders, F. S. Vines, and M. Y. Chen, "Size and shape of the pituitary gland during pregnancy and post partum: measurement with MR imaging," *Radiology*, vol. 181, no. 2, pp. 531–535, 1991.

13

"Primary Hyperparathyroidism (PHPT) in Children: Two Case Reports and Review of the Literature"

Gerdi Tuli, [1,2] **Jessica Munarin**, [1,2] **Daniele Tessaris**, [1,2] **Raffaele Buganza**, [1,2] **Patrizia Matarazzo**, [1,2] **and Luisa De Sanctis** [1,2]

[1] *Department of Pediatric Endocrinology, Regina Margherita Children's Hospital of Turin, Turin, Italy*
[2] *Department of Sciences of Public Health and Pediatrics, University of Turin, Turin, Italy*

Correspondence should be addressed to Gerdi Tuli; gerdi.tuli@unito.it

Academic Editor: Lucy Mastrandrea

Primary hyperparathyroidism (PHPT) is a rare disorder in children and adolescents. Typical biochemical features are hypercalcemia and hypophosphatemia, but the clinical features can be heterogeneous, and in some cases, symptoms are vague and nonspecific, leading to misdiagnosis or late diagnosis. Herein, we report two cases of PHPT in pediatric age with different presenting symptoms, pain in the foot, and progressive alteration of the gait in the first case and recurrent abdominal pain with emotional lability in the second. Biochemical and radiological assessment confirmed PHPT. Both cases were treated surgically as definitive treatment, but in the second case, previous medical treatment with cinacalcet, a calcimimetic agent, was required to reduce serum PTH and calcium levels. After surgery, despite conventional treatment with calcium and calcitriol, case 1 developed a hungry bone syndrome. The analysis of the MEN-1 (Multiple Endocrine Neoplasia) gene was negative in both cases. A diagnosis of PHPT should be considered when children or adolescents present bone pain with radiological imaging of osteolytic lesion and biochemical feature of hypercalcemia associated with hypophosphatemia. In PHPT, the gold standard treatment is represented by surgery followed by strict postoperative endocrine monitoring to maintain adequate homeostasis of calcium and bone metabolism.

1. Introduction

Primary hyperparathyroidism (PHPT), a rare disorder in pediatric age, with an estimated incidence of 2–5 cases in 100,000 live births, is characterized by excessive secretion of parathyroid hormone (PTH), responsible for hypercalcemia and hypophosphatemia [1–3]. Most cases of PHPT are not hereditary, and the familial PHPT accounts for 10–20% of cases [4–7].

The main clinical features involve the skeleton and the kidney. Bone pain, skeleton deformities, and the increased fracture risk at any skeleton sites are the most important symptoms. Rarely, the first manifestation of PHPT can be rickets or osteomalacia, associated with short stature [1,7]. Nephrocalcinosis and nephrolithiasis are the main complications of PHPT, and hypercalciuria is the most common risk factor for renal stone development.

Other clinical features related to PHPT include neurological symptoms (attention-deficit disorders, irritable behaviours, depression, weakness, seizures, proximal myopathy, and lethargy), gastrointestinal symptoms (vomiting, nausea, diarrhea, and acute pancreatitis), and cardiovascular complications, including prolonged QT interval (7–10).

Radiological assessment includes parathyroid and thyroid ultrasound and 99mTC-sestamibi scintigraphy, total body bone scintiscan, jaw X-ray, and X-ray evaluation of the skeletal site with bone pain.

The gold standard treatment in children is surgery [8, 9]. In the presence of severe hypercalcemia, parenteral isotonic solutions or calciomimetic agents such as cinacalcet, which lower serum calcium and PTH, but do not improve bone mass density (BMD), are required [10]. An alternative presurgical therapeutic option includes the use of bisphosphonates that improve BMD and lower biochemical markers of bone turnover in patients with PHPT, but have less effect on lowering calcium and PTH [7].

Similarly to adults, solitary parathyroid adenoma is the most common finding in children with sporadic PHPT [2, 11], but unlike in adult patients, PHPT symptoms are frequently present at diagnosis in pediatric age. However, in the absence of a family history of PHPT, since PHPT symptoms can be vague and nonspecific, the disease may be misdiagnosed or delayed in the diagnosis [8, 9, 11], especially in pubertal age, when rapid bone growth may unmask certain skeletal manifestations of PHPT [1, 2].

We report the clinical history of two female adolescents with PHPT who differed in clinical presentation at diagnosis, both referred to the pediatric endocrinologist 12 months after the onset of symptoms. In the first case, skeletal manifestations of osteolytic lesion at the right calcaneus were present, whereas in the second case, the main symptoms were abdominal pain and irritability.

2. Case Reports

2.1. Case 1. A 16-year-old girl of Philippine origin was referred to our department as she complained of right foot pain and progressive gait abnormalities in the last 12 months. Auxological parameters showed short stature (141.1 cm, <3° Tanner percentile), within a familial short stature context, and normal weight (48 kg, 10° Tanner percentile) and BMI (24.1 kg/m^2).

Radiographic evaluation of the lower limb demonstrated an osteolytic lesion to the right heel and a concomitant lesion of unclear interpretation to the left cuboid bone, both then confirmed at CT scan and MRI.

Biochemical investigations revealed elevated serum PTH levels (598 pg/ml; normal range 15–57), elevated serum calcium concentration (3.02 mmol/L; normal range 2.2–2.7), and low serum phosphate levels (0.56 mmol/L; normal range 1–1.8), as shown in Table 1. The urinary calcium to creatinine ratio was 0.25 mg/mg, and renal ultrasound and ECG were normal.

Total body bone scintiscan with 99Tc-oxidronate revealed increased absorption at the right heel, consistent with a brown tumor finding.

Parathyroid ultrasound did not show any significant pathological signs, but the Tc99/sestaMIBI parathyroid scan revealed an abnormal and persistent focal retention of the tracer in the right inferior thyroid pole, consistent with the hyperactivity of the right inferior parathyroid.

Therefore, the biochemical and radiological features indicated a PHPT condition; to rule out MEN-1, pituitary function was analyzed and showed normal hormonal profile. Fasting glucose, insulin, and calcitonin levels were normal; no lipoma, angiofibroma, or jaw tumors were present; both parents and siblings had normal serum PTH levels. Genetic analysis of the MEN-1 gene was negative for mutations.

The girl underwent right inferior parathyroidectomy through a minimally invasive approach, after intraoperative evaluation of the parathyroid hormone. Histological examination confirmed the presence of an adenoma (dimension 3.3 × 1.7 × 0.5 cm, weight 3 gr). To control the hypocalcemia caused by the transient hypoparathyroidism of the remaining parathyroid glands previously inhibited by the adenoma, conventional treatment with oral administration of calcitriol (0.75 mcg/day) and calcium carbonate was started; the latter was initially given at 2 g/day and then increased up to 3 g/day for numbness; finger paraesthesia and positive Chvostek and Trousseau signs were associated with low serum calcium despite high parathyroid hormone levels (Ca 1.85 mmol/L, PTH 113 ng/ml). Subsequently, the patient no longer presented signs or symptoms of hypocalcemia; laboratory analyses showed adequate calcium-phosphate metabolism and normal serum PTH levels (31 pg/ml).

Three months after surgery, biochemical evaluation again showed an increase in the PTH value (146 pg/ml), with sightly low serum calcium levels (2.02 mmol/L), configuring a hungry bone syndrome (HBS) condition, characterized by an elevated uptake of calcium by the bones after a prolonged period of hypercalcemia due to hyperparathyroidism. The oral calcium carbonate dose was, therefore, increased to 4 g/day, with normalization of serum calcium level (2.4 mmol/L) and partial response of PTH levels (67 pg/ml).

2.2. Case 2. A 14-year-old girl was referred to our department, having complained of recurrent abdominal pain and emotional lability for the last 12 months. Auxological parameters showed normal height (153.7 cm, 10–25° Tanner percentile), weight (47 kg, 10–25° Tanner percentile), and BMI (19.9 kg/m^2). Biochemical investigations revealed high serum calcium concentration (3.36 mmol/L, normal range 2.2–2.7), low phosphate level (0.6 mmol/L; normal range 1–1.8), and elevated PTH levels (320 pg/ml; normal range 15–57), as shown in Table 1.

The parathyroid ultrasound evaluation showed the presence of a hypoechoic nodule in the right inferior thyroid pole (22 × 12 mm), confirmed by the Tc99/sestaMIBI scan which revealed an abnormal and persistent retention of the tracer in the same area, therefore compatible with hyperactivity of the right inferior parathyroid.

To rule out the presence of multiple endocrine neoplasia, pituitary function was investigated and showed normal hormone secretion. Fasting glucose, insulin, and calcitonin levels were normal, and no lipoma, angiofibroma, or jaw tumors were present; parents and siblings had normal serum PTH levels. Genetic analysis for MEN-1 mutations was negative.

The urinary calcium/creatinine ratio was 0.35 mg/mg, and abdominal ultrasound displayed the presence of a small hyperechoic image (5 mm) in the upper pole of the right kidney, consistent with nephrolithiasis, although asymptomatic. Spinal X-ray showed generalized bone rarefaction, evident in all vertebral bodies, and the whole-body bone scan revealed regular ^{99}Tc-oxidronate uptake.

Biochemical and radiological investigations confirmed the diagnosis of PHPT. Prior to surgery, as high serum calcium levels represented a high intraoperative risk, treatment with a calcimimetic agent (cinacalcet) was started,

TABLE 1: Laboratory data of cases reported at diagnosis, after surgery, and at the last evaluation.

		Case 1	Case 2
Serum calcium (mmol/l)	Diagnosis	3.02	3.36
	After surgery	1.85	2.35
	Last evaluation	2.3	2.3
Phosphate (mmol/l)	Diagnosis	0.56	0.6
	After surgery	0.84	1.04
	Last evaluation	0.84	1.13
PTH (pg/ml)	Diagnosis	598	320
	After surgery	113	131
	Last evaluation	67	46
25-hydroxyvitamin D (ng/ml)	Diagnosis	6.8*	16.2*
	After surgery	—	61.9*
	Last evaluation	—	43*
CaU/CrU	Diagnosis	0.25	0.35
	After surgery	0.06	0.1
	Last evaluation	0.01	0.05
Adenoma weight (gr)		3	2.5

at 60 mg/day dose for three months, with an improvement in calcium and phosphate metabolism (Ca 2.97 mmol/L, P 0.6 mmol/L), with still elevated PTH levels (457.9 pg/mL). Since cinacalcet is an off-label drug in pediatric age, permission of the local Ethics Committee and informed consent from the parents were obtained prior to its administration.

The girl, therefore, underwent right inferior parathyroidectomy through a mini-invasive approach, with intraoperative monitoring of the PTH; histological examination confirmed the presence of adenomatous tissue (dimension 2,5 × 1.4 × 0.5 cm, weight 2.5 gr). Biochemical investigations after surgery showed a rapid decrease in calcium level (2.35 mmol/L), with lowering of PTH levels (131 pg/ml); subsequently, as the girl had lip and finger tremors with mild hypocalcemia (Ca 2.01 mmol/L), conventional treatment with oral administration of calcium carbonate (1 g/day) and oral calcitriol (62.5 mcg/day) was started, with no further signs or symptoms of hypocalcemia and normalization of calcium-phosphate homeostasis and normal level of PTH (46 pg/ml) on biochemical monitoring. Calcium treatment was stopped after one month, while calcitriol after two years; currently, after 6 years from the onset of primary hyperparathyroidism, there is no recurrence of the disease and calcium-phosphate metabolism is adequate.

3. Discussion

PHPT is a very rare condition among children and adolescents; Table 2 indicates the data emerging from the literature describing pediatric cohorts with at least 5 subjects [1–25, 27].

The two cases of PHPT reported here showed a different clinical onset at diagnosis, with bone pain in the first case and vague symptoms such as abdominal pain and behavioural problems in the second. Both patients were referred to the pediatric endocrinologist 12 months after the onset of symptoms.

The first presented case highlights that, in case of laboratory data suggestive for PHPT, even in the presence of US of the neck negative for pathological findings, a Tc^{99}/sestaMIBI parathyroid scan has to be performed [9]. Once PHPT is confirmed, if bone pain is present, an X-ray of the syntomatic skeletal site and of the jaw and whole-body scintiscan should be performed, as well as an ECG evaluation.

Parathyroid adenoma represents the most frequent PHPT etiology in pediatric age, with higher aggressive behaviour than adults and higher serum and urinary calcium levels.

It is noteworthy that, in the presence of significant hypercalcemia, especially if associated with cardiac arrhythmia, the intraoperative risk is high; therefore, in such cases, the utilization of a calcimimetic agent, i.e., cinacalcet (Mimpara) or bisphosphonates, for short periods could allow to lower calcium levels, despite high levels of PTH, and to act in a safer surgical context, although few data on their use as calcium-lowering agents in pediatric age are present in the literature so far.

After successful removal of one or more hyperfunctioning parathyroid glands, patients with PHPT show a rapid transient decrease in serum calcium levels due to functional inhibition of healthy parathyroid glands. This hypocalcemia is generally mild, lasts a maximum of 2–4 days after surgery, and is independent of the size of the hyperactive glands [26, 28]. Conventional treatment with oral calcium and calcitriol is the gold standard for this condition. However, in case of long-standing PHPT, hungry bone syndrome (HBS) can occur, as shown in the first case presented. This term has been coined to represent the deep (Ca < 2.1 mmol/l) and prolonged (longer than four days after operation) hypocalcemia, following parathyroidectomy in severe hyperparathyroidism [29].

At the time of presentation, nearly 80% of children are symptomatic and have end-organ damage, mostly involving the bone and kidney [2]. The condition can manifest with various signs and symptoms related to hypercalcemia, involving the gastrointestinal, musculoskeletal, renal, and neurological systems; such nonspecific clinical presentation may, therefore, be responsible for misdiagnosis or delayed diagnosis. In the presence of such symptoms, pediatricians should be aware of monitoring bone metabolism, evaluating serum calcium and phosphate levels, as well as PTH, when bone pain or nephrocalcinosis is also present.

Once PHPT is diagnosed in pediatric age, genetic analysis for Multiple Endocrine Neoplasia (MEN) syndromes and PTH assessment, as well as X-ray of jaw and urinary calcium to creatinine ratio, in parents and siblings should be carried out to search for genetic or familial conditions [30].

In conclusion, PHPT is a rare disease in pediatric age that can be misdiagnosed; the presence of PHPT should be considered if children or adolescents present with bone pain or nephrocalcinosis, radiological imaging of osteolytic lesions, or vague gastrointestinal or neurological not otherwise explained.

Table 2: Main papers reporting patients with PHPT in the pediatric age.

Author	Year	No. of pediatric patients	Main results
Allo et al. [12]	1982	53	Adenoma in 64.2% of studied patients; hyperplasia in 30.2%, overall in <18 y.o. (38%) vs. >18 y.o. (18.5%) patients
Lawson et al. [13]	1996	11	All sporadic PHPT. Delayed diagnosis in children; at diagnosis, 91% patients were symptomatic (renal stones 45%, abdominal pain 18%, learning difficulties 18%, musculoskeletal abnormalities 9%, and fatigue 9%). Mean serum Ca^{++}: 3.39 mmol/l at diagnosis
Cronin et al. [14]	1996	8	Pediatric cohort with PHPT due to parathyroid adenoma, presenting mostly with hypercalcemic crisis (50%). Mean serum Ca^{++}: 3.5 mmol/l at diagnosis
Loh et al. [15]	1998	22	Pediatric cohort with PHPT due to parathyroid adenoma, presenting mostly with fatigue (77%) or weakness (64%). Mean serum Ca^{++}: 3.07 mmol/l; mean serum PTH 131 pg/ml at diagnosis
Harman et al. [16]	1999	33	Pediatric cohort with PHPT due to parathyroid adenoma, symptomatic in 94% of cases, mostly renal stones (7/33) and bone disease (9/33). Mean serum Ca^{++}: 3.02 mmol/l at diagnosis; mean adenoma weight 0.96 gr
Hsu and Levine [17]	2002	16	Single adenomas in 11 patients; multiple-gland disease in 2 patients, including 1 with MEN2
Kollars et al. [2]	2005	52	Symptomatic in 79% of cases; end-organ damage (nephrocalcinosis or lithiasis, acute pancreatitis, or bone involvement) in 44%. Mean serum Ca^{++}: 3.1 mmol/l; mean serum P 1.8 mmol/l; mean serum PTH 76.3 pg/ml at diagnosis
Bhadada et al. [18]	2008	14	Single parathyroid adenoma in 85.7%, 1 patient with four-gland hyperplasia and 1 MEN-1. Main reported symptoms were bone disease, recurrent nephrolithiasis, and pancreatitis. Mean serum Ca^{++}: 2.77 mmol/l; mean P 0.9 mmol/l; mean serum PTH 781 pg/ml at diagnosis
Libansky et al. [19]	2008	10	Pediatric cohort with parathyroid adenoma and 1 ectopic adenoma. Mean serum Ca^{++}: 3.21 mmol/l; mean serum PTH 217.6 pg/ml at diagnosis
Mallet E [4]	2008	55	31 adenomas and 11 hyperplasias underwent surgery. Medical management (i.v. diphosphonates) in 11 neonates. Mean serum Ca^{++}: 3.64 mmol/l; mean serum P 1.3 mmol/l; mean serum PTH 536 pg/ml at diagnosis
Al-shanafey et al. [20]	2010	5	Surgical management in neonates with severe hyperparathyroidism, all symptomatic with lethargy, poor feeding, and irritability. In all patients, surgical treatment was curative. Mean serum Ca^{++}: 3.84 mmol/l; mean serum PTH 3607 pg/ml at diagnosis
George et al. [5]	2010	15	Single parathyroid adenoma in 100% of patients. Main reported symptoms were bone pain, fractures, proximal myopathy, and renal calculi; 33.3% had postoperative HBS. Mean serum Ca^{++}: 3.35 mmol/l; mean serum P 0.98 mmol/l; mean serum PTH 801 pg/ml at diagnosis; mean adenoma weight 3.84 gr
Shah et al. [21]	2012	19	Pediatric cohort with adenoma, presenting mostly bone pain (68%), weakness (68%), or fractures (52.6%)
Li et al. [22]	2012	12	Parathyroid adenoma in 100% (4/12 ectopic adenoma), presenting mostly urinary and bone tissue impairment. Mean serum Ca^{++}: 3.82 mmol/l; mean serum P 1.18 mmol/l; mean serum PTH 1016 pg/ml at diagnosis
Belcher et al. [8]	2013	230	Literature review of studies regarding PHPT in the youth and adolescents. Single adenomas in 80% of patients, multiple-gland hyperplasia in 16.5% (MGH), double adenomas in 0.9%, and normal parathyroid gland in 2.6%. Of MGH, 50% were MEN I, MEN II, or familial non-MEN. Tc(99m)-sestamibi and ultrasound were 86% (37/43) and 74.5% (70/94) sensitive
Burke et al. [27	2013	19	Study aiming to enhance the radioguided parathyroidectomy. Adenoma in 74% and hyperplasia in 26%. No complications were noted in the pediatric patients after surgery. Mean serum Ca^{++}: 3.05 mmol/; mean serum PTH 177 pg/ml at diagnosis. Mean serum Ca^{++}: 2.35 mmol/; mean serum PTH 33 pg/ml after the surgery. Mean adenoma weight 0.44 gr
Alagaratnam S and Kurzawinski [9]	2014	29	Pediatric cohort with adenoma presenting mostly gastrointestinal symptoms (41%) and skeletal manifestations (20.7%)
Roizen and Levine [6]	2014	268	A meta-analysis comparing biochemical profiles in the youth and adults: greater hypercalcemia and hypercalciuria in youths at similar concentrations of serum intact PTH. Mean serum Ca^{++}: 3.2 mmol/; mean serum P 0.9 mmol/l; mean serum PTH 331 pg/ml; mean ALP 995 UI/l at diagnosis. Mean gland weight 2 gr
Mancilla et al. [23]	2017	16	Pediatric cohort with parathyroid and thymic (2/16) adenoma, mostly symptomatic (75%). Mean serum Ca^{++}: 3.02 mmol/; mean serum PTH 177.3 pg/ml at diagnosis

Table 2: Continued.

Author	Year	No. of pediatric patients	Main results
Lou et al. [11]	2017	40	Pediatric cohort with different patterns at diagnosis; increasing rate of diagnosis in asymptomatic subjects, higher postoperative complications, and disease recurrence in patients with positive familial history. Mean serum Ca^{++}: 2.91 mmol/; mean serum PTH 152.5 pg/ml at diagnosis
Vannucci et al. [24]	2018	22	Pediatric cohort with MEN-1 mutation presenting PHPT in 50% of cases, mostly asymptomatic (10/11)
Saponaro et al. [25]	2018	31	Young and adult population with PHPT: significantly lower PTH, higher serum in the younger group. Nephrolithiasis, fragility, fracture, and densitometric parameter rates did not differ between groups. Mean serum Ca^{++}: 2.73 mmol/; mean serum P 0.77 mmol/l; mean serum 25-hydroxyvitamin D 19.6 ng/ml, mean serum PTH 111 pg/ml; mean ALP 232 UI/l at diagnosis
Wang et al. [7]	2018	59	Pediatric cohort reporting bone pain as the most common manifestation, high rate of rickets (45.8%) compared to adults (23.7%), and an important correlation to short stature. Hypercalciuria, more frequent in pediatrics, hypophosphatemia, and urolithiasis among adults. Mean serum Ca^{++}: 3.01 mmol/; mean serum PTH 177 pg/ml; mean serum ALP 374 UI/l; mean serum 25-hydroxyvitamin D 12.9 ng/ml at diagnosis
Rampp et al. [26]	2020	86	Pediatric cohort with parathyroid and thymic (22/86) adenoma presenting systemic and neurocognitive symptoms in 64% and nephrolithiasis in 20%. Mean serum Ca^{++}: 2.93 mmol/; mean serum PTH 110 pg/ml at diagnosis. Mean gland weight 0.3 gr. Mean serum Ca^{++}: 2.42 mmol/l after the surgery
Jovanovic et al. [3]	2020	14	Adults and youth comparison; bone disease in the youth (42.9%) and asymptomatic disease in adults (39.3%). Preoperative serum calcium and PTH significantly higher in the youth than in adults. Mean serum Ca^{++}: 3.47 mmol/; mean serum P 0.8 mmol/l; mean serum PTH 572.6 pg/ml at diagnosis. Mean serum Ca^{++}: 2.42 mmol/; mean serum P 0.92 mmol/l; mean serum PTH 22.8 pg/ml; 25-hydroxyvitamin D 39.5 ng/ml after the surgery

References

[1] A. A. Khan, D. A. Hanley, R. Rizzoli et al., "Primary hyperparathyroidism: review and recommendations on evaluation, diagnosis, and management. A Canadian and international consensus," *Osteoporosis International*, vol. 28, no. 1, pp. 1-19, 2017.

[2] J. Thakker, A. E. Zarroug, J. Van Heerden et al., "Primary hyperparathyroidism in pediatric patients," *Pediatrics*, vol. 115, no. 4, pp. 974–980, 2005.

[3] M. Moir, I. Paunovic, V. Zdravkovic et al., "Case-control study of primary hyperparathyroidism in juvenile vs. adult patients," *International Journal of Pediatric Otorhinolaryngology*, vol. 131, Article ID 109895, 2020.

[4] E. Slijepcevic, "Primary hyperparathyroidism in neonates and childhood," *Hormone Research in Paediatrics*, vol. 69, no. 3, pp. 180–188, 2008.

[5] J. George, S. V. Acharya, T. R. Bandgar, P. S. Menon, and N. S. Shah, "Primary hyperparathyroidism in children and adolescents," *The Indian Journal of Pediatrics*, vol. 77, no. 2, pp. 175–17810, 2010.

[6] J. Roizen and M. A. Levine, "A meta-analysis comparing the biochemistry of primary hyperparathyroidism in youths to the biochemistry of primary hyperparathyroidism in adults," *The Journal of Clinical Endocrinology & Metabolism*, vol. 99, no. 12, pp. 4555–4564, 2014.

[7] W. Wang, J. Kong, M. Nie et al., "Primary hyperparathyroidism in Chinese children and adolescents: a single-centre experience at peking union medical college hospital," *Clinical Endocrinology*, vol. 87, no. 6, pp. 865–873, 2017.

[8] R. Meng, A. M. Metrailer, D. L. Bodenner, and B. C. Stack, "Characterization of hyperparathyroidism in youth and adolescents: a literature review," *International Journal of Pediatric Otorhinolaryngology*, vol. 77, no. 3, pp. 318–322, 2013.

[9] S. Alagaratnam and T. R. Kurzawinski, "Aetiology, diagnosis and surgical treatment of primary hyperparathyroidism in children: new trends," *Hormone Research in Paediatrics*, vol. 83, no. 6, pp. 365–37510, 2015.

[10] P. Schwarz, J. J. Body, J. Cáp et al., "The PRIMARA study: a prospective, descriptive, observational study to review cinacalcet use in patients with primary hyperparathyroidism in clinical practice," *European Journal of Endocrinology*, vol. 171, no. 6, pp. 727–73510, 2014.

[11] I. Lou, D. F. Schneider, R. S. Sippel, H. Chen, and D. M. Elfenbein, "The changing pattern of diagnosing primary hyperparathyroidism in young patients," *The American Journal of Surgery*, vol. 213, no. 1, pp. 146–15010, 2017.

[12] M. Kuhn, N. W. Thompson, J. K. Harness, and R. H. Nishiyama, "Primary hyperparathyroidism in children, adolescents, and young adults," *World Journal of Surgery*, vol. 6, no. 6, pp. 771–77510, 1982.

[13] M. L. Lawson, S. F. Miller, G. Ellis, R. M. Filler, and S. W. Kooh, "Primary hyperparathyroidism in a paediatric hospital," *QJM: An International Journal of Medicine*, vol. 89, no. 12, pp. 921–932, 1996.

[14] C. Cronin, T. Reeve, B. Robinson, P. Clifton-Bligh, A. Guinea, and L. Delbridge, "Primary hyperparathyroidism in childhood and adolescence," *Journal of Paediatrics and Child Health*, vol. 32, no. 5, pp. 397–39910, 1996.

[15] K.-C. Loh, Q.-Y. Duh, D. Shoback, L. Gee, A. Siperstein, and O. H. Clark, "Clinical profile of primary hyperparathyroidism in adolescents and young adults," *Clinical Endocrinology*, vol. 48, no. 4, pp. 435–443, 1998.

[16] C. R. Harman, J. A. van Heerden, D. R. Farley, C. S. Grant, G. B. Thompson, and K. Curlee, "Sporadic primary hyperparathyroidism in young patients," *Archives of Surgery*, vol. 134, no. 6, pp. 651–655, 1999.

[17] S. C. Hsu and M. A. Levine, "Primary hyperparathyroidism in children and adolescents: the Johns Hopkins Children's Center experience," *Journal of Bone and Mineral Research*, vol. 17, no. 2, pp. N44–N50, 2002.

[18] S. K. Bhadada, A. Bhansali, P. Dutta, A. Behera, G. V. Chanukya, and B. R. Mittal, "Characteristics of primary hyperparathyroidism in adolescents," *Journal of Pediatric Endocrinology and Metabolism*, vol. 21, no. 12, pp. 1147–1153, 2008.

[19] P. Libánský, J. Astl, S. Adámek et al., "Surgical treatment of primary hyperparathyroidism in children: report of 10 cases," *International Journal of Pediatric Otorhinolaryngology*, vol. 72, no. 8, pp. 1177–1182, 2008.

[20] S. Foltán, R. Al-Hosaini, A. Al-Ashwal, and A. Al-Rabeeah, "Surgical management of severe neonatal hyperparathyroidism: one center's experience," *Journal of Pediatric Surgery*, vol. 45, no. 4, pp. 714–717, 2010.

[21] V. N. Shah, S. K. Bhadada, A. Bhansali, A. Behera, B. R. Mittal, and V. Bhavin, "Influence of age and gender on presentation of symptomatic primary hyperparathyroidism," *Journal of Postgraduate Medicine*, vol. 58, no. 2, pp. 107–111, 2012.

[22] C.-C. Li, C. Yang, S. Wang, J. Zhang, X.-R. Kong, and J. Ouyang, "A 10-year retrospective study of primary hyperparathyroidism in children," *Experimental and Clinical Endocrinology & Diabetes*, vol. 120, no. 04, pp. 229–233, 2012.

[23] E. E. Mancilla, M. A. Levine, and N. S. Adzick, "Outcomes of minimally invasive parathyroidectomy in pediatric patients with primary hyperparathyroidism owing to parathyroid adenoma: a single institution experience," *Journal of Pediatric Surgery*, vol. 52, no. 1, pp. 188–191, 2017.

[24] L. Vannucci, F. Marini, F. Giusti, S. Ciuffi, F. Tonelli, and M. L. Brandi, "MEN1 in children and adolescents: data from patients of a regional referral center for hereditary endocrine tumors," *Endocrine*, vol. 59, no. 2, pp. 438–448, 2018.

[25] F. Saponaro, C. Marcocci, F. Cacciatore et al., "Clinical profile of juvenile primary hyperparathyroidism: a prospective study," *Endocrine*, vol. 59, no. 2, pp. 344–352, 2018.

[26] R. D. Materazzi, E. E. Mancilla, N. S. Adzick et al., "Single gland, ectopic location: adenomas are common causes of primary hyperparathyroidism in children and adolescents," *World Journal of Surgery*, vol. 44, no. 5, pp. 1518–1525, 2020.

[27] J. F. Burke, K. Jacobson, A. Gosain, R. S. Sippel, and H. Chen, "Radioguided parathyroidectomy effective in pediatric patients," *Journal of Surgical Research*, vol. 184, no. 1, pp. 312–317, 2013.

[28] J. E. Iyer, S. Van Thiel, J. A. Romijn, and N. A. T. Hamdy, "Therapy OF endocrine disease: hungry bone syndrome: still a challenge in the post-operative management of primary hyperparathyroidism: a systematic review of the literature," *European Journal of Endocrinology*, vol. 168, no. 3, pp. R45–R5310, 2013.

[29] J. Westerdahl, P. Lindblom, S. Valdemarsson, S. Tibblin, and A. Bergenfelz, "Risk factors for postoperative hypocalcemia after surgery for primary hyperparathyroidism," *Archives of Surgery*, vol. 135, no. 2, pp. 142–147, 2000.

[30] C. D. C. Kamilaris and C. A. Stratakis, "Multiple endocrine neoplasia type 1 (MEN1): an update and the significance of early genetic and clinical diagnosis," *Front Endocrinol (Lausanne)*, vol. 11, 2019.

14

Late-Onset Isolated Corticotrope Deficiency in a Woman with Down Syndrome

Ibtissem Oueslati, Marwa Ben Jemaa, Meriem Yazidi, Fatma Chaker, and Melika Chihaoui

Department of Endocrinology, La Rabta University Hospital, University of Tunis-El Manar, Faculty of Medicine, Tunis, Tunisia

Correspondence should be addressed to Ibtissem Oueslati; ouesibtissem@gmail.com

Academic Editor: Osamu Isozaki

Isolated corticotrope deficiency is a rare cause of secondary adrenocortical insufficiency. Its occurrence in patients with Down syndrome is exceptional. Herein, we report a case of an isolated corticotrope deficiency diagnosed at the age of 33 years in a woman with Down syndrome and discuss its possible mechanisms. A 33-year-old woman with Down syndrome was referred to our department for the investigation of low blood pressure. She complained of asthenia, dizziness, and palpitation with arterial hypotension for the past 4 years. The thyroid function was normal and anti-thyroperoxidase antibodies were negative. The peak of cortisol level in response to the insulin-induced hypoglycemia test was 9.4 μg/dl. ACTH level was normal, indicating corticotrope deficiency. Other pituitary hormones were normal. Magnetic resonance imaging scan revealed a partially empty sella turcica. Genetic analysis showed no mutations and no copy number variants of the TBX19 and NFKB2 genes. The mechanism of isolated corticotrope deficiency is unclear, but it may be induced by autoimmune mechanism in similar to other disorders of patients with Down syndrome.

1. Introduction

Down syndrome (DS) is the most common genetic abnormality resulting from the trisomy of chromosome 21. It affects one in 500 to one in 1,000 live births. Patients with Down syndrome present with morphological abnormalities, a varying degree of intellectual disability, and other comorbidities such as congenital heart disease, celiac disease, and endocrinopathies. The most common endocrine dysfunctions in patients with Down syndrome are Hashimoto's thyroiditis, Graves' disease, obesity, and diabetes mellitus [1].

Isolated corticotrope deficiency is a rare cause of secondary adrenocortical insufficiency. It is defined as low or absent adrenocorticotropic hormone (ACTH) production with normal secretion of other pituitary hormones and the absence of structural defects within the pituitary gland [2]. To the best of our knowledge, its occurrence in patients with Down syndrome was reported in only one case [3].

Herein, we report a case of an isolated corticotrope deficiency diagnosed at the age of 33 years in a woman with Down syndrome and discuss its possible mechanisms.

2. Case Presentation

A 33-year-old woman with Down syndrome was referred to our department for the investigation of low blood pressure. She was born, at term, to nonconsanguineous parents with no history of birth trauma, neonatal hypoglycemia, and prolonged jaundice. Her past medical history was unremarkable apart from surgery for tympanic imperforation. Her age at menarche was 12 years and she had regular periods. Her family history was notable for type 2 diabetes mellitus and arterial hypertension without any history of autoimmune diseases or congenital hypopituitarism.

The patient complained of asthenia, dizziness, and palpitation with arterial hypotension for the past 4 years. Concomitant capillary glucose levels were about 0.82 and

0.85 g/L. Neither bodyweight loss nor polyuria were reported. She was not taking any drugs.

On physical examination, she had a bodyweight of 64 kg, a height of 153 cm corresponding to a body mass index of 27.3 kg/m^2, a blood pressure of 90/60 mmHg, and a regular pulse of 75 bpm. The skin was pale without hyperpigmentation. The hydration state and thyroid, abdominal, and neurological examinations were normal.

The results of biological investigations are shown in Table 1. The thyroid function was normal and anti-thyroperoxidase antibodies were negative. The peak of the cortisol level in response to the insulin-induced hypoglycemia test was 9.4 μg/dl. The ACTH level was normal indicating corticotrope deficiency. Other pituitary hormones were normal, consisting with the diagnosis of an isolated corticotrope deficiency.

Magnetic resonance imaging (MRI) scan revealed a small and homogeneous anterior pituitary gland with a partially empty sella turcica. There was no tumor and the posterior lobe bright spot was normal. The pituitary stalk was median and thin (Figure 1).

Genetic analysis using high-throughput sequencing showed no mutations and no copy number variants of the TBX19 and NFKB2 genes. Pituitary antibodies were not available.

Lifelong replacement therapy with an oral hydrocortisone dose of 20 mg per day was prescribed to our patient. The other pituitary hormones remained normal over the course of follow-up.

Table 1: Blood biological and hormonal parameters.

	Values	Reference ranges
Fasting glucose (mmol/L)	4.95	3.84–5.44
Creatinine (μmol/L)	61.8	61–106
Sodium (mmol/L)	137	136–145
Potassium (mmol/L)	4	3,5–5,1
Calcium (mg/L)	87	85–105
Phosphorus (mg/L)	29	23–47
White blood cells(mm^3)	7060	4000–10,000
Lymphocytes	1360	1500–4000
Neutrophils	5210	1500–7000
Hemoglobin (g/dL)	13.1	12–16
TSH (mIU/L)	1.97	0.35–4.95
FT4 (ng/dL)	0.91	0.7–1.5
8h cortisol (μg/dL)	8.4	4–20
Pic cortisol (μg/dL)	9.4	≥18
ACTH (pg/ml)	21.4	10–48
Prolactin (ng/ml)	20	<25
FSH (IU/L)	1.7	3.35–12.6
LH (IU/L)	6.53	2.39–6.6
IGF1 (ng/ml)	290	109–358

3. Discussion

ACTH that is derived from the cleavage of the precursor polypeptide pro-opiomelanocortin (POMC) is produced by the anterior pituitary gland after stimulation by hypothalamic corticotropin-releasing hormone (CRH). ACTH stimulates the adrenal glands to produce glucocorticoids and adrenal androgens. Corticotrope deficiency results from the decrease or the absence of ACTH production. It is most often associated with other pituitary hormone deficiencies. Isolated corticotrope deficiency is uncommon, especially in adults. Its prevalence is underestimated as it is often misdiagnosed for a long time. In adults, the mean age at disease diagnosis is 50 years and there is a male predominance [4]. In our case, the diagnosis was established at the age of 33 years and the symptoms started at the age of 29 years.

The clinical presentation of isolated corticotrope deficiency is variable and nonspecific. It is insidious in the majority of cases. The acute adrenal crisis is rare. The common chief symptoms are fatigue, weakness, anorexia, and weight loss [5]. Other complaints such as hypoglycemia, hypotension, depression, apathy, and some neurological and musculoskeletal symptoms were also reported [4, 6]. Our patient complained of asthenia, dizziness, and palpitation with arterial hypotension.

Isolated corticotrope deficiency can be caused by several etiologies that can be classified into congenital or acquired forms. In some cases, the etiology remains unknown and the ACTH deficiency is called idiopathic isolated corticotrope deficiency.

The congenital form is more frequent in childhood. Two forms were described. The early-onset form which appears before the age of one or two years and the late-onset form after 3 years [7]. A case of congenital isolated corticotrope deficiency was diagnosed at the age of 29 years [5].

The development of the hypothalamic-pituitary axis depends on the sequential expression of numerous transcription factors and signaling molecules. Genetic mutations in some of these factors can lead to an isolated corticotrope deficiency. The T-box pituitary restricted transcription factor (TBX19) is a member of the T-box gene family that is required for the expression of the POMC gene. Individuals with mutations in TBX19 have a neonatal-onset ACTH deficiency [8]. These mutations were not reported in late-onset forms of isolated corticotrope deficiency.

Corticotrope deficiency can also result from mutations in the POMC gene, and it is in this case associated with early-onset obesity and red hair pigmentation [9]. Moreover, isolated corticotrope deficiency may be associated with variable immune deficiencies in the context of DAVID syndrome (deficit in anterior pituitary function and variable immunodeficiency) due to heterozygous mutations in the *NFKB2* gene [10]. Its pathogenesis in this syndrome remains unclear. In our case, the genetic analysis showed neither mutations nor copy number variants on the *TBX19* and *NFKB2* genes.

The acquired forms of isolated corticotrope deficiency are more frequent in adults. In the absence of steroid-induced adrenal insufficiency, autoimmunity is considered as the primary underlying mechanism for isolated corticotrope deficiency in adults [10, 11]. In our patient, regarding the age of onset, the Down syndrome condition, and the MRI aspect, the most probably incriminated etiology is an autoimmune disorder.

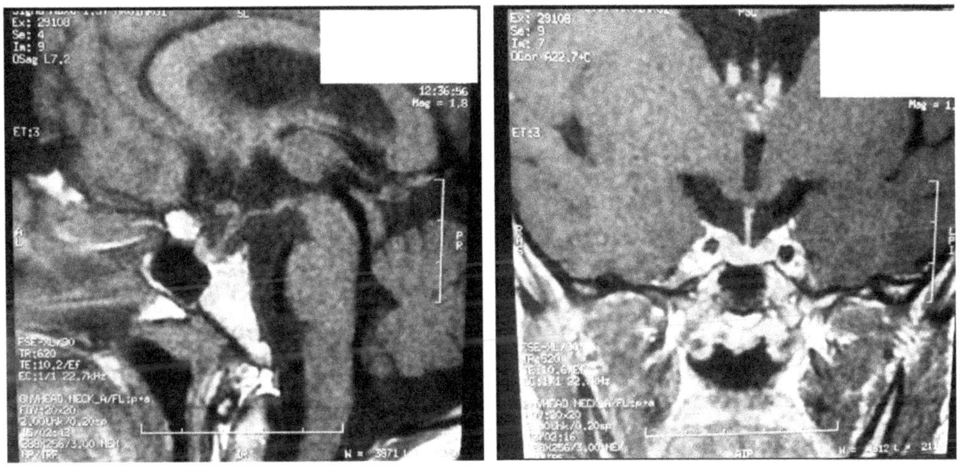

FIGURE 1: MRI scan showing a small and homogeneous anterior pituitary gland with a partially empty sella turcica.

Autoimmune diseases are more frequent in patients with Down syndrome than in the rest of the population. Thyroid autoimmune disorders such as Hashimoto's thyroiditis or Grave's disease are the commonest. These patients are also more predisposed to develop early-onset type 1 diabetes, Addison disease, celiac disease, alopecia areata, chronic autoimmune hepatitis, and primary sclerosing cholangitis [12]. According to many authors, these patients share clinical features, such as autoimmune manifestations and specific autoantibodies, with patients suffering from autoimmune polyendocrine syndrome type 1 [13]. This syndrome results from inactivating mutations in the autoimmune regulator (AIRE) gene, located on chromosome 21. The AIRE acts as a transcriptional regulator that promotes immunological central tolerance by inducing the ectopic thymic expression of many tissue-specific antigens [14]. Its mutations are associated with a huge spectrum of phenotypes. Two major forms were identified. The classical autoimmune polyendocrinopathy candidiasis ectodermal dystrophy (APCED) is an autosomal recessive disease defined by the presence of at least two of the major components including chronic mucocutaneous candidiasis, chronic hypoparathyroidism, and autoimmune Addison's disease [15]. The nonclassical form is caused by dominant heterozygous mutations mainly in the first plant homeodomain (PHD1) zinc finger of AIRE and is characterized by late-onset, milder phenotype, and reduced penetrance [15]. The pituitary involvement in autoimmune polyendocrine syndrome type 1 is a rare condition. Growth hormone deficiency, central diabetes insipidus, gonadotropin deficiency, and ACTH deficiency were reported.

In patients with Down syndrome, Skogberg et al. demonstrated that the AIRE gene is overexpressed, which may alter thymic selection processes and affect the susceptibility for autoimmune diseases [13]. On the contrary, other authors reported that the level of AIRE expression in the thymus of patients with Down syndrome is reduced [16,17].

Corticotrope cells are often the first to be affected in lymphocytic hypophysitis, and adult isolated corticotrope deficiency was suggested to have a link with an autoimmune process [18]. De Bellis et al. demonstrated higher pituitary and hypothalamic antibody titers, respectively, in 14.8 and 18.5% of patients with isolated corticotrope deficiency [19]. Among corticotrope cell antibodies, Tpit antibodies are involved in the development of lymphocytic hypophysitis [20]. Tpit is an essential transcription factor for the development of corticotrope cells. However, this antibody is not specific to lymphocytic hypophysitis, as it was also detected in other autoimmune endocrine diseases [21]. Kiyota et al. identified a novel anterior pituitary autoantigen candidate, Rab GDI alpha, in patients with isolated corticotrope deficiency [22].

To the best of our knowledge, the coexistence of Down syndrome and isolated corticotrope deficiency was reported in only one case [3]. It was an 8-year-old boy with Down syndrome, congenital primary hypothyroidism, and central precocious puberty who presented with fatigue. The basal cortisol level was 7.6 μg/dl, the stimulated cortisol level was 10.2 μg/dl, and the ACTH level was 41.6 pg/ml. The pituitary MRI revealed pituitary gland hypoplasia. The etiology of the isolated corticotrope deficiency was not determined in this case.

4. Conclusion

In the absence of steroid-induced adrenal insufficiency, isolated corticotrope deficiency is a rare condition. Genetic forms are most often diagnosed in childhood, whereas in adults it is mainly secondary to an autoimmune disorder. The occurrence of an isolated corticotrope deficiency in patients with Down syndrome is exceptional. Its mechanism is still unclear. It may be induced by an autoimmune disorder.

Acknowledgments

The authors thank Dr. Alexandru Saveanu and Pr Anne Barlier (Laboratory of Molecular Biology, Hospital La Conception, Marseille, France) for their help in the molecular study.

References

[1] Y. Hawli, M. Nasrallah, and G. E.-H. Fuleihan, "Endocrine and musculoskeletal abnormalities in patients with Down syndrome," *Nature Reviews Endocrinology*, vol. 5, no. 6, pp. 327–334, 2009.

[2] J. Kinoshita, S. Higashino, S. Fushida et al., "Isolated adrenocorticotropic hormone deficiency development during chemotherapy for gastric cancer: a case report," *Journal of Medical Case Reports*, vol. 8, p. 90, 2014.

[3] A. Guven and A. Cebeci, "A rare endocrine manifestation of Down syndrome: central precocious puberty: three cases report," *European Journal of Medical Case Reports*, vol. 4, no. 11, pp. 404–407, 2020.

[4] Y. Goto, K. Tatsuzawa, K. Aita et al., "Neurological symptoms in a patient with isolated adrenocorticotropin deficiency: case report and literature review," *BMC Endocrine Disorders*, vol. 16, p. 2, 2016.

[5] Q. Guo, J. Lu, Y. Mu, K. Chen, and C. Pan, "Adult idiopathic isolated ACTH deficiency: a short series and literature review," *Neuro Endocrinology Letters*, vol. 34, no. 7, pp. 693–700, 2013.

[6] C. Hoshino, N. Satoh, M. Narita, A. Kikuchi, and M. Inoue, "Painful hypoadrenalism," *BMJ Case Reports*, vol. 2011, Article ID bcr0120113735, 2011.

[7] L. L. Pham, C. Garot, T. Brue et al., "Clinical, biological and genetic analysis of 8 cases of congenital isolated adrenocorticotrophic hormone (ACTH) deficiency," *PLoS One*, vol. 6, no. 10, Article ID e26516, 2011.

[8] T. K. Ghosh, J. D. Brook, and A. Wilsdon, "T-Box Genes in human development and disease," *Current Topics in Developmental Biology*, vol. 122, pp. 383–415, 2017.

[9] M. S. Mendiratta, Y. Yang, A. E. Balazs et al., "Early onset obesity and adrenal insufficiency associated with a homozygous POMC mutation," *International Journal of Pediatric Endocrinology*, vol. 2011, no. 1, p. 5, 2011.

[10] T. Brue, M. H. Quentien, K. Khetchoumian et al., "Mutations in NFKB2 and potential genetic heterogeneity in patients with DAVID syndrome, having variable endocrine and immune deficiencies," *BMC Medical Genetics*, vol. 15, p. 139, 2014.

[11] C. Shi, F. Wang, A. Tong et al., "NFKB2 mutation in common variable immunodeficiency and isolated adrenocorticotropic hormone deficiency: a case report and review of literature," *Medicine (Baltimore)*, vol. 95, no. 40, Article ID e5081, 2016.

[12] T. Aversa, M. Valenzise, A. Corrias et al., "In children with autoimmune thyroid diseases the association with Down syndrome can modify the clustering of extra-thyroidal autoimmune disorders," *Journal of Pediatric Endocrinology and Metabolism*, vol. 29, no. 9, pp. 1041–1046, 2016.

[13] G. Skogberg, V. Lundberg, S. Lindgren et al., "Altered expression of autoimmune regulator in infant Down syndrome thymus, a possible contributor to an autoimmune phenotype," *The Journal of Immunology*, vol. 193, no. 5, pp. 2187–2195, 2014.

[14] L. De Martino, D. Capalbo, N. Improda et al., "Novel findings into AIRE genetics and functioning: clinical implications," *Frontiers in Pediatrics*, vol. 4, p. 86, 2016.

[15] B. E. Oftedal, A. Hellesen, M. M. Erichsen et al., "Dominant mutations in the autoimmune regulator AIRE are associated with common organ-specific autoimmune diseases," *Immunity*, vol. 42, no. 6, pp. 1185–1196, 2015.

[16] M. Giménez-Barcons, A. Casteràs, M. d. P. Armengol et al., "Autoimmune predisposition in Down syndrome may result from a partial central tolerance failure due to insufficient intrathymic expression ofAIREand peripheral antigens," *The Journal of Immunology*, vol. 193, no. 8, pp. 3872–3879, 2014.

[17] F. A. Lima, C. A. Moreira-Filho, P. L. Ramos et al., "Decreased AIRE expression and global thymic hypofunction in Down syndrome," *The Journal of Immunology*, vol. 187, no. 6, pp. 3422–3430, 2011.

[18] F. M. Alabdrabalnabi, Z. A. Al Saeed, and Y. A. Elamin, "Hypoglycemia as initial presentation in patient with isolated ACTH deficiency," *AACE Clinical Case Reports*, vol. 6, no. 6, pp. e338–e341, 2020.

[19] A. De Bellis, E. Pane, G. Bellastella et al., "Detection of antipituitary and antihypothalamus antibodies to investigate the role of pituitary or hypothalamic autoimmunity in patients with selective idiopathic hypopituitarism," *Clinical Endocrinology*, vol. 75, no. 3, pp. 361–366, 2011.

[20] Y. Takahashi, "Mechanisms in endocrinology: autoimmune hypopituitarism: novel mechanistic insights," *European Journal of Endocrinology*, vol. 182, no. 4, pp. R59–R66, 2020.

[21] C. J. A. Smith, S. Bensing, C. Burns et al., "Identification of TPIT and other novel autoantigens in lymphocytic hypophysitis; immunoscreening of a pituitary cDNA library and development of immunoprecipitation assays," *European Journal of Endocrinology*, vol. 166, no. 3, pp. 391–398, 2012.

[22] A. Kiyota, S. Iwama, Y. Sugimura et al., "Identification of the novel autoantigen candidate Rab GDP dissociation inhibitor alpha in isolated adrenocorticotropin deficiency," *Endocrine Journal*, vol. 62, no. 2, pp. 153–160, 2015.

15

A Nonfunctioning Pituitary Macroadenoma Presenting as Cyclical Vomiting and Severe Hyponatremia in a Young Female

Dinuka S. Warapitiya,[1] Dimuthu Muthukuda,[2] W. A. H. P. Sanjeewa,[1] Kushalee Poornima Jayawickreme,[1] and Shyama Subasinghe[3]

[1]*Postgraduate Institute of Medicine, University of Colombo, Colombo, Sri Lanka*
[2]*Diabetes and Endocrinology Unit, Sri Jayewardenepura General Hospital, Nugegoda, Colombo, Sri Lanka*
[3]*Sri Jayewardenepura General Hospital, Nugegoda, Colombo, Sri Lanka*

Correspondence should be addressed to Dinuka S. Warapitiya; dswarapitiya@gmail.com

Academic Editor: Wayne V. Moore

Introduction. Recurrent vomiting is a commonly overlooked debilitating symptom which causes significant impact on the quality of life. There are several causes for vomiting, ranging from commonly known causes to rare causes. Nonfunctioning pituitary macroadenomas generally present with visual disturbances, headache, and symptoms due to anterior pituitary hormone deficiencies. This case report is about an atypical presentation of a nonfunctioning pituitary macroadenoma in which the patient presented with cyclical vomiting with severe hyponatremia. *Case Report.* A 23-year-old girl presented with four to five episodes of vomiting per day for two days duration. She had a history of similar episodes of vomiting since 2016, with each episode generally lasting for 4-5 days and occurring in every four to six months. All episodes exhibited similar symptomatology and she was free of symptoms in-between. Generalized body weakness, postural dizziness, reduced appetite, and secondary amenorrhea were other symptoms she has had since 2016. Examination findings showed a low body mass index (BMI) (16 kg/m^2) with normal system examination. Investigations showed severe hyponatremia (110 mmol/L) with hypokalemia (3.2 mmol/L) and hypochloremia (74 mmol/L). Her urinary excretion of potassium, sodium, and serum osmolality was low. Urine osmolality was mildly elevated compared to serum osmolality. Blood urea was normal. Severe hyponatremia with minimal hyponatremic symptoms was suggestive of chronic hyponatremia, which was accentuated by ongoing vomiting and possible reduced intake of salt. Further investigations showed evidence of secondary hypoadrenalism, central hypothyroidism, hypogonadotropic hypogonadism, and mild hyperprolactinemia. Magnetic resonance imaging (MRI) revealed a pituitary macroadenoma with mass effect on the optic chiasma. Hydrocortisone and levothyroxine were started, and she underwent transsphenoidal resection of the pituitary tumor. She recovered from cyclical vomiting. *Conclusion.* There can be multiple overlapping aetiologies for every observed symptom, sign, and abnormal investigation finding. Therefore, aetiological diagnosis is challenging, especially in the presence of an atypical clinical presentation. Cyclical vomiting and severe hyponatremia are atypical presentations of nonfunctioning pituitary macroadenomas.

1. Introduction

Clinically nonfunctioning pituitary adenoma is a common type of tumor in the sellar region [1]. The prevalence of nonfunctioning pituitary adenomas varies between 60 and 100 cases per million population [1, 2]. It has a bimodal peak incidence between the ages of 25–45 years and 60–70 years and the incidence rate is 1.02–1.08 per 100000 [1, 2]. There is an equal incidence among both genders [1, 2].

These lesions are usually found incidentally (mainly microadenoma) or diagnosed based on symptoms and signs of anterior pituitary hormone deficiency and compressive symptoms such as headache and visual field defects [1].

We are presenting an atypical presentation of non-functioning pituitary macroadenomas.

This case is of a Sri Lankan law student with various psychosocial problems. She presented with cyclical vomiting for 3 years duration. There can be multiple causes for vomiting. Vomiting usually disturbs the acid base and electrolyte balance of the body. Our case illustrates that uncommon aetiology could be the reason for common clinical presentations and investigation abnormalities. Identifying the correct aetiology is lifesaving.

A few case reports have shown that patients with adrenal insufficiency present with intractable nausea and vomiting [3]. However, this is an atypical rare clinical presentation of a nonfunctioning pituitary macroadenoma in which the patient presented with cyclical vomiting. This case also highlights that, despite having several psychosocial issues, an organic pathology should always be sought before attributing the unexplained symptoms to a psychological illness. Hence, we decided to report this case in order to share our clinical experience.

2. Case History

A 23-year-old Sri Lankan female university student presented to the medical casualty ward with several episodes of vomiting for two days duration. She had vomited 5-6 episodes per day, which was associated with burning-type chest pain and regurgitation. Vomiting was a nonprojectile, nonbilious, and nonfecal in nature. There was no hematemesis. Vomiting was preceded by nausea and she had tried to induce vomiting by digital stimulation of the throat. There was no history of fever, abdominal pain, dysuria, abdominal distention, or altered bowel habits. However, she complained of reduced appetite and generalized body weakness for 3 years duration and postural dizziness for the last 2 days. She denied associated headache, photophobia, visual disturbances, and weight loss. Further questioning of her past history revealed frequent hospital visits due to similar type of recurrent episodes of vomiting over the last 3 years. These episodes always followed the same pattern with sudden onset of vomiting preceded by nausea lasting for 4-5 days. There were 4-5 episodes of vomiting per day. In each episode of vomiting, she was managed as having gastroesophageal reflux disease with proton pump inhibitors and prokinetics as an outpatient without being investigated thoroughly. In between these episodes, she was perfectly normal and engaged in her usual day-to-day activities. The first episode occurred 3 years earlier. She attributed its onset to the breakup of her relationship. Initially, the vomiting frequency was less, around 1-2 episodes in every 6 months. However, the frequency had increased recently. Last hospital visit due to recurrent vomiting took place 3 months earlier. However, we were unable to find her past medical records of her previous hospital visits.

On further inquiring, she denied excessive exercise and use of appetite suppressants and diuretics which are common with eating disorders. She did not have ideas of body-image distortion. She denied intake of large volume of water. There was no history of polyuria, polydipsia, or nocturia.

She had attained menarche at the age of 14 years and developed secondary amenorrhea since the age of 20 years. She denied galactorrhea. She was on anxiolytics for acute stress reaction following her relationship breakup 5 years earlier. Anxiolytics was taken only for one-month duration.

Onset of recurrent episodes of cyclical vomiting and amenorrhea all had occurred in 2016, soon after she started her university life.

She disclosed that her mother had died from an astrocytoma 7 years ago. She lived with her siblings, father, and stepmother.

On examination, her Glasgow coma scale was 15/15. She had a low BMI, 16 kg/m^2. Her pulse rate was 78 beats/minute and blood pressure was 95/60 mmHg. There were no signs suggestive of an eating disorder such as dental caries, erosions over knuckles of hands, parotid enlargement, or brittle hair. Rest of her system examination was normal.

2.1. Investigations. She had normal capillary blood glucose level on admission (80 mg/dl). Her white cell count, haemoglobin, platelet, liver transaminases, alkaline phosphate, serum albumin, serum amylase level, and total bilirubin level were normal. Her chest X-ray, electrocardiogram, and urine analysis were normal. Her total serum beta HCG level was normal. C-reactive protein was 5 mg/l and ESR was 10 mm.

However, she had markedly deranged serum electrolyte levels. Her serum sodium was 110 mmol/L (136–145 mmol/L). Serum potassium and chloride were 3.2 mmol/L (3.5–5.3 mmol/L) and 74 mmol/L (97–111 mmol/L), respectively. Repeated serum electrolyte showed similar low values. Arterial blood gas analysis showed respiratory alkalosis (PH, 7.481; PCO_2, 24 mmHg; PO_2, 125 mmHg; and bicarbonate level, 17 mmol/L) probably due to stress-induced hyperventilation. Her blood urea was normal (14 mg/dl). Serum creatinine was 44.9 μmol/L. Serum osmolality was found to be 223 mOsm/kg and urine osmolality was 266 mOsm/kg. Her average urine output was 1050/day. Urinary electrolyte studies showed low urinary potassium and sodium levels, 5.3 mmol/L and 14 mmol/L, respectively. Urine chloride level was 24 mmol/L.

Observed electrolyte abnormalities were evaluated thoroughly. Her random serum cortisol level (105 nmol/l) which was taken on admission day at 1 a.m. was low. Vomiting is an acute stress to the body. It usually causes high cortisol level in the body. This result contradicted it. She also had low thyroid stimulating hormone (TSH) of 0.209 μIU/ml (0.55–4.78 μIU/ml), low free triiodothyronine (T_3) of 1.32 pg/ml (2.30–4.20 pg/ml), and low normal free tetraiodothyronine (T_4) level of 0.98 ng/dl (0.93–1.7 ng/dl).

With the background history of generalized body weakness, reduced appetite, and secondary amenorrhea, she was investigated further. Her both follicular stimulating hormone (FSH, 1.4 mIU/ml) and luteinizing hormone (LH, 0.4 mIU/ml) were found to be low. Ultrasound abdomen scan showed a hypoplastic uterus. There were no other abnormalities in the ultrasound scan of abdomen. Her prolactin level was found to be mildly elevated. Serum prolactin level was 81 ng/ml (nonpregnant range, 2–29.2 ng/ml) and with 5 : 1 dilution it was 90.8 ng/ml. Summary of blood and urine investigation findings is shown in Table 1.

She had biochemical evidence of hypoadrenalism, possible central hypothyroidism, hypogonadotropic hypogonadism, and mild hyperprolactinemia.

Table 1: Summary of blood and urine investigation findings.

Name of the investigation	Value	Name of the investigation	Value
White cell count	6000 cells/mm3	Serum creatinine	44.9 μmol/L
Neutrophil	81%	PH	7.481
Lymphocyte	16%	PCO_2	24 mmHg
Haemoglobin	12.3 g/dl	PO_2	125 mmHg
Platelet	244 000/mm3	Bicarbonate level	17 mmol/L
		Blood urea	14 mg/dl
Serum sodium	110 mmol/L (136–145 mmol/L)		
Serum potassium	3.2 mmol/L (3.5–5.3 mmol/L)	Her random serum cortisol level	105 nmol/l
Serum chloride	74 mmol/L (97–111 mmol/L)	TSH	0.209 μIU/ml (0.55–4.78 μIU/ml)
Plasma osmolality	223 mOsm/kg	T3 level	1.32 pg/ml (2.30–4.20 pg/ml)
Urine osmolality	266 mOsm/kg	T4 level	0.98 ng/dl (0.93–1.7 ng/dl).
Urine sodium	14 mmol/L	LH level	0.4 mIU/ml
Urine potassium	5.3 mmol/L	FSH level	1.4 mIU/ml
Urine chloride	24 mmol/L	Serum prolactin level	81 ng/ml (nonpregnant range, 2.–29.2 ng/ml)
		Serum prolactin level (5 : 1 dilution)	90.8 ng/ml.
Alanine transaminase	23.4 U/l (7–35 U/l)	Total serum beta HCG	<2 mIU/ml (<10)
Aspartate transaminase	20.3 U/l (0–31 U/l)		
Alkaline phosphatase	68.2 U/l (30–120 U/l)	Urine full report	Normal
Total protein	6.5 g/dl (6–8 g/dl)		
Serum albumin	4.1 g/dl (3.7-5 g/dl)		
Adjusted calcium	8.7 mg/dl (8.6–10 mg/dl)		
Serum magnesium	0.9 mmol/L (0.7–1 mmol/l)		
Serum inorganic phosphorous	3 mg/dl (2.7–4.5 mg/dl)		
Serum amylase	32 U/l (30–110 U/l)		
C-reactive protein	5 mg/l		
ESR	10 mm		

To assess her hypothalamic-pituitary axis further, magnetic resonance imaging (MRI) of pituitary was done. MRI scan showed 2.4 cm × 2 cm × 2 cm sized lobular mass occupying sellar and suprasellar area with mass effect on optic chiasma, optic tracts, and AI segment of bilateral anterior cerebral arteries. There was enlargement of sellar by the lesion caudally and the mass has bulged into the sphenoid sinus. There were scattered hemorrhages on the mass (Figure 1). Humphrey field analyzer threshold plot demonstrated bitemporal hemianopia. The diagnosis of a pituitary nonfunctioning macroadenoma with mass effect causing hypoadrenalism, central hypothyroidism, hypogonadotropic hypogonadism, and hyperprolactinemia due to stalk effect was made.

2.2. Differential Diagnosis. The differential diagnosis made on admission is illustrated in Table 2.

2.3. Management, Outcome, and Follow-Up. On admission, she was managed with antiemetics. Volume loss due to vomiting was replaced with equal volumes of oral rehydration fluid. Since the patient tolerated very low level of serum sodium, she was managed as having chronic hyponatremia worsened further by recurrent vomiting and reduced intake of salt. Therefore, aggressive management was not done to correct hyponatremia. Intravenous hydrocortisone 100 mg bolus dose was given suspecting hypoadrenalism and continued intravenous hydrocortisone 50 mg every 6 hours. Low serum potassium and chloride levels were thought to be due to vomiting, which got corrected after oral hydration. She had respiratory alkalosis due to stress-induced hyperventilation.

After making a diagnosis of a nonfunctioning pituitary macroadenoma with hormonal deficiency and mass effect, the patient was started on levothyroxine 50 μg daily while continuing intravenous hydrocortisone 50 mg every 6 hours. Four days after hormonal replacement, her serum sodium level became stable around 132 mmol/L. Her vomiting improved. There was marked improvement of her generalized body weakness and appetite. The intravenously administered hydrocortisone was then converted to oral hydrocortisone and after 2 weeks of treatment there was further improvement. One month later, her serum-free T4 was 0.81 ng/dl (0.93–1.7 ng/dl).

Transsphenoidal resection of the pituitary tumor was performed one month after the diagnosis. Histology revealed a pituitary adenoma. The first twenty-four hours of postoperative period were covered with intravenous hydrocortisone 100 mg every 6 hours and the same dose of

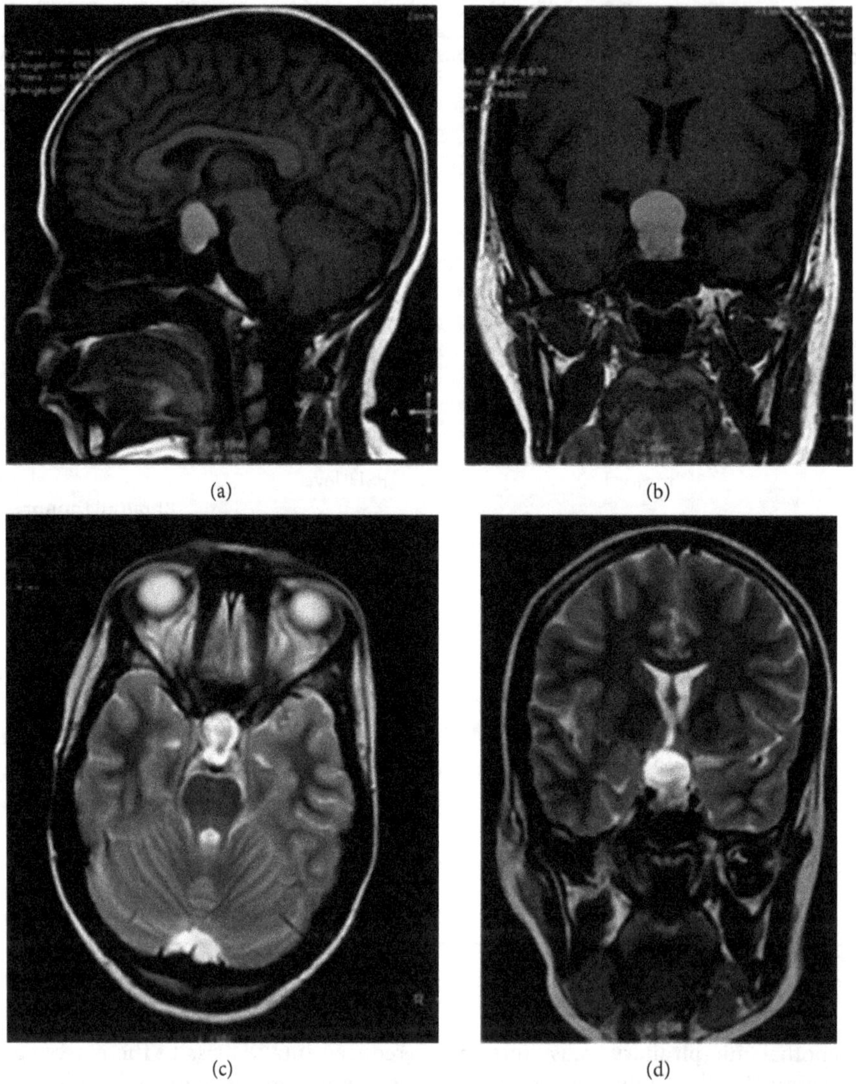

Figure 1: MRI of this patient showing lobular tumor occupying sellar and suprasellar region measuring 2.4 cm × 2.0 cm × 2.0 cm. Caudal part of the lesion showed intermediate signal intensity in T2-weighted images. Superior mass effect is seen on the optic chiasma, optic tract, and AI segments of bilateral anterior cerebral arteries. Mass is bulged into the sphenoid sinuses. ((a, b)) T1-weighted, gadolinium-enhanced sagittal and coronal views. ((c, d)) T2-weighted axial and coronal views.

Table 2: Differential diagnosis.

(1) Recurrent vomiting due to gastroesophageal reflux disease or any other abdominal pathology in the abdomen
(2) Chronic infection, e.g., pyelonephritis
(3) Eating disorder, e.g., anorexia nervosa
(4) Syndrome of inappropriate antidiuretic hormone secretion (SIADH)
(5) Adrenal insufficiency
(6) Cyclical vomiting syndrome
(7) Psychogenic vomiting

levothyroxine. The postoperative period was complicated with transient diabetes insipidus, which was managed with intravenous vasopressin followed by desmopressin nasal spray.

She was discharged with 50 μg of levothyroxine and orally administered total 20 mg daily dose of hydrocortisone. Currently, her general condition is stable with serum sodium 136 mmol/L and free T_4 0,96 ng/dl. She was free of symptoms suggestive of hypoadrenalism. MRI pituitary performed five months after the surgery showed no residual tumor. Interestingly, she recovered from her episodes of recurrent vomiting following hormone replacement and pituitary surgery.

3. Discussion

Pituitary tumors account for 15.5% of all central nervous system (CNS) neoplasms [1, 5]. In young adults (20–34 years), 30% of CNS tumors are due to pituitary adenomas [1, 5]. Nonfunctioning pituitary adenomas account for a mean of 33% of all pituitary adenomas, which are lower than those of prolactinomas, which account for 47% of all pituitary adenomas [1, 6]. Nonfunctioning pituitary adenomas commonly appear as pituitary macroadenomas [1]. Their symptoms and signs are usually due to anterior pituitary hormone deficiency and mass effect on adjacent structure, especially on optic chiasma, occurring in 60%–80% of cases [1, 2].

Most of patients with nonfunctioning pituitary adenomas have one or more anterior pituitary hormone deficiencies [1, 7, 8]. More than 20% of patients with nonfunctioning pituitary adenoma have two or more hormone deficiencies [1, 7]. 40%–75% of patients with nonfunctioning pituitary adenoma can have hypogonadotropic hypogonadism, and 20%–40% of cases develop central hypothyroidism and hypocortisolism [1, 7]. There can be mild hyperprolactinemia (<100 mg/ml) due to the compression of pituitary stalk by the tumor interrupting the descending dopaminergic effects [1].

8%–10% of pituitary adenomas can present as pituitary apoplexy [7]. Pituitary apoplexy is due to infarction or hemorrhage of the pituitary tumor that is characterized by sudden onset headache, vomiting, altered level of consciousness, hemodynamic instability, and visual abnormalities [1, 7].

In this case, the patient presented with atypical symptoms of nonfunctioning pituitary macroadenoma, though she had biochemical evidence supportive of a pituitary macroadenoma. She presented with recurrent vomiting in the background of cyclical episodes of vomiting with intermittent vomiting-free periods. She complained of generalized body weakness and reduced appetite, which might be nonspecific symptoms associated with hypoadrenalism. She had secondary amenorrhea suggestive of involvement of the hypothalamic-pituitary axis. Our patient's presentation is different from the typical presentation seen in pituitary apoplexy, although there were scattered hemorrhages in the lesion in MRI study.

Our patient had various psychosocial issues such as loss of the mother at young age, relationship breakup, and stresses from university life. The patient attributed onset of all her symptoms following her relationship breakup which occurred soon after she entered the university. Having several psychosocial problems could mislead the doctors from the correct diagnosis pathway by attributing all nonspecific, unexplained symptoms to a psychological illness. Although could have been having coexistent psychological issues, before making a psychological diagnosis, it is mandatory to exclude organic causes. This case highlights the importance of excluding organic causes before arriving at a psychological diagnosis.

Severe hyponatremia was another rare presentation of a nonfunctioning pituitary macroadenoma, which was observed in this case. With the history of recurrent vomiting, it is likely that one can mistakenly take vomiting as the sole cause for the observed electrolyte imbalance. This case highlights the importance of evaluating an electrolyte imbalance thoroughly because there can be multiple underlying aetiologies.

Only a few case reports have shown severe hyponatremia as a presenting symptom of a pituitary macroadenoma as in this case [4]. Therefore, high index of suspicion is needed when evaluating chronic or persistent hyponatremia [4].

Hyponatremia is defined as a serum sodium level less than 135 mmol/L. Severe hyponatremia is when serum sodium is below 125 mmol/L, which is associated with increased morbidity and mortality [4]. An approach to the evaluation of hyponatremia involves history taking, examination of each system of body, taking history of diuretics or any other drug use, serum, and urine biochemical tests. It is necessary to evaluate volume status, osmolality levels of the body, and urinary sodium level.

Hyponatremia due to hypopituitarism is usually due to secondary hypoadrenalism rather than central hypothyroidism [9]. Hyponatremia due to secondary hypoadrenalism is caused by impaired electrolyte-free water excretion in the absence of normal cortisol activity in the kidney [9]. Also, there is increased secretion of arginine vasopressin, a secondary ACTH secretagogue, which results in urinary concentration and can further impair hyponatremia [9].

Alteration in renal perfusion and reduced glomerular filtration are seen in hypothyroidism. Hyponatremia due to hypothyroidism is due to inability to excrete free water. There is effect of arginine vasopressin on dilution of urine. Reduced glomerular filtration rate in hypothyroidism diminishes free water excretion by reducing water delivery to the tubules, which causes hyponatremia [9].

Unlike in primary hypoadrenalism, in secondary hypoadrenalism, since there is no mineralocorticoid deficiency, it is unlikely that patients develop hyperkalemia.

Protracted vomiting without replacement of fluid ideally should cause volume depletion and hypernatremia [9]. However, if the patient takes fluid and food low in sodium content and in conjunction with a baroreceptor mediated stimulus to arginine vasopressin secretion which is an antidiuretic hormone, this can result in hyponatremia with vomiting and diarrhea [9]. History and examination are needed in evaluating hyponatremia due to vomiting and diarrhea. Symptoms and signs of volume depletion can be seen [9]. The urine sodium will be low with volume depletion but, with ongoing vomiting, it can be high due to urinary loss of bicarbonate, which causes excretion of an accompanying cation [9]. However, low urinary chloride level is a reliable indicator of volume depletion with vomiting [9].

It is clinician's duty to find correct aetiology of hyponatremia. Our patient had severe hyponatremia with minimal hyponatremic symptoms due to its chronic nature. However, having low serum potassium and serum chloride level with low urinary sodium and potassium levels highlighted that her hyponatremia was worsened by ongoing vomiting episodes and by reduced intake of salts due to reduced appetite. She denied polydipsia and polyuria, and her urine output was normal. She had low plasma osmolality with mildly elevated urine osmolality. Her blood urea level was normal. This led to the evaluation to find aetiology for hidden euvolemic chronic hyponatremia. This led to the diagnosis of underlying pituitary macroadenoma. Observed low serum potassium and chloride were attributed due to vomiting and reduced intake of salt.

This is a very atypical presentation of a patient with a nonfunctioning pituitary adenoma who presented with cyclical vomiting with severe hyponatremia. After correcting her hormone deficiencies and undergoing pituitary surgery, she did not develop any episode of recurrent vomiting.

4. Conclusion

Although nonfunctioning pituitary macroadenomas generally present with symptoms and signs of anterior pituitary hormone deficiencies and mass effect on adjacent structures, they can also have unusual presentations. Cyclical vomiting and severe hyponatremia are atypical presentations of nonfunctioning pituitary macroadenomas. Overlapping multiple aetiologies can be found in a patient with recurrent vomiting and hyponatremia. Identification of the correct aetiology is lifesaving. Therefore, high level of suspicion is needed when evaluating recurrent vomiting and hyponatremia.

Consent

Written informed consent was obtained from the patient for the publication of this case report.

References

[1] M. Mercado, V. Melgar, L. Salame, and D. Cuenca, "Clinically non-functioning pituitary adenomas: pathogenic, diagnostic and therapeutic aspects," *Endocrinología, Diabetes Y Nutrición (English ed.)*, vol. 64, no. 7, pp. 384–395, 2017.

[2] M. E. Molitch, "Pituitary incidentalomas," *Best Practice & Research Clinical Endocrinology & Metabolism*, vol. 23, no. 5, pp. 667–675, 2009.

[3] S. Mandadi, S. Sattar, B. Towfiq, and G. Bachuwa, "A case of nausea and vomiting to remember," *BMJ Case Reports*, vol. 2015, 2015.

[4] B. V. K. M. Bopeththa, S. M. M. Niyaz, and C. Medagedara, "Pituitary macroadenoma presenting as severe hyponatremia: a case report," *Journal of Medical Case Reports*, vol. 13, no. 1, p. 40, 2019.

[5] Q. T. Ostrom, H. Gittleman, J. Fulop, M. Liu, R. Blanda, and C. Kromer, "CBTRUS statistical report: primary brain and central nervous system tumors diagnosed in the United States in 2008–2012," *Neuro-Oncology*, vol. 17, no. 4, pp. iv1–iv62, 2015.

[6] A. Raappana, J. Koivukangas, T. Ebeling, and T. Pirilä, "Incidence of pituitary adenomas in Northern Finland in 1992–2007," *The Journal of Clinical Endocrinology & Metabolism*, vol. 95, no. 9, pp. 4268–4275, 2010.

[7] G. Vargas, B. Gonzalez, C. Ramirez, A. Ferreira, E. Espinosa, and V. Mendoza, "Clinical characteristics and treatment outcome of 485 patients with nonfunctioning pituitary macroadenomas," *International Journal of Endocrinology*, vol. 2015, Article ID 756069, , 2015.

[8] M. E. Molitch, "Diagnosis and treatment of pituitary adenomas," *JAMA*, vol. 317, no. 5, pp. 516–524, 2017.

[9] J. G. Verbalis, S. R. Goldsmith, A. Greenberg et al., "Diagnosis, evaluation, and treatment of hyponatremia: expert panel recommendations," *The American Journal of Medicine*, vol. 126, no. 10, pp. S1–S42, 2013.

16

Adrenal and Hepatic Venous Sampling in a Case of Aldosterone-Producing Adrenocortical Carcinoma with Hepatic Metastasis

Toru Sugiyama,[1] **Yuriko Sasahara**,[1] **Hironobu Sasano**,[2] **and Eri Hayakawa**[1]

[1]*Division of Endocrinology and Metabolism, Japanese Red Cross Musashino Hospital, Tokyo, Japan*
[2]*Department of Pathology, Tohoku University School of Medicine, Sendai, Miyagi, Japan*

Correspondence should be addressed to Toru Sugiyama; tsugiyama@musashino.jrc.or.jp

Academic Editor: Lucy Mastrandrea

Background. Adrenocortical carcinoma (ACC) is a rare and highly aggressive malignancy. ACCs often secrete adrenal steroid hormones including cortisol and androgens; however, aldosterone-producing ACC is very rare. Although adrenal production of aldosterone is assessed by adrenal venous sampling, the use of sampling from the relevant vein to assess aldosterone production from a tumor arising from ACC metastasis has not been previously reported. *Case Presentation.* We report the case of a 69-year-old Japanese man with aldosterone-producing ACC with hepatic metastasis. He presented with a history of treatment-resistant hypertension and hypokalemia. Endocrinological examination showed markedly increased plasma aldosterone concentration and suppressed plasma renin activity. Serum cortisol concentration was not suppressed by administration of dexamethasone 1 mg, and normal circadian variation of cortisol secretion was disrupted. Abdominal computed tomography showed a large tumor in the left adrenal gland and multiple tumors in the liver. Together, these results strongly suggested ACC with multiple liver metastases causing primary aldosteronism and subclinical Cushing syndrome. Adrenal and hepatic venous sampling showed markedly increased aldosterone concentration in the left adrenal vein but no increase in the hepatic vein, despite a pathological diagnosis of ACC with hepatic metastasis, with immunohistochemical investigation showing both primary and secondary tumors to have synthetic capability for aldosterone. The patient received mitotane but declined combination chemotherapy and died 2 months later. *Conclusion.* This is the first report of adrenal and hepatic venous sampling in a case of aldosterone-producing ACC with hepatic metastasis. The case suggests that hepatic venous sampling is unable to detect aldosterone production from liver metastases arising from ACC.

1. Introduction

Adrenocortical carcinoma (ACC) is a rare, highly aggressive malignancy with an estimated annual incidence of 0.7–2.0 cases per million population. It has a heterogeneous clinical presentation, and prognosis is generally poor. Approximately 60–70% of ACCs secrete hormones, mostly glucocorticoids or androgens. Less than 10% of hormone-secreting ACCs produce aldosterone, in which cases the excessive production can cause primary aldosteronism [1–3].

Common causes of primary aldosteronism are an aldosterone-producing adenoma or bilateral idiopathic adrenal hyperplasia. The condition frequently results in difficult-to-treat arterial hypertension, sodium retention, and hypokalemia.

In cases of primary aldosteronism, adrenal venous sampling (AVS) is considered the gold standard test for determining whether the excessive aldosterone production is uni- or bilateral and identifying the adrenal gland responsible [4]. However, there have been no reports of the use of sampling from the relevant vein to assess aldosterone production from a tumor arising from ACC metastasis.

Here, we report what we believe to be the first case of aldosterone-producing ACC with hepatic metastasis in which adrenal and hepatic venous sampling were carried out to assess the production of aldosterone from the primary and secondary tumor, respectively.

2. Case Presentation

A 69-year-old man with an 8-month history of treatment-resistant hypertension and hypokalemia was referred to our hospital for investigation of suspected secondary hypertension. On physical examination, the only abnormal finding was hypertension (178/105 mmHg); there were no signs of Cushing syndrome (e.g., moon facies, central obesity, and buffalo hump).

Laboratory findings showed hypokalemia (2.3 mEq/L) (Table 1). The results of endocrine examination (Table 2) showed a markedly increased plasma aldosterone concentration (PAC; 1710 pg/mL) and suppressed plasma renin activity (PRA: 0.2 ng/mL/h). Serum DHEA-S (35 μg/dL) was within the normal range (12–133 μg/dL). Fasting plasma concentrations of the adrenocorticotropic hormone (ACTH) and serum cortisol were 2.1 pg/mL (below the lower limit of normal, 7.2 pg/mL) and 9.4 μg/dL (within the normal range, 4.0–18.2 μg/dL), respectively. Serum cortisol concentration was not suppressed in response to an overnight low-dose (1 mg) dexamethasone suppression test, and normal circadian variation of cortisol secretion was disrupted. Both urinary aldosterone concentration and cortisol concentration were increased: 549 μg/24 h (normal, $<$10 μg/24 h) and 328 μg/24 h (upper limit of normal, 80.3 μg/24 h), respectively.

Abdominal computed tomography (CT) showed a left adrenal tumor (diameter, 7 cm) and multiple liver tumors (diameter, ~4 cm) (Figure 1).

The combined examination and investigation results strongly suggested ACC with multiple liver metastases causing primary aldosteronism and subclinical Cushing syndrome. Such cases are classified as clinical stage IV and therefore ineligible for surgery to remove the adrenal tumor. However, the patient hoped to have the adrenal tumor removed, so he requested investigation of the liver tumors to confirm that they had arisen from the ACC.

Adrenal and hepatic venous sampling were carried out. Aldosterone concentration was markedly increased in the left adrenal vein (64,500 μg/dL) but not in the right adrenal or hepatic vein (4870 and 1210 μg/dL, respectively) (Table 3). These findings suggested that the liver tumors were not secreting aldosterone; therefore, biopsies of tissue from both the left adrenal tumor and the liver tumors were carried out to enable pathological diagnosis. Based on the Weiss criteria, the biopsy results for the left adrenal and liver tumors were pathologically consistent with the diagnosis of ACC with hepatic metastasis. Immunohistochemical investigation showed strong positive staining for SF-1, P450c17, P450c21, 3βHSD2, CYP11B1, and CYP11B2 and partial positive staining for P450scc and 3βHSD1 in both the ACC and the liver metastases (Figure 2); these findings indicated synthetic capability for aldosterone and cortisol. The DHEA-ST test result was negative for both the ACC and the liver metastases.

The patient received mitotane (1500 mg/day) but declined combination chemotherapy. Hypoalbuminemia and severe edema of the lung and lower extremities developed rapidly despite administration of high doses of spironolactone, and he died 2 months later.

3. Discussion

To our knowledge, this is the first report of a case of aldosterone-producing ACC with hepatic metastasis in which adrenal and hepatic venous sampling were carried out to assess the production of aldosterone from metastasis of ACC. This was an unusual case because hypersecretion of aldosterone from ACC is rare; in the majority of cases (approximately 60–70%), ACCs present with an excess of adrenal hormone (mostly glucocorticoids or androgens) [1–3].

Although AVS is considered the gold standard test for determining whether the right, the left, or both adrenal glands are responsible for the aldosterone excess in cases of primary aldosteronism, to our knowledge, there have been no reports of the use of sampling from the relevant vein to assess aldosterone production from a tumor suspected to have arisen from ACC metastasis. In the case presented in this report, we used hepatic venous sampling to try to help determine whether the liver tumors were ACC metastases or other hepatic tumors (e.g., hepatocellular carcinoma). However, aldosterone concentration in the hepatic veins was not increased, despite the pathological diagnosis of hepatic metastasis of ACC and its synthetic capability for aldosterone.

In cases of insulinoma, hepatic venous sampling after selective intra-arterial injections of calcium into the relevant hepatic artery is carried out to exclude hepatic metastasis of insulinoma [5–8]. In a similar way, liver metastases arising from ACC might be expected to be detected by hepatic venous sampling. Because aldosterone is a lipophilic steroid hormone, it should be released into the blood circulation once synthesized. Our experience in this case suggests that hepatic venous sampling is unsuitable for diagnosis of ACC with hepatic metastasis. Although the liver tumors were found by immunohistochemical investigation to have synthetic capability for aldosterone and cortisol, aldosterone concentration in the hepatic veins was found not to be increased. This might be explained by the limited transportation of aldosterone to the hepatic vein or degradation of aldosterone during its passage through the liver. Further basic research is required to explain this finding.

Adrenocortical carcinoma has a generally poor prognosis, with overall 5-year survival ranging from 60–80% in patients with stage I disease to 13% in those with stage IV. Clinical outcomes vary greatly due to differences in tumor biology, disease presentation, and management options [1, 2, 9, 10]. The results of a recent systematic review and meta-analysis show that cortisol-secreting ACCs are associated with worse overall survival [11]. This higher mortality rate could be explained by negative effects of cortisol on the immune and cardiovascular systems. In cases of aldosterone-secreting ACCs, scarcity of data means that prognosis is uncertain. In the case presented here, the marked hyperaldosteronism could have negatively affected the cardiovascular system and electrolyte balance and thus contributed to the poor outcome.

TABLE 1: Laboratory findings.

Blood cell count		Biochemistry			
WBC (/μL)	6000	TP (g/dL)	7.0	UN (mg/dL)	11.5
Neutrophil (%)	62.2	Alb (g/dL)	4.2	Cr (mg/dL)	0.59
Lymphocyte (%)	28.3	LDH (IU/L)	330	UA (mg/dL)	4.1
Monocyte (%)	8.3	AST (IU/L)	22	Na (mEq/L)	147
Eosinophil (%)	0.7	ALT (IU/L)	39	K (mEq/L)	2.3
Basophil (%)	0.5	γ-GT (IU/L)	31	Cl (mEq/L)	95
RBC ($\times 10^6$/μL)	4.47	T-Bil (mg/dL)	0.8	Ca (mg/dL)	8.7
Hemoglobin (g/dL)	13.0	ALP (IU/L)	308	P (mg/dL)	2.6
Hematocrit (%)	38.2	Plasma glucose (mg/dL)	95	T-chol (mg/dL)	167
Platelet ($\times 10^4$/μL)	24.5	CK (IU/L)	216	HDL-c (mg/dL)	60.7
		CRP (mg/dL)	0.17	LDL-c (mg/dL)	95.6
				TG (mg/dL)	95

TABLE 2: Endocrinological examination.

Hormonal profile			Normal range	
Plasma ACTH (pg/mL)	2.1		7.2–63.3	
Serum cortisol (μg/dL)	9.4		4.0–18.3	
Plasma renin activity (ng/mL/h)	0.2		0.3–2.9	
PAC (pg/mL)	1710		140–1030	
Serum DHEA-S (μg/dL)	35		12–133	
Urinary free cortisol (μg/24 h)	328		11.2–80.3	
Urinary free aldosterone (μg/24 h)	549		<10	
Circadian variation of plasma ACTH and serum cortisol and low-dose (1 mg) DST results				
Time	06:00	16:00	23:00	1 mg DST
Plasma ACTH (pg/mL)	<1.0	<1.0	<1.0	<1.0
Serum cortisol (μg/dL)	9.8	11.3	11.6	12.0

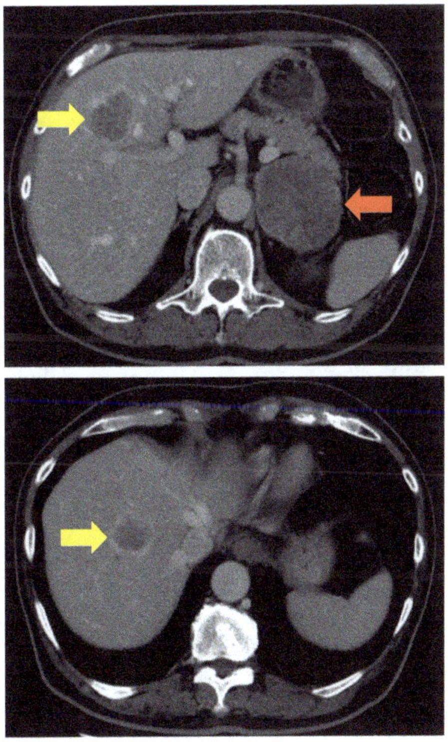

FIGURE 1: Abdominal computed tomography scan. The red arrow indicates the left adrenal tumor (diameter, 7 cm). The yellow arrows indicate multiple liver tumors (diameter, ~4 cm).

TABLE 3: Adrenal and hepatic venous sampling.

	Sampling point	PAC (pg/mL)	Cortisol (μg/dL)	PAC : cortisol ratio
Before ACTH loading	Inferior vena cava	3890	18.3	21.3×10^{-3}
	Left adrenal vein	35,000	44.7	78.3×10^{-3}
	Right adrenal vein	3310	23.2	14.3×10^{-3}
	Hepatic vein	1360	18.8	7.2×10^{-3}
After ACTH loading	Inferior vena cava	4260	21.4	19.9×10^{-3}
	Left adrenal vein	64,500	58.2	110.8×10^{-3}
	Right adrenal vein	4870	132	3.7×10^{-3}
	Hepatic vein	1210	21.2	5.7×10^{-3}

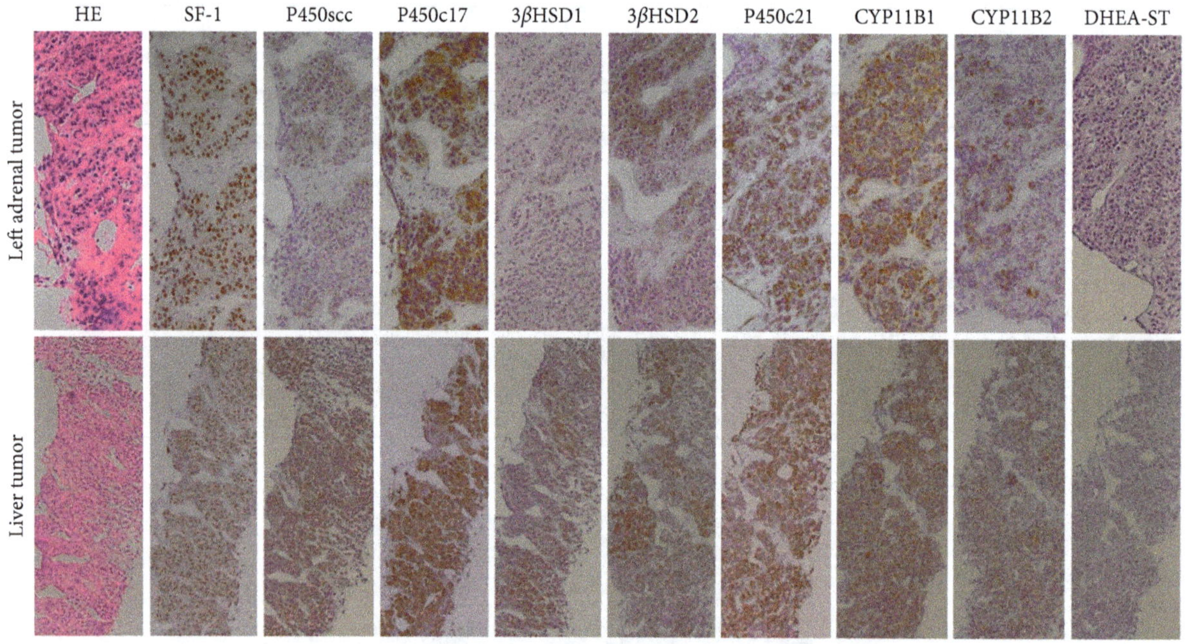

FIGURE 2: Results of histopathological and immunohistochemical investigation of left adrenal and liver biopsy specimens (magnification, ×200). Microscopic appearance (hematoxylin and eosin, HE, staining) showed eosinophilic tumor cell cytoplasm, nuclear atypia, diffuse architecture, and sinusoidal invasion. Immunohistochemical staining showed strong positive reactivity for SF-1, P450c17, 3βHSD2, P450c21, CYP11B1, and CYP11B2 and partial positive reactivity for P450scc and 3βHSD1 in both the left adrenal tumor (upper panel) and the liver tumor (lower panel). The DHEA-ST test result was negative for both specimens.

Management of ACC remains challenging due to the heterogeneous and often unpredictable nature of this disease. If our patient's liver metastases had not produced excessive aldosterone, surgical resection of the primary tumor might have resolved the hyperaldosteronism, and this might have led to a better outcome.

4. Conclusion

We report the first case of adrenal and hepatic venous sampling in a patient with aldosterone-producing ACC with hepatic metastasis. Hepatic venous sampling did not detect aldosterone production from the liver tumors.

Abbreviations

3βHSD: 3β-Hydroxysteroid dehydrogenase
ACC: Adrenocortical carcinoma
ACTH: Adrenocorticotropic hormone
Alb: Albumin
ALP: Alkaline phosphatase
ALT: Alanine aminotransferase
AST: Aspartate aminotransferase
CK: Creatine kinase
Cr: Creatinine
CRP: C-reactive protein
CYP: Cytochrome P450
DHEA-ST: Dehydroepiandrosterone sulfotransferase
DST: Dexamethasone suppression test
HDL-c: High-density lipoprotein cholesterol
HE: Hematoxylin and eosin
LDH: Lactase dehydrogenase
LDL-c: Low-density lipoprotein cholesterol
P450c17: Cytochrome P450 17
P450c21: Cytochrome P450 21
P450scc: Cytochrome P450 side-chain cleavage

PAC: Plasma aldosterone concentration
RBC: Red blood cell
SF-1: Steroidogenic factor 1
T-Bil: Total bilirubin
T-chol: Total cholesterol
TG: Triglycerides
TP: Total protein
UA: Uric acid
UN: Urea nitrogen
WBC: White blood cell
γ-GT: γ-Glutamyltranspeptidase.

Ethical Approval

The need for ethical approval and consent to the submission of case reports were waived by the ethics review committee of Japanese Red Cross Musashino Hospital. We followed the principles of the Declaration of Helsinki and paid careful attention to protecting the patient's identity.

Consent

The patient's family provided their informed consent to publication of this case report, including the figures.

Authors' Contributions

TS was the main author to treat this patient and wrote the manuscript. YS cared for the patient when he was admitted to the hospital. HS carried out the pathological and immunohistochemical investigation. EH provided professional opinions regarding the patient's care and commented on the manuscript. All authors read and approved the final submitted version of the manuscript.

Acknowledgments

The authors would like to thank the Tama Society of Clinical Endocrinology and Metabolism, whose members participated in helpful discussions.

References

[1] T. Else, A. C. Kim, A. Sabolch et al., "Adrenocortical carcinoma," *Endocrine Reviews*, vol. 35, no. 2, pp. 282–326, 2014.
[2] M. Fassnacht, M. Kroiss, and B. Allolio, "Update in adrenocortical carcinoma," *The Journal of Clinical Endocrinology & Metabolism*, vol. 98, no. 12, pp. 4551–4564, 2013.
[3] T. M. Seccia, A. Fassina, G. G. Nussdorfer, A. C. Pessina, and G. P. Rossi, "Aldosterone-producing adrenocortical carcinoma: an unusual cause of Conn's syndrome with an ominous clinical course," *Endocrine-Related Cancer*, vol. 12, no. 1, pp. 149–159, 2005.
[4] G. P. Rossi, "Primary aldosteronism," *Journal of the American College of Cardiology*, vol. 74, no. 22, pp. 2799–2811, 2019.
[5] J.-M. Guettier, A. Kam, R. Chang et al., "Localization of insulinomas to regions of the pancreas by intraarterial calcium stimulation: the NIH experience," *The Journal of Clinical Endocrinology & Metabolism*, vol. 94, no. 4, pp. 1074–1080, 2009.
[6] P. Moreno-Moreno, M. R. Alhambra-Expósito, A. D. Herrera-Martínez et al., "Arterial calcium stimulation with hepatic venous sampling in the localization diagnosis of endogenous hyperinsulinism," *International Journal of Endocrinology*, vol. 2016, Article ID 4581094, 6 pages, 2016.
[7] M. Imamura, K. Takahashi, H. Adachi et al., "Usefulness of selective arterial secretin injection test for localization of gastrinoma in the zollinger-ellison syndrome," *Annals of Surgery*, vol. 205, no. 3, pp. 230–239, 1987.
[8] P. L. Pereira, A. J. Roche, G. W. Maier et al., "Insulinoma and islet cell hyperplasia: value of the calcium intraarterial stimulation test when findings of other preoperative studies are negative," *Radiology*, vol. 206, no. 3, pp. 703–709, 1998.
[9] S. Jasim and M. A. Habra, "Management of adrenocortical carcinoma," *Current Oncology Reports*, vol. 21, no. 3, p. 20, 2019.
[10] T. Else, A. R. Williams, A. Sabolch, S. Jolly, B. S. Miller, and G. D. Hammer, "Adjuvant therapies and patient and tumor characteristics associated with survival of adult patients with adrenocortical carcinoma," *The Journal of Clinical Endocrinology & Metabolism*, vol. 99, no. 2, pp. 455–461, 2014.
[11] T. Vanbrabant, M. Fassnacht, G. Assie, and O. M. Dekkers, "Influence of hormonal functional status on survival in adrenocortical carcinoma: systematic review and meta-analysis," *European Journal of Endocrinology*, vol. 179, no. 6, pp. 429–436, 2018.

17

Ectopic Cushing's Syndrome Secondary to Metastatic Paraganglioma

R. Daya,[1,2] C. Wingfield,[1] P. Sotshononda,[1] F. Seedat,[1,2] S. Bulbulia,[1,2] M. D. Simmons,[3] M. Louw,[3] and Z. Bayat[1,2]

[1]*Division of Endocrinology and Metabolism, Department of Internal Medicine, Helen Joseph Hospital, 1 Perth Road, Rossmore, Johannesburg, South Africa*
[2]*Division of Endocrinology and Metabolism, Department of Internal Medicine, Faculty of Health Sciences, School of Clinical Medicine, University of the Witwatersrand, Johannesburg, South Africa*
[3]*Department of Anatomical Pathology, School of Pathology, University of the Witwatersrand, Johannesburg, South Africa*

Correspondence should be addressed to R. Daya; reyna.daya13@gmail.com

Academic Editor: Désirée Deandreis

Paraneoplastic or ectopic Cushing's syndrome (CS) is a rare cause of endogenous hypercortisolism. It is due to ectopic adrenocorticotropic hormone (ACTH) secretion and has been reported in association with a variety of neuroendocrine tumors such as small-cell lung carcinoma, carcinoid tumors, and medullary carcinoma of the thyroid. Paragangliomas (PGLs) are rare neuroendocrine tumors that can secrete catecholamines. Case reports and reports of ectopic ACTH secretion from metastatic PGLs causing CS are exceedingly rare. We present a case of a 38-year-old female, who presented with typical signs, symptoms, and complications of CS, secondary to a PGL with widespread metastases, which eventually led to her demise.

1. Introduction

Pheochromocytomas (PCCs) and paragangliomas (PGLs) are rare neuroendocrine tumors, collectively termed pheochromocytoma–paraganglioma (PPGL). PCCs usually arise from the adrenal medulla, whilst PGLs arise from chromaffin tissue outside of the adrenal medulla and can secrete neuropeptides and catecholamines so are also referred to as extra-adrenal PCC.

Cushing's syndrome (CS) is a collection of signs and symptoms due to prolonged exposure to either endogenous or exogenous excess glucocorticoids (GCs) resulting in a disruption of the normal hypothalamic-pituitary-adrenal axis [1]. CS is broadly categorised as adrenocorticotropic hormone (ACTH) dependent (70–80%) or ACTH independent (20–30%) [2]. ACTH-dependent CS occurs most commonly secondary to a pituitary corticotrophic adenoma (Cushing's disease), whilst less frequently, it may be caused by an extrapituitary tumor (ectopic ACTH secretion) or rarely a tumor secreting corticotropin-releasing hormone (CRH) [2].

Ectopic CS is a rare cause of endogenous hypercortisolism accounting for 5–20% of all CS cases and 10–20% of ACTH-dependent CS patients [2]. It is due to ectopic ACTH secretion and has been reported in association with a variety of neuroendocrine tumors such as small-cell lung carcinoma, carcinoid tumors, and medullary carcinoma of the thyroid. Ectopic ACTH secretion from PGLs is rare and limited to case reports. Case reports and reports of metastatic PGL causing CS are exceedingly rare.

2. Case

A 38-year-old female presented to hospital with a longstanding history of progressive abdominal pain and distension. Functional inquiry revealed complaints of amenorrhoea, worsening malaise, proximal muscle weakness, insomnia, weight gain, and persecutory delusions.

She had a background history of Human Immunodeficiency Virus (HIV) infection, for which she was on second-line antiretroviral therapy (ARV) (tenofovir, lamivudine, and dolutegravir) due to previous virological failure, with no history of any prior opportunistic infections. In addition, she was diagnosed with hypertension and type 2 diabetes mellitus a few years prior, which was insufficiently controlled (glycated haemoglobin (HbA1 c) level of 7.6%) on admission. She had no micro- or macrovascular complications. Her medication included amlodipine and metformin; however, she was not on any medication for her mental health complaints. There was no history of headaches, palpitations, or hyperhidrosis. She denied any symptoms of sleep apnoea. She was a nonsmoker and denied any history of exogenous corticosteroid use (oral, nasal, topical, or injectable). There was no family history of Cushing's syndrome/disease or pheochromocytoma.

Her body weight and height were 183 pounds (83 kg) and 5 foot 4 inches (165 cm), respectively, with a body mass index of 30.5 kg/m^2. Physical examination revealed typical cushingoid features including moon facies, facial plethora, and prominent truncal, facial, and nuchal adiposity, as well as multiple areas of bruising. Abdominal distention was noted, with visible violaceous striae and no palpable masses. The rest of the clinical examination was normal.

Her latest CD4 lymphocyte count was 131 cells/mm^3 with an undetectable viral load. Fasting blood glucose levels were elevated. Biochemical investigations revealed an elevated random serum cortisol level of 1118 nmol/L (133–537 nmol/L), with an inappropriately normal adrenocorticotrophic hormone (ACTH) level of 4.6 pmol/L (1.6–13.9 pmol/L) (Table 1). In addition, there was an elevated 24-hour urinary free cortisol level of 10447 nmol/24 hours (10–124 nmol/24 hours). A repeat sample confirmed an elevated urinary free cortisol level. Low- (1 mg) and high-dose (8 mg) dexamethasone suppression tests were conducted, and both showed an inability to suppress plasma cortisol levels (Table 2). The rest of the biochemical investigations are shown in Table 1.

Based on her history, clinical examination, and investigations, a diagnosis of CS was made. To determine the underlying etiology, further imaging was carried out.

Abdominal sonography showed hepatomegaly (span of 188 mm) with multiple hypodense hepatic lesions suggestive of metastatic disease. The adrenal glands, pancreas, spleen, and kidneys were normal. In addition, the pituitary gland was normal on imaging. Contrast-enhanced computed tomography (CT) of the chest and abdomen confirmed the liver lesions and multiple lesions in the pancreas and lungs, with no significant abdominal or thoracic lymphadenopathy (Figures 1 and 2).

Based on the radiologic investigations, the etiology of her CS was strongly suspected to be due to ectopic ACTH secretion from an advanced malignancy of uncertain primary origin.

Before we could complete the workup, the patient developed urosepsis, complicated by septic shock, leading to her unfortunate demise. Her autopsy findings revealed a large tumor in the lower lobe of the left lung (40 × 35 × 25 mm). Numerous tumor deposits were noted in the liver, with smaller deposits seen in the thyroid, heart (endocardium), liver, pancreas, spleen, left kidney, and peritoneal lymph nodes. The brain (pituitary) and adrenal glands were normal. Right kidney pyelonephritis was confirmed as the source of sepsis.

On histology, all the metastatic tumor deposits, including the tumor in the left lung, were similar to the tumor in the liver. The liver section showed a nesting (Zellballen) pattern of cells within a prominent vascular network (Figure 3). The cells were round with granular eosinophilic cytoplasm. Nuclear atypia and mitotic figures were also evident.

Immunohistochemistry stained positive for chromogranin (Figure 4) and synaptophysin and negative for cytokeratin 7 and 20. ACTH staining was not shown in both the lung and liver lesions. Immunostaining for CRH is not available in our setting, nor are we able to measure CRH levels in plasma.

Based on the histological and immunohistochemistry findings, a diagnosis of metastatic paraganglioma with paraneoplastic phenomena resulting in CS was made. The cause of death was deemed as systemic sepsis.

3. Discussion

Pheochromocytomas (PCCs) and paragangliomas (PGLs) are rare neuroendocrine tumors, collectively termed pheochromocytoma-paraganglioma (PPGL). PGLs are grouped based on their origin in the parasympathetic or the sympathetic nervous system. Sympathetic PGLs are most commonly found in the para-aortic region of the abdomen, pelvis, and chest [3, 4]. Parasympathetic PGLs typically arise from the head and neck region, including the carotid body, vagus nerve, and jugular foramen, of which less than 5% are malignant [5].

The most common sites for PGLs with catecholamine hypersecretion are localized in the abdomen and pelvis. The catecholamine secretion causes paroxysmal episodic hypertension, often accompanied by palpitations, headache and/or hyperhidrosis. Nonfunctional or silent PGLs most commonly manifest as abdominal pain or an incidentally found mass.

25–40% of PPGLs have an underlying germline mutation, of which a mutation in the succinate dehydrogenase (SDH) family is most common. Patients with a mutation in the B subunit of SDH (SDHB) are more likely to have metastatic disease. Other frequent syndrome-associated PPGLs secondary to germline mutations include Von Hippel–Lindau disease (VHL), Multiple Endocrine Neoplasia 2 (MEN2), and Neurofibromatosis type 1 (NF1) [5, 6].

The histological features of PGLs are similar to those of adrenal PCCs. The tumor cells usually show chief cells arranged in nests, alveolar-like, and stereo-like structures surrounded by sustentacular cells partly or entirely with delicate fibrovascular stroma (a Zellballen pattern), although they may also grow in a diffuse pattern [7].

Synaptophysin is an integral membrane protein of small synaptic vesicles in the brain and endocrine cells and is

TABLE 1: Summary of biochemical results.

Variable	Result	Reference range
White cell count	8.45	3.90–12.60 × 109/L
Hemoglobin	**9.0**	11.6–16.4 g/dl
Mean cell volume	89.6	78.9–98.5 fL
Platelet count	311	186–454 × 109/L
Sodium	145	136–145 mmol/L
Potassium	**3.2**	3.5–5.1 mmol/L
Urea	5.6	2.1–7.1 mmol/L
Creatinine	65	49–90 umol/L
eGFR (estimated glomerular filtration rate)	104	>89 mL/mim/1.73 m^2
HbA1 C (glycated hemoglobin)	**7.6**	<6.5%
Fasting blood glucose	**11.6**	3.3–6.0 mmol/L
Calcium	2.28	2.15–2.50 mmol/L
Magnesium	0.87	0.63–1.05 mmol/L
Inorganic phosphate	0.75	0.78–1.42 mmol/L
ALP (alkaline phosphatase)	58	42–98 U/L
GGT (gamma-glutamyl transferase)	40	<40 U/L
TSH (thyroid-stimulating hormone)	0.84	0.35–5.50 mIU/L
8 am cortisol	**1118**	133–537 nmol/L
ACTH (adrenocorticotropic hormone)	4.6	1.6–13.9 pmol/L
24-hour urinary free cortisol (1st sample)	**10447**	10–124 nmol/24 hours
24-hour urinary free cortisol (2nd sample)	**9856**	10–124 nmol/24 hours
Midnight cortisol	**1042**	<50 nmol/L
Chromogranin A	**750.3**	0.0–84.7 ng/mL

TABLE 2: Low- and high-dose dexamethasone suppression test.

Dexamethasone suppression	1 mg	8 mg
Time of administration	0 : 00	0 : 00
Midnight cortisol	1042	1750
8 am cortisol	796	1253

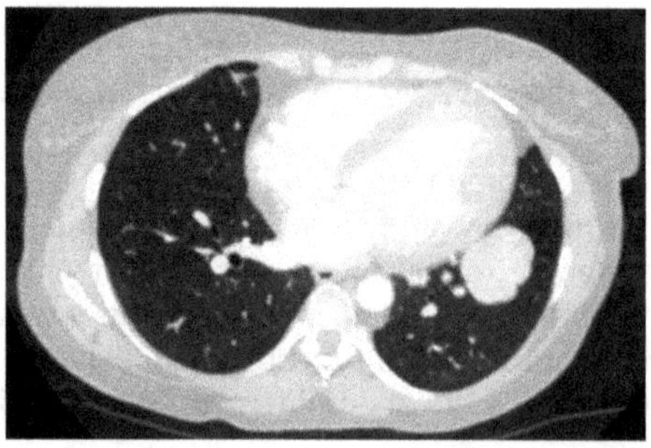

FIGURE 1: Contrast-enhanced computed tomography (CT) of the chest showing a lung mass measuring 4.4 × 4.0 × 4.0 cm.

abundant in neuroendocrine cells of diffuse origin and tumor tissues with neuroendocrine function [8, 9]. Chromogranin A is the precursor to several functional peptides, which negatively modulate neuroendocrine function in an autocrine and paracrine manner. It is produced by chromaffin cells of the adrenal medulla, paraganglia, and beta cells of the pancreas and is found to be significantly elevated in serum in patients with neuroendocrine tumors [10]. In addition, it can be assessed on immunohistochemistry in neuroendocrine tissue.

Cytokeratins are keratin proteins found in the intracytoplasmic cytoskeleton of epithelial tissue [11]. They are an important component of intermediate filaments. Immunohistochemistry staining for cytokeratin is helpful in the diagnostic differentiation of metastatic lesions and assists in determining the site of origin [12].

The combination of cytokeratin negativity and chromogranin and synaptophysin positivity on immunohistochemistry is required for a definitive diagnosis of PGLs.

The natural history of PPGLs varies from a benign tumor cured with surgery to the development of rapidly progressive metastatic disease with approximately 10% of PCCs and 25% of PGLs being malignant [4]. The overall 5-year survival rate ranges between 20 and 70% in patients with metastatic disease in comparison to those without metastatic disease whose survival is 90% [13]. Malignancy is defined by the presence of metastatic lesions at sites where neuroendocrine tissue is not normally present, e.g., the lymph nodes, bone, lung, and liver [14].

Our patient's immunohistochemistry stained positive for both chromogranin and synaptophysin and negative for cytokeratin. The combination of Zellballen pattern on histology, a cytokeratin negative stain, and positive chromogranin and synaptophysin staining on immunohistochemistry confirm that our patient had a PGL. On morphological examination, all the tumor deposits in the various organs were identical. The finding of tumor deposit in sites where neuroendocrine tissue is not usually present confirmed the diagnosis of disseminated malignant PGL in our patient.

CS is a rare endocrine condition with an estimated incidence of 2-3 cases per million people per year [15, 16]. CS compromises a group of signs and symptoms that reflects prolonged and inappropriately high exposure of glucocorticoids (endogenous or exogenous) to various tissues. Whilst

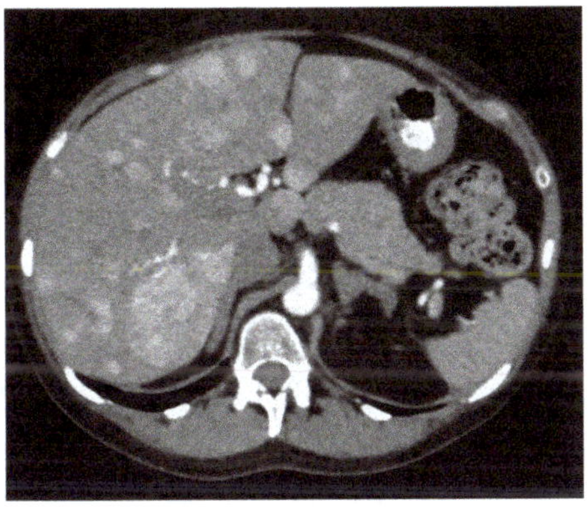

Figure 2: CT of the abdomen showing multiple irregular lesions in the liver, with the largest measuring 6.0 × 6.0 cm (white arrow).

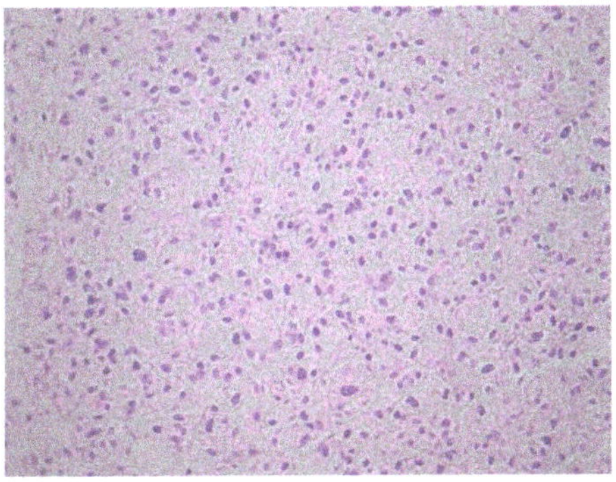

Figure 3: Haematoxylin-and-eosin- (H&E-) stained section of the liver showing a characteristic nesting pattern ("Zellballen") of cells (400× magnification).

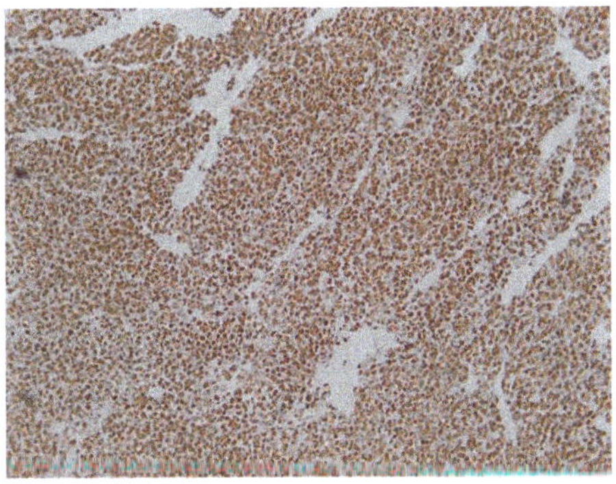

Figure 4: Photomicrograph (100×) of the liver showing strong diffuse staining of tumor cells with a chromogranin.

classical CS is clinically unmistakable, the spectrum of clinical features is broad and nonspecific, often overlapping with a variety of medical conditions including type 2 diabetes mellitus, obesity, and polycystic ovarian syndrome. The unique clinical features of CS include violaceous striae, facial plethora, proximal muscle weakness, easy bruisability, and unexplained osteoporosis [17]. Symptoms are determined by the level of hypercortisolemia and not by the duration of exposure or the size of the tumor [18–21].

Whilst the clinical features of CS may be subtle, the metabolic abnormalities are more upfront. Hypokalemia may be present in up to 58% of cases [22]. Other common metabolic abnormalities include metabolic alkalosis and hyperglycemia.

The exact biological mechanism of ectopic ACTH secretion is unknown [2]. Whilst clinical features of CS due to ectopic ACTH secretion are similar to those due to pituitary ACTH secretion, they tend to have a more rapid onset and progression. Common causes of ectopic ACTH secretion include small-cell lung carcinoma (SCLC), bronchial carcinoid, and neuroendocrine tumor of the lung, small intestines, and the pancreas [23]. Thymic carcinoid and medullary carcinoma of the thyroid may also secrete ACTH, but these are rare [24–26].

Prior to this case, only a few cases of ectopic ACTH secretion associated with PGLs have been described in the literature [27, 28]. As with our patient, in the majority of PGL cases with ectopic ACTH production, patients are female and have metabolic features (hypertension, hyperglycemia, and hypokalemia) [27, 28]. However, very few have shown catecholamine hypersecretion [27]. Most patients with PGL who secrete ACTH have significantly elevated plasma cortisol and ACTH levels [27, 28]. However, there is one case described with a normal plasma ACTH level and another with low ACTH levels [27].

In our case, biochemistry failed to demonstrate excess ACTH in serum. This may suggest that the tumor cells produced a small amount of ACTH, which stimulated the synthesis of cortisol. Excessive cortisol would then inhibit the secretion of ACTH in the pituitary as a negative feedback. A normal ACTH level in the face of an extremely elevated cortisol level is inappropriate and suggests ACTH secretion independent of the control of the hypothalamic-pituitary axis (HPA).

In our patient, postmortem specimens failed to stain for ACTH. This may have been due to the severe necrosis and autolysis of the tumor. Normal pituitary and adrenal glands on autopsy (both macroscopic and histological), elevated serum cortisol, elevated 24-hour urinary free cortisol level and ACTH levels, and failure to suppress on a high-dose dexamethasone suppression test support the diagnosis of ectopic ACTH production. Immunostaining for CRH is not available in our setting, nor are we able to measure CRH levels in plasma.

4. Conclusions

We present a 38-year-old female, with widespread metastatic PGL, with CS due to ectopic ACTH secretion. Whilst the diagnosis of CS was confirmed while the patient was alive, the diagnosis of metastatic PGL was made on postmortem as the patient demised whilst still being investigated. Autopsy findings showed multiple tumor deposits with histological examination revealing a Zellballen pattern in keeping with a PGL. Positive immunohistochemistry staining for chromogranin and synaptophysin combined with negative staining for cytokeratin sealed the diagnosis of a PGL. The nondemarcated, widespread autolytic degradation of the tissue is likely responsible for the loss of demonstrable hormone expression (ACTH staining).

It is possible that our patient may have had an underlying genetic mutation predisposing her to develop metastatic PGL; however, due to her demise prior to the diagnosis; we were unable to offer her genetic testing. Her prognosis was poor in view of such widespread disease. The hypersecretion of cortisol may have resulted in hyperglycemia and suppression of her immune system, which predisposed her to severe infections, leading to her demise. Whilst her underling HIV may have contributed, we considered this unlikely due to her undetectable viral load.

This case represents a very rare cause of ectopic CS, most likely caused by an ACTH-producing metastatic PGL.

Abbreviations

PGL: Paraganglioma
PPGL: Pheochromocytoma-paraganglioma
CS: Cushing's syndrome
ACTH: Adrenocorticotropic hormone
CT: Computed tomography.

Ethical Approval

Ethical approval was granted by the Human Research Ethics Committee (Medical) from the University of the Witwatersrand (M2011154), and this study was performed in accordance with the ethical standards as laid down in the 1964 Declaration of Helsinki and its later amendments or comparable ethical standards.

Consent

The patient gave verbal and written consent for this case report prior to her demise.

Disclosure

This work was performed as part of the employment of the authors in the Gauteng Department of Health, South Africa.

Acknowledgments

The authors acknowledge Mr. E. Liebenberg, from the Department of Anatomical Pathology, University of the Witwatersrand.

References

[1] L. K. Nieman, B. M. K. Biller, J. W. Findling et al., "The diagnosis of Cushing's syndrome: an endocrine society clinical practice guideline," *The Journal of Clinical Endocrinology & Metabolism*, vol. 93, no. 5, pp. 1526–1540, 2008.

[2] A. Lacroix, R. A. Feelders, C. A. Stratakis, and L. K. Nieman, "Cushing's syndrome," *The Lancet*, vol. 386, no. 9996, pp. 913–927, 2015.

[3] P. Li and D. Zhao, "A rare case of retroperitoneal paraganglioma—case report and literature review," *Translational Gastroenterology and Hepatology*, vol. 1, 2016.

[4] H. Wang and C. Jepegnanam, "Recognition and management of phaeochromocytoma and paraganglioma," *Anaesthesia & Intensive Care Medicine*, vol. 18, no. 10, pp. 496–501, 2017.

[5] D. E. Benn, B. G. Robinson, and R. J. Clifton-Bligh, "15 years of paraganglioma: clinical manifestations of paraganglioma syndromes types 1–5," *Endocrine-related Cancer*, vol. 22, no. 4, pp. T91–T103, 2015.

[6] F. Khatami, M. Mohammadamoli, and S. M. Tavangar, "Genetic and epigenetic differences of benign and malignant pheochromocytomas and paragangliomas (PPGLs)," *Endocrine Regulations*, vol. 52, no. 1, pp. 41–54, 2018.

[7] K. Kovacs, D. Bell, G. W. Gardiner, R. J. Honey, J. Goguen, and F. Rotondo, "Malignant paraganglioma of the urinary bladder: immunohistochemical study of prognostic indicators," *Endocrine Pathology*, vol. 16, no. 4, pp. 363–370, 2005.

[8] W. Saeger, M. Fassnacht, R. Chita et al., "High diagnostic accuracy of adrenal core biopsy: results of the German and Austrian adrenal network multicenter trial in 220 consecutive patients," *Human Pathology*, vol. 34, no. 2, pp. 180–186, 2003.

[9] A. M. Isidori, G. A. Kaltsas, C. Pozza et al., "The ectopic adrenocorticotropin syndrome: clinical features, diagnosis, management, and long-term follow-up," *The Journal of Clinical Endocrinology & Metabolism*, vol. 91, no. 2, pp. 371–377, 2006.

[10] D. Cotesta, C. Caliumi, P. Alò et al., "High plasma levels of human chromogranin A and adrenomedullin in patients with pheochromocytoma," *Tumori Journal*, vol. 91, no. 1, pp. 53–58, 2005.

[11] H. Herrmann, H. Bär, L. Kreplak, S. V. Strelkov, and U. Aebi, "Intermediate filaments: from cell architecture to nanomechanics," *Nature Reviews Molecular Cell Biology*, vol. 8, no. 7, pp. 562–573, 2007.

[12] S. Kummar, M. Fogarasi, A. Canova, A. Mota, and T. Ciesielski, "Cytokeratin 7 and 20 staining for the diagnosis of lung and colorectal adenocarcinoma," *British Journal of Cancer*, vol. 86, no. 12, pp. 1884–1887, 2002.

[13] O. Hamidi, W. F. Young Jr, L. Gruber et al., "Outcomes of patients with metastatic phaeochromocytoma and paraganglioma: a systematic review and meta-analysis," *Clinical Endocrinology*, vol. 87, no. 5, pp. 440–450, 2017.

[14] R. Ilona Linnoila, H. R. Keiser, S. M. Steinberg, and E. E. Lack, "Histopathology of benign versus malignant sympathoadrenal paragangliomas: clinicopathologic study of 120 cases including unusual histologic features," *Human Pathology*, vol. 21, no. 11, pp. 1168–1180, 1990.

[15] J. Etxabe and J. A. Vazquez, "Morbidity and mortality in Cushing's disease: an epidemiological approach," *Clinical Endocrinology*, vol. 40, no. 4, pp. 479–484, 1994.

[16] J. Lindholm, S. Juul, J. O. L. Jørgensen et al., "Incidence and late prognosis of Cushing's syndrome: a population-based Study1," *The Journal of Clinical Endocrinology & Metabolism*, vol. 86, no. 1, pp. 117–123, 2001.

[17] E. Ross and D. Linch, "Cushing's Syndrome?killing disease: discriminatory value of signs and symptoms aiding early diagnosis," *The Lancet*, vol. 320, no. 8299, pp. 646–649, 1982.

[18] S. Ejaz, R. Vassilopoulou-Sellin, N. L. Busaidy et al., "Cushing syndrome secondary to ectopic adrenocorticotropic hormone secretion," *Cancer*, vol. 117, no. 19, pp. 4381–4389, 2011.

[19] I. Ilias, D. J. Torpy, K. Pacak, N. Mullen, R. A. Wesley, and L. K. Nieman, "Cushing's syndrome due to ectopic corticotropin secretion: twenty years' experience at the national institutes of health," *The Journal of Clinical Endocrinology & Metabolism*, vol. 90, no. 8, pp. 4955–4962, 2005.

[20] G. T. McMahon, M. A. Blake, and C.-L. Wu, "Case 1-2010," *New England Journal of Medicine*, vol. 362, no. 2, pp. 156–166, 2010.

[21] A. M. Isidori and A. Lenzi, "Ectopic ACTH syndrome," *Arquivos Brasileiros de Endocrinologia & Metabologia*, vol. 51, no. 8, pp. 1217–1225, 2007.

[22] D. J. Torpy, N. Mullen, I. Ilias, and L. K. Nieman, "Association of hypertension and hypokalemia with Cushing's syndrome caused by ectopic ACTH secretion," *Annals of the New York Academy of Sciences*, vol. 970, no. 1, pp. 134–144, 2002.
[23] N. Kanaji, N. Watanabe, N. Kita et al., "Paraneoplastic syndromes associated with lung cancer nobuhiro kanaji, naoki watanabe, nobuyuki kita, shuji bandoh, akira tadokoro, tomoya ishii, hiroaki dobashi, takuya matsunaga," *World Journal of Clinical Oncology*, vol. 5, no. 3, p. 197, 2014.
[24] M. J. M. Garrido, C. G. Ponce, S. M. Escalante, V. P. Sanz, and A. C. Mena, "Cushing's paraneoplastic syndrome as first manifestation of an adenocarcinoma of unknown origin," *Clinical and Translational Oncology*, vol. 8, no. 8, pp. 621–623, 2006.
[25] K. Yoh, K. Kubota, M. Nomura et al., "Cushing's syndrome associated with adenocarcinoma of the lung," *Internal Medicine*, vol. 42, no. 9, pp. 831–833, 2003.
[26] V. Parsons and B. Rigby, "Cushing's syndrome associated with adenocarcinoma of the ovary," *The Lancet*, vol. 272, no. 7054, pp. 992–994, 1958.
[27] S. Liu, Z. Liu, F. Chen, W. Xu, and G. Yuan, "Adrenocorticotropic hormone-producing paraganglioma with low plasma ACTH level: a case report and review of the literature," *Frontiers in Endocrinology*, vol. 10, p. 936, 2020.
[28] J. E. Paleń-Tytko, E. M. Przybylik-Mazurek, E. J. Rzepka et al., "Ectopic ACTH syndrome of different origin—diagnostic approach and clinical outcome. Experience of one Clinical Centre," *Plos One*, vol. 15, no. 11, Article ID e0242679, 2020.

18

Low Grade Islet but Marked Exocrine Pancreas Inflammation in an Adult with Autoimmune Pre-Diabetes

Hiroshi Nomoto,[1] Tatyana Gurlo,[1] Madeline Rosenberger,[1] Mark D. Girgis,[2] Sarah Dry,[3] and Peter C. Butler [1]

[1]*David Geffen School of Medicine at UCLA, Larry L. Hillblom Islet Research Center, Los Angeles, CA, USA*
[2]*David Geffen School of Medicine at UCLA, Department of Surgery, Los Angeles, CA, USA*
[3]*David Geffen School of Medicine at UCLA, Department of Pathology, Los Angeles, CA, USA*

Correspondence should be addressed to Peter C. Butler; pbutler@mednet.ucla.edu

Academic Editor: Wayne V. Moore

There is unexplained deficit in size and function of the exocrine pancreas in type 1 diabetes (T1D). We obtained pancreas from an individual with pre-T1D obtained at surgery and addressed the question, what is the relative inflammation in the exocrine and endocrine pancreas in pre-T1D in the absence of the potential confounding changes at autopsy or in brain dead organ donors. Pancreas was removed surgically from a 36 year woman for benign neuroendocrine tumors (NET). The patient had gestational diabetes at age 29 and has a 23 year old sister with T1D. Pre-operative fasting glucose of 109 mg/dl and HbA1C 5.8% revealed prediabetes with an anti-GAD 1,144 (5–250 U/ml) together with family history implying pre-T1D. There was patchy low grade immune infiltration in some, but not all, islets that met criteria for autoimmune insulitis. The exocrine pancreas showed more abundant inflammation with areas of chronic pancreatitis and acinar to ductal metaplasia, and with other areas of atrophy and fatty infiltration. In pre-T1D inflammation may be more prominent in the exocrine than the endocrine pancreas, calling into question the sequence of events and assumed islet centric basis of autoimmunity leading to T1D.

1. Introduction

Type 1 diabetes (T1D) is an autoimmune disease with an eventual near complete loss of beta cells [1]. In adult onset T1D (in those with slow progressing beta cell dysfunction sometimes referred to as latent autoimmune disease in adults, or LADA and by others as slowly progressive insulin dependent diabetes mellitus, or SPIDDM) [2, 3] there may be as much as a 5–10 year prediabetes phase following the detection of autoantibodies and clinical diabetes onset. Considerable effort has been expended on arresting disease progression during the prediabetes phase of T1D, but with limited success. This is partly due to a limited understanding of the sequence of events leading to loss of beta cell function in T1D. Recent studies of the endocrine pancreas of individuals with pre-T1D reveal a surprisingly low grade inflammatory infiltrate [4]. It is possible that this is due to the high dose glucocorticoid therapy typically administered to reduce cerebral edema prior to organ retrieval from brain dead organ donors. Also, brain death is known to be a potential confounder of immunopathology [5, 6]. The present reported case provided the rare opportunity to examine pancreas obtained at surgery from an ambulatory patient with pre-T1D in the absence of massive glucocorticoid therapy or effects of brain death.

It has also long been appreciated that there is an unexplained decrease in both size and function of the exocrine pancreas in T1D [3, 7, 8] with abnormalities in the ductal anatomy [9]. The small pancreatic size has recently been found to be already present in individuals with pre-T1D [10, 11]. The exocrine pancreas in both slowly progressive and fulminant forms of T1D have increased inflammatory cells that are comparable in subtypes to those observed in islets in the same individuals [12–14] as well as activation of the pancreatic duct compartment (PDG) [15], a regenerative compartment that is activated by pancreatitis. Taken together these studies have raised the possibility that inflammation originating in the exocrine pancreas may play a role in the pathophysiology of insulitis. It was therefore also of particular interest in the present case where surgically resected pancreas became available from an individual with pre-T1D to evaluate the exocrine and endocrine pancreas in the pre-T1D phase.

2. Case Presentation

A 36 year old woman presented to the UCLA medical center with abdominal pain. Previously at age 27 bilateral pheochromocytoma were resected surgically with biochemical and clinical resolution of catecholamine excess. There was no family history of endocrine neoplasia, and she was screened negatively for MEN1 and RET mutations associated with multiple endocrine neoplasia. The blood glucose on the day of surgery ranged from 95 to 126 mg/dl, and on discharge 5 days later fasting blood glucose was 104 mg/dl on no glucose lowering therapy. At age 29, the patient developed gestational diabetes. Diabetes resolved on delivery of a healthy baby girl. The patient's 23 year old sister has T1D treated with insulin. On examination she was well nourished (BMI 27 kg/m^2). There was no clinical or biochemical evidence of recurrence of pheochromocytoma but a CT scan of the abdomen revealed 4 hypervascular well demarcated nodular lesions in the head and uncinate of the pancreas with marked fatty replacement of the pancreatic body and tail. The pancreas volume was approximately 50% of normal for age and gender. Cytological evaluation of an ERCP fine needle aspirant of a mass in head of pancreas was consistent with a neuroendocrine tumor. The hemoglobin 13.1 g/dL (11.6–15.2 g/dL), red cell count $4.22 \times 10^6/\mu L$ ($3.97–5.09 \times 10^6/\mu L$) and white blood cell count $5.05 \times 10^3/\mu L$ ($4.16–9.95 \times 10^3/\mu L$) were normal. Fasting blood glucose was 109 mg/dl increasing to 181 mg/dl with simultaneous plasma C-peptide 7.6 ng/ml 2 hours after a 75 g glucose tolerance test. HbA1C was 5.8%. Plasma lipase, liver function tests and renal function were normal. Anti-GAD was strongly positive 1,144 (5–250 U/ml), but autoantibodies to ICA-512, IA-2 and Zn8 (all evaluated more than two months preoperatively) were not detected. The HLA type of the patient was DRB1∗ 07:01:01, DRB1∗ 16:01:01, DRB4∗ 01:03:01, DRB5∗ 02:02, DQB1∗02:02:01, DQA1∗01:02, DQA1∗02:01:01.

A Whipple resection contained mass 2×4 cm in size that was composed of multiple neuroendocrine tumors. The mass had a tan-white semi-firm cut surface. The mass was less than 0.1 cm from the uncinate margin. The pancreatic duct 0.2 cm in diameter was identified within the Whipple resection and was clear of the tumor. Histologically the mass was a well differentiated neuroendocrine tumor (Supplementary Figure 1) with a Ki-67 labeling index of <1%. All margins of the neuroendocrine tumor tissue were clear with no necrosis, lymphatic or neural invasion identified. 25 regional lymph nodes were examined and none contained tumor. The tumor stained strongly positively for synaptophysin, weakly for chromogranin, negatively for insulin, glucagon, pancreatic polypeptide, somatostatin and glutamate decarboxylase (Supplementary Figure 1). Residual tail of pancreas was noted at surgery to be small and firmly adherent to surrounding structures consistent with the CT scan evaluation of the pancreas. The patient made an uneventful recovery post operatively. Diabetes was managed with 3–5 units of insulin glargine QHS with fasting glucose values in the 90–105 mg/dl range and corresponding C-peptide values of 0.7 and 2.5 ng/ml. One year later diabetes remains well controlled with insulin glargine 5 units.

Having obtained IRB approval (IRB#17-001712) resected pancreas remote from the NETs was examined histologically as previously described [16, 17]. Tumor free pancreas (Figures 1 and 2) showed relatively normal islets with a pancreatic beta cell fractional area measured in sections stained for C-peptide being 0.57 ± 0.09%. There was a low grade and immune cell islet infiltrate that varied between islets that had no immune infiltrate to others that occasionally met the criteria of insulitis [18]. The mean immune infiltrate (illustrated in Figures 1 and 3) was 1.95 ± 0.21 CD45$^+$, 1.47 ± 0.18 CD3$^+$, 1.14 ± 0.14 CD8$^+$, and 0.04 ± 0.00 CD68$^+$ cells/islet section, with 3.4% of islets being negative for insulin (pseudo-atrophic islets, Figure 4(c)). Beta cell replication by Ki67 was not detected but areas of increased cell replication were present in areas of acinar to ductal metaplasia (Figure 2(d)). Beta cell apoptosis was not detected but increased TUNEL staining in areas of exocrine immune infiltration served as a positive control.

The exocrine pancreas showed more abnormalities than the endocrine pancreas with regions of chronic pancreatitis characterized by acinar to ductal metaplasia (Figures 2, 4(b) and 4(d), 4(e)), inflammation and fibrosis with areas of exocrine atrophy (Figure 2). These regions of inflammation were lobular in distribution as previously reported for recent onset T1D in humans and with no evidence of local ductal dilatation. CD45+ and CD3+ cells were frequently detected within exocrine pancreas parenchyma either as scattered single cells or as focal dense infiltrates (Figures 1(c) and 4(a)), and often associated with areas of acinar-to-ductal metaplasia (Figures 4(b) and 3(d), 3(e)). In relation to islets, CD45+ and CD3+ cells were mostly present in the islet periphery (peri-insulitis). Macrophages were less frequent in pancreatic parenchyma (Figure 3(b)), but were occasionally detected in the islet periphery (Figures 3(a) and 3(b)) and as a cluster inside islets (Figure 3(c)).

3. Discussion

The present case provided the opportunity to evaluate pancreas procured at surgery from an adult individual with pre-T1D (also potentially referred to as pre-LADA or pre-SPIDDM). It remains unresolved whether there is a distinct type of autoimmune mediated diabetes termed LADA originally described to distinguish adults that develop autoimmune mediated diabetes from type 2 diabetes when it was not widely recognized that T1D may occur at any age of life [2], as occurs in other autoimmune endocrinopathies such as Hashimoto's thyroiditis. The present case does not have a high risk HLA type for T1D [19], a finding that used to be considered a characteristic of LADA, but was subsequently challenged [20].

The point of particular interest in this case is that, to our knowledge, uniquely we had access to freshly procured pancreas from an individual with autoimmune pre-diabetes without the potential confounding effects of brain death, the ICU

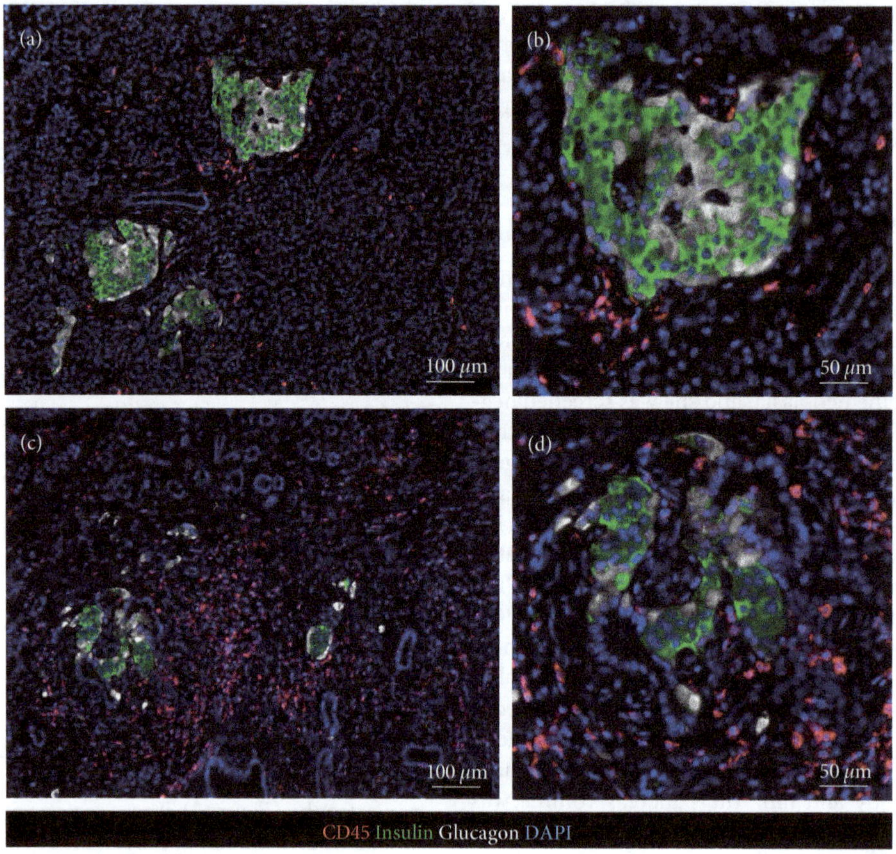

FIGURE 1: Representative immunofluorescence images of a pancreatic section stained for leucocyte common antigen CD45 (red), C-peptide (green), glucagon (white), nuclei DAPI (blue), illustrating variable immune infiltration of pancreatic parenchyma and islets. (b) and (d) are high magnification images of islets in (a) and (c) respectively. (b) shows the focal aggregation of CD45+ cells at one pole of the islet typical in early T1D and referred to as peri-insulitis.

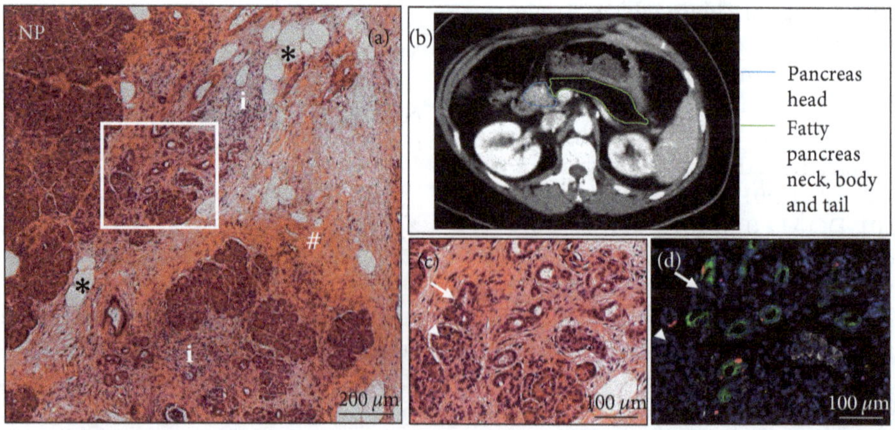

FIGURE 2: (a) Representative image of pancreatic section stained with H&E: NP-normal parenchyma, *—fat deposition, # — fibrosis, i —a site of inflammation next to the area of acinar-to-ductal metaplasia (box). (b) Cross-sectional view of CT scan slice of the pancreas showing normal density of the head of the pancreas while the neck, body and tail show low density consistent with fatty replacement acinar tissue. (c) High magnification of the boxed area (in (a)) illustrating acinar to ductal metaplasia (arrow) versus normal acinar tissue (arrow head). (d) Image of the same area in the adjacent section immunostained with anti-cytokeratin (green), Ki67 (red) and C-peptide (white).

environment and massive corticosteroid therapy typically administered prior to retrieval of organs from brain dead organ donors. The latter might attenuate the inflammatory infiltrate in an autoimmune setting. Brain death has been reported to induce changes that impact islet vasculature and function, potentially introducing confounding effects on exocrine or endocrine pancreas through massive release of cytokines [5, 6]. We should mention that the pancreatic neuroendocrine

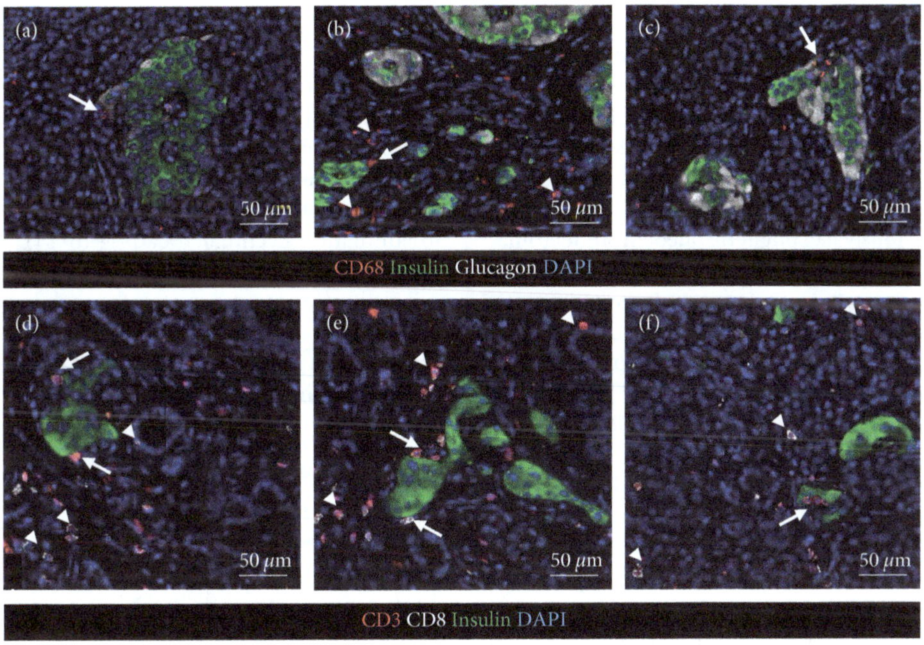

Figure 3: Representative immunofluorescence images of the pancreatic sections stained for macrophage marker CD68 (red), insulin (green), glucagon (white) in panels (a–c), or for T cell markers CD3 and CD8 (red and white respectively) and insulin (green) in panels (d and e); blue -nuclei (DAPI). Macrophages were found in peri-islet area (a–c, arrows) or pancreatic parenchyma (b, arrow head). CD8+CD3+ T cells were frequent throughout the parenchyma (d and e, arrow heads), in the areas of acinar-to-ductal metaplasia (d, e, arrow heads), and in the peri-islet area (d–f, arrows).

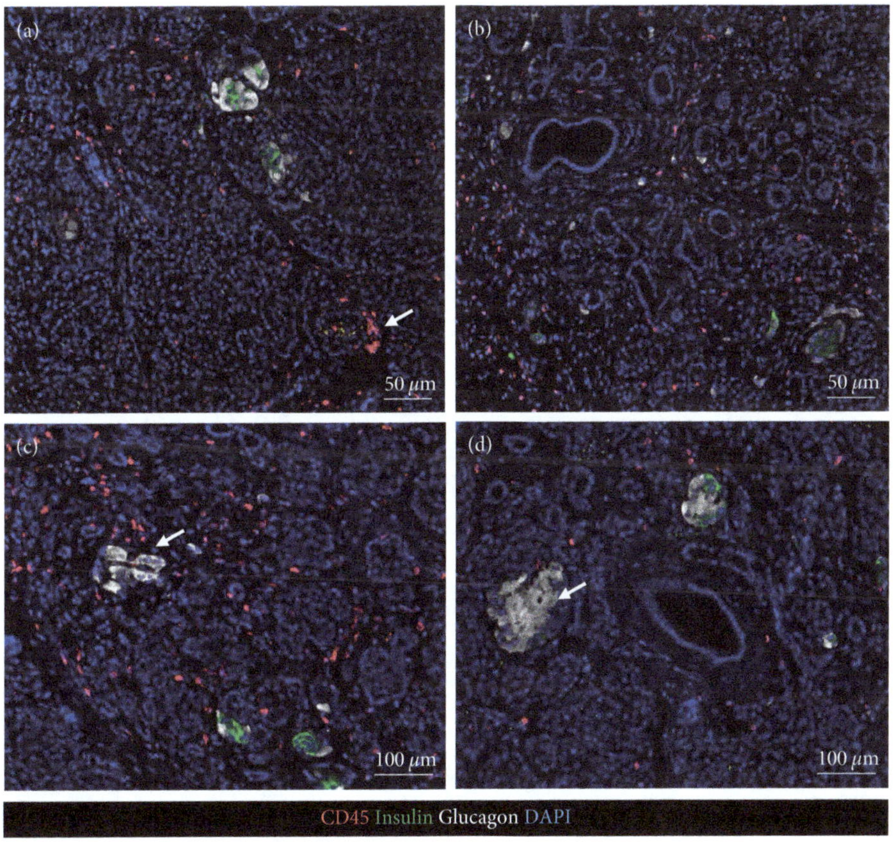

Figure 4: Representative immunofluorescence images of a pancreatic section stained for leucocyte common antigen CD45 (red), insulin (green), glucagon (white), nuclei DAPI (blue). Leucocytes are presented scattered throughout the exocrine pancreas as well as in occasional focal aggregates (a, arrow). Leucocytes are also present in areas of acinar-to-ductal metaplasia illustrated in (b). While most islets in this case had beta cells present, as expected in evolving type 1 diabetes, occasional islets were present with no detectable beta cells (c, arrow) or a few beta cells with minimally insulin immunoreactivity (d, arrow).

tumors in this case also present a potential confounding influence on the exocrine pathology. While the tumor cluster did not involve the main pancreatic duct, and lipase levels were consistently normal, it is plausible that some of the exocrine changes might be a consequence of the tumors rather than autoimmunity. Also, while the patient screened negatively for the known genetic variants for multiple endocrine neoplasia, the fact that she previously had biliateral pheochromocytomas before developing a complex of neuroendocrine tumors in the pancreas implies she may have an as yet undescribed genetic predisposition to endocrine tumors. Anti-GAD antibodies have been reported in individuals with GAD expressing neuroendocrine tumors and stiff man syndrome [21]. The tumor in the present patient did not express GAD and the patient had no features consistent with stiff man syndrome.

The patient had a fasting blood glucose and HbA1C in the prediabetes range but marked glucose intolerance. Uniquely in the present patient, we were able to document that the impaired fasting glucose and glucose intolerance was already present despite minimal beta cell loss and low grade islet inflammation. Prospective clinical trials have noted a progressive decline in glucose tolerance in the pre-T1D phase [22], characterized by both a progressive defect in insulin secretion [23, 24] and increasing insulin resistance characteristic of T1D, plausibly due to declining pulsatility of insulin secretion [25, 26].

The present case also provided a unique opportunity to evaluate the exocrine pancreas in pre-T1D. Radiological findings and subsequent direct observation at surgery revealed a relatively atrophic pancreas of ~50% volume expected for age with fatty infiltration in the tail. There is exocrine pancreas atrophy with increased pancreatic fat with advanced age [17] but this does not impact the endocrine pancreas that remains well preserved. Increased pancreatic fat in type 2 diabetes is attributable to associated obesity, but since pancreatic fat is comparable in obese individuals with and without type 2 diabetes [27], pancreatic fat does not appear sufficient to cause diabetes. Therefore the accumulation of fat and exocrine atrophy do not seem likely mediators of beta cell failure in the presented case. There was lobular low grade chronic pancreatitis confirmed histologically. While it is possible that the areas of exocrine pancreas immediately adjacent to the NETs in the head of the pancreas might be impacted by the tumors, it was notable that by palpation the tail of the pancreas was firm, atrophic and adherent to surrounding structures consistent with chronic low grade pancreatitis. Also, plasma lipase levels were normal on multiple occasions that would be unusual for obstructive pancreatitis and that there was no discernable pancreatic duct dilatation macroscopically or histologically as would be expected with obstructive pancreatitis.

Finally, the exocrine pancreatic findings in this case mirror those reported in pre-T1D from brain dead organ donors [10] in the absence of tumors.

4. Conclusion

In conclusion, in the present case of apparent pre-T1D, the low level of insulitis reported in autoantibody positive brain dead organ donors with and without T1D is reproduced, assuring that this finding is not an artifact consequent on high doses glucocorticoids given prior to organ procurement. Also, the finding of prominent exocrine changes of immune inflammation, acinar to ductal metaplasia and acinar atrophy in the pre-T1D phase are supportive of studies that implied that exocrine inflammation may contribute to development of islet inflammation eventually leading to T1D [3, 9, 12–14]. The present case supports those findings of low grade islet immune cell infiltration but more prominent changes in exocrine pancreas extended here to pre-T1D consistent with loss of pancreas volume in pre-T1D [11]. As yet the origin of the exocrine inflammation in T1D and its role in the eventual loss of beta cell function and mass remains unknown.

Abbreviations

NET:	Neuroendocrine tumor
T1D:	Type 1 diabetes
Anti-GAD:	Antibody against glutamic acid decarboxylase
PDG:	Pancreatic duct gland
LADA:	Latent autoimmune disease in adults.

Authors' Contributions

H.N. performed the histological studies and undertook the microscopy and morphological analysis with assistance from TG. MR assisted in histology staining and analysis. SD reviewed the microscopic slides along with H.N., T.G., and P.C.B. M.D.G. performed the surgery and along with P.C.B. researched data, wrote, reviewed, and edited the manuscript, in addition to contribution to the discussion.

Acknowledgments

This work was supported by the NIH/NIDDK (Grant #DK059579) and the Larry L. Hillblom Foundation (Grant #2014-D-001-NET) to PCB. We thank Bonnie Lui for editorial assistance.

Supplementary Materials

Supplementary Figure 1: no insulin, glucagon, pancreatic polypeptide, somatostatin or glutamate decarboxylase (GAD) was detected in the tumor. (A) Representative bright field image of resected tumor with the margin of the pancreas parenchyma containing islets of Langerhans stained for insulin (brown). Dotted line identifies the tumor margin. (B) Representative immunofluorescence image of the area shown in panel A on the adjacent section stained for glucagon (white), pancreatic polypeptide (red) and somatostatin (green); blue — nuclei (DAPI). (C) Ki67 staining in tumor (brown, arrow). (D) Representative immunofluorescence image of the tumor section stained for synaptophysin (green) and chromogranin A (CHGA, red). (*Supplementary Materials*)

References

[1] M. A. Atkinson, G. S. Eisenbarth, and A. W. Michels, "Type 1 diabetes," *The Lancet*, vol. 383, no. 9911, pp. 69–82, 2014.

[2] G. Stenstrom, A. Gottsater, E. Bakhtadze, B. Berger, and G. Sundkvist, "Latent autoimmune diabetes in adults: definition, prevalence, beta-cell function, and treatment," *Diabetes*, vol. 54, no. Suppl 2, pp. S68–S72, 2005.

[3] T. Kobayashi, K. Aida, T. Fukui et al., "Pancreatic ductal hyperplasia/dysplasia with obstructive chronic pancreatitis: an association with reduced pancreatic weight in type 1 diabetes," *Diabetologia*, vol. 59, no. 4, pp. 865–867, 2016.

[4] M. Campbell-Thompson, A. Fu, J. Kaddis et al., "Insulitis and beta-cell mass in the natural history of type 1 diabetes," *Diabetes*, vol. 65, no. 3, pp. 719–731, 2016.

[5] J. L. Contreras, C. Eckstein, C. A. Smyth et al., "Brain death significantly reduces isolated pancreatic islet yields and functionality in vitro and in vivo after transplantation in rats," *Diabetes*, vol. 52, no. 12, pp. 2935–2942, 2003.

[6] R. Obermaier, E. von Dobschuetz, T. Keck et al., "Brain death impairs pancreatic microcirculation," *American Journal of Transplantation*, vol. 4, no. 2, pp. 210–215, 2004.

[7] M. Lohr and G. Kloppel, "Residual insulin positivity and pancreatic atrophy in relation to duration of chronic type 1 (insulin-dependent) diabetes mellitus and microangiopathy," *Diabetologia*, vol. 30, no. 10, pp. 757–762, 1987.

[8] B. M. Frier, J. H. Saunders, K. G. Wormsley, and I. A. Bouchier, "Exocrine pancreatic function in juvenile-onset diabetes mellitus," *Gut*, vol. 17, no. 9, pp. 685–691, 1976.

[9] K. Nakanishi, T. Kobayashi, H. Miyashita et al., "Exocrine pancreatic ductograms in insulin-dependent diabetes mellitus," *American Journal of Gastroenterology*, vol. 89, no. 5, pp. 762–766, 1994.

[10] M. L. Campbell-Thompson, J. S. Kaddis, C. Wasserfall et al., "The influence of type 1 diabetes on pancreatic weight," *Diabetologia*, vol. 59, no. 1, pp. 217–221, 2016.

[11] M. L. Campbell-Thompson, S. L. Filipp, J. R. Grajo et al., "Relative pancreas volume is reduced in first-degree relatives of patients with type 1 diabetes," *Diabetes Care*, vol. 42, no. 2, pp. 281–287, 2019.

[12] T. Rodriguez-Calvo, O. Ekwall, N. Amirian, J. Zapardiel-Gonzalo, and M. G. von Herrath, "Increased immune cell infiltration of the exocrine pancreas: a possible contribution to the pathogenesis of type 1 diabetes," *Diabetes*, vol. 63, no. 11, pp. 3880–3890, 2014.

[13] K. Aida, T. Fukui, E. Jimbo et al., "Distinct inflammatory changes of the pancreas of slowly progressive insulin-dependent (Type 1) diabetes," *Pancreas*, vol. 47, no. 9, pp. 1101–1109, 2018.

[14] M. Takita, E. Jimbo, T. Fukui et al., "Unique Inflammatory changes in exocrine and endocrine pancreas in enterovirus-induced fulminant type 1 diabetes," *The Journal of Clinical Endocrinology & Metabolism*, vol. 104, no. 10, pp. 4282–4294, 2019.

[15] A. S. Moin, P. C. Butler, and A. E. Butler, "Increased proliferation of the pancreatic duct gland compartment in type 1 diabetes," *Journal of Clinical Endocrinology & Metabolism*, vol. 102, no. 1, pp. 200–209, 2017.

[16] A. E. Butler, R. Galasso, J. J. Meier, R. Basu, R. A. Rizza, and P. C. Butler, "Modestly increased beta cell apoptosis but no increased beta cell replication in recent-onset type 1 diabetic patients who died of diabetic ketoacidosis," *Diabetologia*, vol. 50, no. 11, pp. 2323–2331, 2007.

[17] Y. Saisho, A. Butler, E. Manesso, D. Elashoff, R. A. Rizza, and P. C. Bulter, "Beta-cell mass and turnover in humans: effects of obesity and aging," *Diabetes Care*, vol. 36, no. 1, pp. 111–117, 2013.

[18] M. L. Campbell-Thompson, M. A. Atkinson, A. E. Butler et al., "The diagnosis of insulitis in human type 1 diabetes," *Diabetologia*, vol. 56, no. 11, pp. 2541–2543, 2013.

[19] T. Tuomi, A. Carlsson, H. Li et al., "Clinical and genetic characteristics of type 2 diabetes with and without GAD antibodies," *Diabetes*, vol. 48, no. 1, pp. 150–157, 1999.

[20] G. Stenstrom, B. Berger, H. Borg, P. Fernlund, J. S. Dorman, and G. Sundkvist, "*HLA-DQ* genotypes in classic type 1 diabetes and in latent autoimmune diabetes of the adult," *American Journal of Epidemiology*, vol. 156, no. 9, pp. 787–796, 2002.

[21] H. Arino, R. Hoftberger, N. Gresa-Arribas et al., "Paraneoplastic neurological syndromes and glutamic acid decarboxylase antibodies," *JAMA Neurology*, vol. 72, no. 8, pp. 874–881, 2015.

[22] J. M. Sosenko, J. S. Skyler, K. C. Herold, and J. P. Palmer, "The metabolic progression to type 1 diabetes as indicated by serial oral glucose tolerance testing in the diabetes prevention trial-type 1," *Diabetes*, vol. 61, no. 6, pp. 1331–1337, 2012.

[23] S. Srikanta, O. P. Ganda, G. S. Eisenbarth, and J. S. Soeldner, "Islet-cell antibodies and beta-cell function in monozygotic triplets and twins initially discordant for type I diabetes mellitus," *New England Journal of Medicine*, vol. 308, no. 6, pp. 322–325, 1983.

[24] S. Srikanta, O. P. Ganda, A. Rabizadeh, J. S. Soeldner, and G. S. Eisenbarth, "First-degree relatives of patients with type I diabetes mellitus. Islet-cell antibodies and abnormal insulin secretion," *New England Journal of Medicine*, vol. 313, no. 8, pp. 461–464, 1985.

[25] A. V. Matveyenko, D. Liuwantara, T. Gurlo et al., "Pulsatile portal vein insulin delivery enhances hepatic insulin action and signaling," *Diabetes*, vol. 61, no. 9, pp. 2269–2279, 2012.

[26] P. J. Bingley, D. R. Matthews, A. J. Williams, G. F. Bottazzo, and E. A. Gale, "Loss of regular oscillatory insulin secretion in islet cell antibody positive non-diabetic subjects," *Diabetologia*, vol. 35, no. 1, pp. 32–38, 1992.

[27] Y. Saisho, A. E. Butler, J. J. Meier et al., "Pancreas volumes in humans from birth to age one hundred taking into account sex, obesity, and presence of type-2 diabetes," *Clinical Anatomy*, vol. 20, no. 8, pp. 933–942, 2007.

19

Possible Iodine-Induced Thyrotoxicosis in a Previously Healthy Adolescent following Administration of Iodinated Contrast Media

Jennifer Apsan and Zoltan Antal

Department of Pediatrics, Division of Endocrinology Weill Cornell Medicine, New York Presbyterian Hospital, New York, NY, USA

Correspondence should be addressed to Jennifer Apsan; jea9136@nyp.org

Academic Editor: Lucy Mastrandrea

Introduction. Jod-Basedow Syndrome refers to a paradoxical phenomenon in which large loads of iodine can cause hyperthyroidism. It is most commonly seen in populations already at risk for thyroid disease or those with underlying kidney disease. *Case Presentation.* We present a case of an acutely ill 17-year-old boy with symptomatic hyperthyroidism following an iodinated contrast CT scan to rule out appendicitis. *Discussion/Conclusion.* This case underscores the importance of recognizing this phenomenon even in the pediatric population and in those with no preexisting history of thyroid disease. Course complications including bronchospasm, hypertension, transaminitis, and bilateral palmar desquamating rash are rare and highlight the complexities involved in the disease state and in managing side effect profiles of treatment.

1. Introduction

Iodine is an essential mineral, necessary for optimal thyroid function. Iodine is commonly found in a variety of foods, such as iodized salt and seafood, and in routinely utilized household items, including nutritional supplements and skin cleaners. In medical settings, iodine is a component of various medications (amiodarone and expectorants), iodine-based swabs used for skin cleaning prior to invasive procedures, and iodinated contrast media (ICM). ICM is an increasingly common source of potential iodine toxicity as CT scans have become an increasingly popular imaging modality in the United States [1]. Recommended adult daily iodine intake is typically set at about 150 μg per day by the Institute of Medicine, United Nations Children's Fund (UNICEF), World Health Organization, and the International Council for the Control of Iodine Deficiency Disorders (ICCIDD) [2]. Contrast media is known to contain about 13,500 μg of free iodine and 15–60 g of bound iodine [3, 4]. Typically, the physiological response to these large iodine loads is a transient hypothyroid state, induced by inhibiting the thyroid peroxidase enzyme involved in thyroglobulin iodination in a phenomenon known as the Wolff–Chaikoff effect. Eventually, equilibrium ensues as downregulation of the Na-I transporters which permit less iodine into the thyroid gland, thus allowing the gland to return to normal function by escaping the Wolff–Chaikoff effect. The escape or adaptation phenomenon can occur in as quickly as 48 hours and allows for adaptation to a high iodide environment without risk of thyroid dysfunction [5, 6]. Inability to escape from this inhibitory effect of large iodine doses can result in clinical or subclinical hypothyroidism. This has been described largely in fetuses, newborns, patients with underlying chronic disease, patients with autoimmune thyroiditis, or in those previously treated with radioimmunoassay (RAI), surgery, or antithyroid drugs, but has also been described in some with no known underlying conditions [7, 8]. In some people, a paradoxical hyperthyroid state is induced after administration of a large iodine load. Typically, this is seen in those with autoimmune thyroiditis, prior thyroid surgical history, prior goiter formation, Graves' disease, or kidney disease, which can impact iodine excretion.

Mainstays of treatment for hyperthyroidism include withdrawal of the offending agent, antithyroid drugs, beta blockade to decrease sympathetic tone, and steroids [5]. Multiple cases of iodine-induced hyperthyroidism are described in the adult population. Many of these patients have underlying thyroid or kidney disease which can predispose them to a state of iodine-induced hyperthyroidism [9 11]. This phenomenon is not described well in the pediatric population. Here, we describe the presentation, diagnosis, and management of a 17-year-old boy with presumed iodine-induced hyperthyroidism.

2. Case Presentation

A previously healthy 17-year-old adolescent presented to the emergency department with 3-4 days of acute and chronic right lower quadrant abdominal pain. He was sent for a protocoled contrast CT scan (78 ml Omnipaque 300) that was suggestive of acute appendicitis. He was taken to the operating room, on postcontrast day 1, where his appendix was removed. Intraoperatively, he experienced a brief episode of bronchospasm with complete resolution and successful extubation following epinephrine administration. The patient was found to be positive for rhinovirus/enterovirus at that time. On postoperative day 2, the patient had an acute episode of flushing, fatigue, fevers, and tachycardia. Infectious workup was pursued, and antibiotics were started. On postoperative day 4, flushing and tachycardia (HR 100–110 bpm) persisted, and further laboratory evaluation was notable for an elevated serum free T4 level of 4.1 ng/dL (reference values: 0.9–1.8 ng/dL) and a serum TSH level of <0.0008 uiu/ml (reference values: 0.6–4.8 uiu/ml), confirming a diagnosis of hyperthyroidism. Burch–Wartofsky score at the time of symptoms was 15, indicating a low risk for thyroid storm. Physical exam revealed that the patient was extremely fatigued, weak, and tremulous. There was no exophthalmos or lid lag, and no palpable thyromegaly or thyroid nodules. Further evaluations revealed negative thyroid stimulating immunoglobulin (TSI), antithyroglobulin, and antithyroperoxidase antibody levels. A significantly elevated serum thyroglobulin level was noted, 274 ng/ml (reference values: 0.8–29.4 ng/ml). Thyroid ultrasound was normal with no evidence of thyroid enlargement, hyperemia, or heterogeneity of the gland. Thyroid scintigraphy was considered but deferred secondary to the recent iodine load given for CT scan.

Methimazole therapy was initiated but appeared to be inadequate as a monotherapy despite increasing dosing, as there was a rapid worsening of clinical symptoms and biochemical hyperthyroidism (Table 1/Figure 1). A mild transient transaminitis was also noted, raising concerns over increasing the methimazole dose. Steroids and propranolol were added to the regimen on postcontrast day 9 which resulted in a rapid and steady decline of serum thyroxine levels over the next 7 days. One week after discharge and 12 days after the initiation of therapy, methimazole was weaned and discontinued secondary to a significant worsening transaminitis and bilateral palmar desquamating rash. Steroid therapy was also stopped after 8 days of treatment due to episodic hypertension. Further evaluation of the potential cause of transaminitis revealed an acute EBV infection. The transaminitis significantly improved within the subsequent 10 days, and thyroid function continued to remain within normal limits. Three months later, transaminitis fully resolved.

Serum iodine studies were obtained during the hospitalization. After contrast day 10, serum iodine levels were found to be 181 ug/L (reference values: 90–92 ug/L), which fully normalized to 79 ug/L (reference values: 52–109 ug/L) on postcontrast day 22, at which time thyroid function tests normalized as well.

3. Discussion/Conclusion

Our patient's clinical and laboratory data confirmed a diagnosis of acute, transient hyperthyroidism. The differential for transient thyroiditis in an adolescent includes Hashitoxicosis (hyperthyroidism caused by inflammation associated with Hashimoto's thyroiditis) and subacute thyroiditis in the setting of acute inflammation secondary to trauma or viral infection. Although autoimmune thyroiditis is the most common underlying cause of acute hyperthyroidism, our patient's autoantibody titers were negative, and thyroid ultrasound findings were not consistent with a diagnosis of autoimmune thyroiditis. He also had no evidence of inflammation, enlargement, or increased vascularity on thyroid ultrasound (Figure 2), and clinically, he had no evidence of pain or enlargement to his thyroid gland, making traumatic injury to thyroid from his intubation or virally induced hyperthyroidism unlikely. A less common cause of acute transient hyperthyroidism is excess iodine administration in a phenomenon known as Jod-Basedow syndrome [5]. The time course of our patient's presentation shortly following administration of iodinated contrast supports iodine-induced hyperthyroidisim or Jod-Basedow syndrome as the most likely cause. At a dose of 78 ml of Omnipapague 300, our patient was exposed to approximately 23 grams organic iodine; many folds more than the International Council for the Control of Iodine Deficiency Disorders (ICCIDD) recommended a tolerable upper level of 1,100 μg per day in adults [1, 12] Significantly increased thyroglobulin levels well above the normal range, as were seen in our patient, support overactivity of the thyroid gland. Thyroglobulin levels are thought to correlate with iodine exposure and may be a potential biomarker of iodine overload [13, 14].

Although the diagnosis of Jod-Basedow Syndrome is not typically dependent on confirmed elevation in serum iodine levels, our patient's elevated iodine levels correlated directly with the change in thyroid functions, further supporting the diagnosis [1]. Although other case reports have noted even higher iodine levels, our initial serum measurement was obtained 10 days after contrast administration and 7 days following initial diagnosis of hyperthyroidism. Thus, the iodine levels were presumed to be higher at the onset of disease.

Jod-Basedow syndrome typically occurs in those who have underlying thyroid disease such as autoimmune thyroiditis, goiter formation, or in those with underlying kidney

Table 1: Thyroid function tests.

	12/28/ 17+	2/23/20 PCD 4	2/24/20 PCD 5*	2/27/20 PCD 8	2/28/20 PCD 9**	2/29/20 PCD 10	3/1/20 PCD11	3/6/20 PCD16***	3/11/20 PCD 21****
TSH (uIU/ml) 0.6–4.8	1.165	<0.0008	<0.0008	0.0009	0.008	0.009	0.008	0.011	0.822
Free T4 (ng/dL) 0.9–1.8 (ng/dL)	1.0	4.1	5.1	6.8	7.4	7.0	5.2	2.4	1.3
Total T4 (ug/dL) 4.5–10.9		15.0	16.5	26.9	26.3	24.7	21.5	8.1	6.4
Total T3 (ng/mL) 0.6–1.8		1.79	1.81	4.06	3.90	2.76	1.91	0.76	1.00
TSI (IU/L) <0.54IU/L			<0.10						
TPO ab (IU/ml) 0.0–9.0			<0.3						
Tg ag (IU/ml) 0.0–4.0			<0.9						

PCD: Post contrast day, +available as baseline from prior GI appointment for poor weight gain, *methimazole started, **hydrocortisone 100 mg q 8/ propranolol 40 mg q 8 hours started, ***methimazole stopped/Hydrocortisone stopped, ****propranolol stopped.

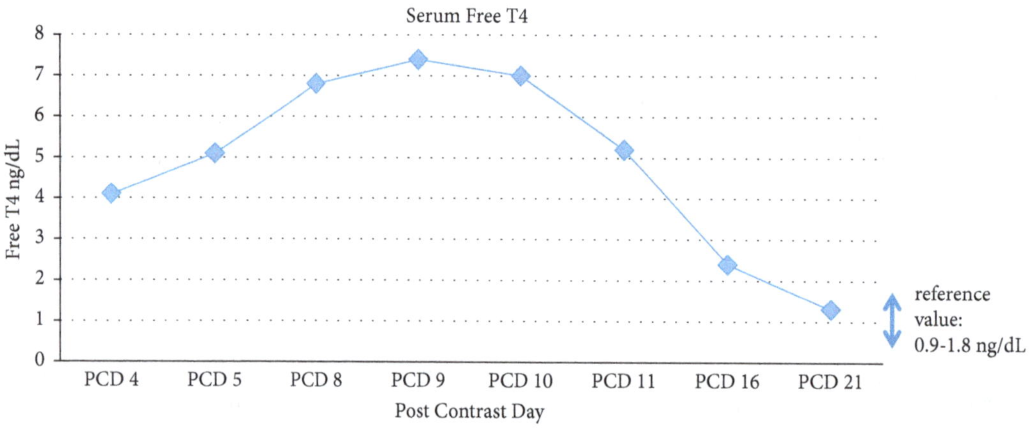

Figure 1: Serum Free T4 level in case study patient.

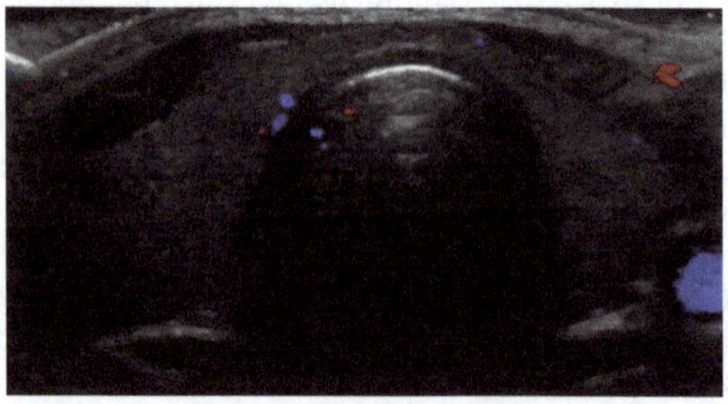

Figure 2: Thyroid ultrasound on post contrast day 7 reveals homogeneous and non enlarged thyroid gland measuring Isthmus: 0.2 cm, Right lobe: 2.3 × 4.3 × 0.9 cm Left lobe: 1.3 × 4.3 × 1.1 cm. Echogenicity is within normal limits with no increased vascularity.

disease as iodine is renally excreted. Our patient had previously documented routinely obtained thyroid function tests for an unrelated reason 2 years prior to this hospitalization (Table 1), decreasing our suspicion of prior underlying thyroid disease. Furthermore, the documented negative thyroid antibody status and normal renal function during the admission further excludes the typical underlying risk factors. We suspect that his underlying rhinovirus/enterovirus and EBV infections may have precipitated this thyroid response to iodinated contrast. The connection between viral infection and impaired thyroid function is well documented [15]. Specifically, EBV has been shown to have immunomodulatory effects and has been linked to autoimmune thyroid disease [16, 17]. In our patient, the exact mechanism of interaction between vial infection and response to iodine is not fully understood.

The reported timeline of contrast-induced hyperthyroidism in other case reports is variable, typically occurring from days to weeks following contrast administration [3, 14, 18]. However, there are reports of hyperthyroidism occurring as early as postcontrast day 1 [4]. While most cases of Jod-Basedow syndrome present as subclinical hyperthyroidism without clinical symptoms, our patient was overtly symptomatic with tremulousness and tachycardia. It not fully clear why the range of reactions to iodine exposure is so varied. Recent data point to a possible genetic predisposition [19]. Bronchospasm is not clearly associated with Jod-Baslow syndrome, and it remains unclear to date if this event in our patient was related to his thyroid disease or a reaction to his anesthesia [3, 4, 18].

This case also highlights the importance of managing side effects once medication is deemed necessary. Our patient developed both transmaminitis and hypertension. Transaminitis poses a clinical conundrum, as it has been described both as part of the natural history of hyperthyroidism [20] as well as a potential adverse effect of thionamides. In our case, the differential diagnosis additionally included EBV infection. Our decision to closely observe and continue methimazole therapy led to a successful outcome, but required a multidisciplinary effort involving other medical disciplines as well as the patient and patient's family. Steroid treatment was initiated in an effort to decrease peripheral conversion of T4 to T3 and to potentially avoid requiring increased Methimazole dosing. Thyroid function tests improved significantly once steroids were started, but our patient became significantly hypertensive at outpatient follow-up, and steroids were discontinued 6 days later. Given the uncertainty of the timeline and duration of our patient's hyperthyroidism, coupled with his significant clinical symptoms, we believe the steroid therapy was a valuable addition to the treatment regimen and was associated with significant clinical and biochemical improvement.

This case highlights the complexity of thyroid physiology and the importance of considering Jod-Basedow syndrome as a differential diagnosis even in previously healthy populations with no overt overlying risk factors. It also highlights the complexities involved in managing side effect profiles of treatment and the need for close follow-up. Although the majority of reported cases are in adults, it is important that pediatric providers are aware of the risk of this condition occurring in children as well.

Consent

Subjects have given their informed consent to publish their case.

Authors' Contributions

Apsan conceptualized the study (equal), wrote the original draft (lead), and reviewed and edited the manuscript (equal). Antal conceptualized the study and (equal) reviewed and edited the manuscript (equal).

References

[1] S. Y. Lee, C. M. Rhee, A. M. Leung, L. E. Braverman, G. A. Brent, and E. N. Pearce, "A review: radiographic iodinated contrast media-induced thyroid dysfunction," *The Journal of Clinical Endocrinology & Metabolism*, vol. 100, no. 2, pp. 376–383, 2015.

[2] H. Bürgi, "Iodine excess," *Best Practice & Research Clinical Endocrinology & Metabolism*, vol. 24, no. 1, pp. 107–115, 2010.

[3] A. J. van der Molen, H. S. Thomsen, and S. K. Morcos, "Contrast media safety committee, european society of urogenital radiology (ESUR). Effect of iodinated contrast media on thyroid function in adults," *European Radiology*, vol. 14, no. 5, pp. 902–907, 2004.

[4] C. M. Rhee, I. Bhan, E. K. Alexander, and S. M. Brunelli, "Association between iodinated contrast media exposure and incident hyperthyroidism and hypothyroidism," *Archives of Internal Medicine*, vol. 172, no. 2, pp. 153–159, 2012.

[5] H. R. Rose, "Jod Basedow syndrome," *in StatPearls, US National Library of Medicine*, Bethesda, MD, USA, 2021, https://www.ncbi.nlm.nih.gov/books/NBK544277/.

[6] K. Sarafoglou, *Pediatric Endocrinology and Inborn Error of Metabolism*, New YorkMcGraw Hill, New York, NY, USA, 2009.

[7] K. Markou, N. Georgopoulos, V. Kyriazopoulou, and A. G. Vagenakis, "Iodine-induced hypothyroidism," *Thyroid*, vol. 11, no. 5, pp. 501–510, 2001, PMID: 11396709.

[8] S. Melmed and R. H. Williams, *Williams Textbook of Endocrinology*, Elsevier/Saunders, Philadelphia, PA, USA, 12th edition, 2011.

[9] K. Lithgow and C. Symonds, "Severe thyrotoxicosis secondary to povidone-iodine from peritoneal dialysis," *Case Reports in Endocrinology*, vol. 2017, Article ID 2683120, 4 pages, 2017.

[10] L. Leuştean, C. Preda, M. C. Ungureanu et al., "Jod-basedow effect due to prolonged use of lugol solution-case report," *Revista Medico-Chirurgicala a Societatii de Medici si Naturalisti din Iasi*, vol. 118, no. 4, pp. 1013–1017, 2014, PMID: 25581962.

[11] E. Brotfain, L. Koyfman, A. Frenkel, A. Smolikov, A. Zlotnik, and M. Klein, "Iodine-induced hyperthyroidism-an old clinical entity that is still relevant to daily ICU practice: a case report," *Case Reports in Endocrinology*, vol. 2013, Article ID 792745, 4 pages, 2013.

[12] "Omnipaque™ (Iohexol) injection 140 180 240 300 350 140 350," 2021, https://www.accessdata.fda.gov/drugsatfda_docs/label/2017/018956s099lbl.pdf.

[13] A. M. Leung and L. E. Braverman, "Consequences of excess iodine," *Nature Reviews Endocrinology*, vol. 10, no. 3, pp. 136–142, 2014.

[14] A. M. El-Shirbiny, S. S. Stavrou, A. Dnistrian, M. Sonenberg, S. M. Larson, and C. R. Divgi, "Jod-basedow syndrome following oral iodine and radioiodinated-antibody administration," *Journal of Nuclear Medicine*, vol. 38, no. 11, pp. 1816-1817, 1997, Erratum in: Journal of Nuclear Medicine 1998 Mar;39(3):489.

[15] R. Desailloud and D. Hober, "Viruses and thyroiditis: an update," *Virology Journal*, vol. 6, no. 1, p. 5, 2009.

[16] A. Dittfeld, K. Gwizdek, M. Michalski, and R. Wojnicz, "A possible link between the epstein-barr virus infection and autoimmune thyroid disorders," *Central European Journal of Immunology*, vol. 41, no. 3, pp. 297–301, 2016.

[17] A. Janegova, P. Janega, B. Rychly, K. Kuracinova, and P. Babal, "The role of epstein-barr virus infection in the development of autoimmune thyroid diseases," *Endokrynologia Polska*, vol. 66, no. 2, pp. 132–136, 2015, PMID: 25931043.

[18] M. Higgs, E. Hull, and E. Lujan, "A case report of post-operative jöd-basedow phenomennon following oral and IV iodine contrast administration," *Case Reports in Endocrinology*, vol. 2014, Article ID 980283, 3 pages, 2014.

[19] M. J. Cha, D. Y. Kang, W. Lee et al., "Hypersensitivity reactions to iodinated contrast media: a multicenter study of 196 081 patients," *Radiology*, vol. 293, no. 1, pp. 117–124, 2019, PMID: 31478801.

[20] S. Khemichian and T. L. Fong, "Hepatic dysfunction in hyperthyroidism," *Gastroenterology & Hepatology*, vol. 7, no. 5, pp. 337–9, 2011.

20

An Extremely Rare *SRD5A2* Gene c.485A>C Mutation in a Compound Heterozygous Newborn with Disorders of Sex Development First Identified in Vietnam

Phan Tuong Quynh Le,[1,2] Thanh Nha Uyen Le,[1] Thi Thanh Binh Nguyen,[3] Minh Thao Nguyen,[4] and Thi Minh Thi Ha[1,2]

[1]*Department of Medical Genetics, University of Medicine and Pharmacy, Hue University, Hue, Vietnam*
[2]*Center of Prenatal and Neonatal Screening-Diagnosis, University of Medicine and Pharmacy Hospital, Hue University, Hue, Vietnam*
[3]*Department of Pediatrics, University of Medicine and Pharmacy, Hue University, Hue, Vietnam*
[4]*Department of Anatomy and Surgical Training, University of Medicine and Pharmacy, Hue University, Hue, Vietnam*

Correspondence should be addressed to Thi Minh Thi Ha; htmthi@hueuni.edu.vn

Academic Editor: Toshihiro Kita

SRD5A2 (steroid 5-alpha-reductase 2) mutation, which impairs 5α-reductase-2 enzyme activity, is among the causes of 46,XY disorders of sex development (DSD). Here, we report a rare pathogenic mutation NM_000348.4:c.485A>C (NP_000339.2: p.His162Pro) of *SRD5A2* gene in a compound heterozygous state first identified in a Vietnamese newborn with 5α-reductase-2 enzyme deficiency. We also first submitted this rare mutation to ClinVar database (VCV000973099.1). The patient presented with hyperpigmented labia-majora-like bifid scrotum, clitoris-like phallus, perineoscrotal hypospadias, and blind-ending vagina. The other mutation NM_000348.4:c.680G>A (NP_000339.2:p.Arg227Gln) was reported previously. This compound heterozygous mutation was first detected by next-generation sequencing. By Sanger sequencing, we confirmed that the c.485A>C mutation was maternal inherited, whereas the c.680G>A mutation was paternal inherited. Up to date, this is the first report of this rare compound heterozygous state of *SRD5A2* c.485A>C and c.680G>A mutations in patients with 46,XY DSD generally as well as in Vietnamese population particularly and is also the second report in the world carrying the pathogenic mutation NM_000348.4: c.485A>C (NP_000339.2:p.His162Pro). Our finding has enriched the understanding of the spectrum of *SRD5A2* variants and phenotypic correlation in Asian patients with 46,XY DSD.

1. Introduction

The 5-alpha-reductase-2 (5αRD2) deficiency (OMIM 264600), first described in 1974 by Imperato-McGinley et al. [1] and Walsh et al. [2], is a rare 46,XY disorder of sex development (DSD). The affected patients might present a wide spectrum of variable clinical manifestations from completely phenotypic females to normal males [3]. Female external genitalia with clitoromegaly or microphallus at birth, various degrees of hypospadias, and unilateral/bilateral cryptorchidism are the most common features [4, 5].

The 5αRD2 enzyme is important for the conversion of testosterone to dihydrotestosterone (DHT), which is more biologically active [6]. Testosterone plays a key function in stimulating the Wolffian ducts during sexual differentiation, whereas DHT controls the virilization of external genitalia, urethra, and prostate during embryogenesis and mediates masculinization at puberty [7].

The *SRD5A2* gene (steroid 5-alpha-reductase 2, OMIM 607306) on chromosome 2 (2p23.1) encodes the 5αRD2 enzyme. To date, approximately 180 variants of *SRD5A2* gene have been identified, with missense and nonsense

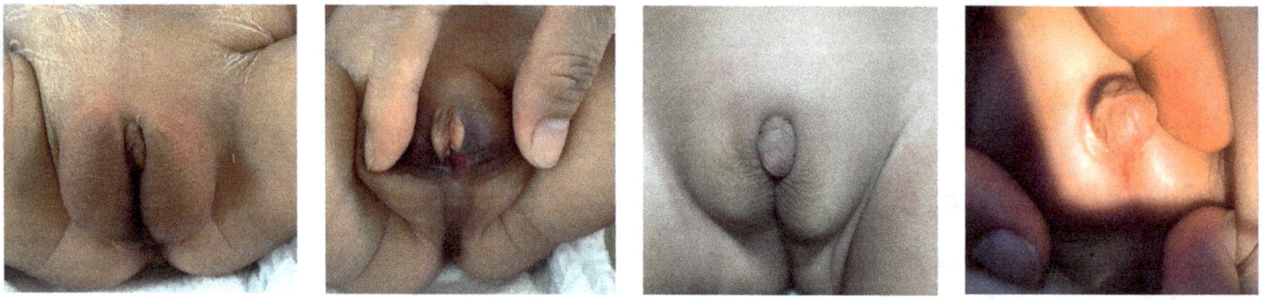

(a) (b) (c) (d)

Figure 1: Patient's abnormal genital phenotype: at the age of three days, (a) labia-majora-like bifid scrotum with clitoris-like microphallus and (b) perineoscrotal hypospadias; at the age of two years and three months, (c, d) microphallus had grown to 1.5 cm in length.

mutations being the most common (Human Gene Mutation Database). The NM_000348.4:c.680G>A mutation (NP_000339.2:p.Arg227Gln) was detected in three Vietnamese patients in a homozygous state [5, 8] and was one of the most frequent mutations in Asians [9]. In 2019, Cheng et al. first reported a novel *SRD5A2* mutation (NM_000348.4:c.485A>C) (NP_000339.2: p.His162Pro) in adult Chinese twins with 5αRD2 enzyme deficiency [10]. However, the authors have not yet submitted this variant to ClinVar database. Herein, we present the data of the world's second report, a Vietnamese newborn with 46,XY DSD, who possesses this rare mutation in a heterozygous compound state. We also submitted this rare variant to ClinVar database for the first time (VCV000973099.1).

2. Case Presentation

The patient is the second child of healthy and non-consanguineous parents, born at the 40th week of gestation. The patient's external genitalia were found to be abnormal at birth. At the age of three days (November, 2019), physical examination showed a hyperpigmented labia-majora-like bifid scrotum with bilateral masses palpable (Figure 1(a)), a microphallus of 0.8 cm with clitoris-like underdeveloped glans, and perineoscrotal hypospadias with short blind-ending vagina (Figure 1(b)). At the age of two years and three months, a second medical examination revealed that the microphallus had grown to 1.5 cm in length (Figures 1(c), and 1(d)) and that the depth of blind-ending vagina was 1 cm (March, 2022). The patient was reared as a female at birth, and the gender was changed from female to male after being diagnosed. There was no history of DSD in the family. The patient's older sister, who is five years old, is developing normally.

Ultrasonography at newborn revealed the absence of Mullerian remnants and the presence of bilateral testes in the labia majora. The right testis was 11.4 × 7 × 6 mm in size, while the left was 11.5 × 9 × 6 mm in size. The rete testis and epididymis were both present. The structures of male urethra were observed. The penis with corpus cavernosa and corpus spongiosum was buried.

The blood samples' biochemical analysis revealed a normal baseline testosterone level of 1.04 ng/mL. There was no DHT level available.

The karyotype of the patient was 46,XY (Figure 2(a)). DNA was extracted from peripheral blood sample. Polymerase chain reaction (PCR) assay with *SRY*-specific primers revealed a result of positive *SRY*. DNA sample was subjected to next-generation sequencing (NGS) (NextSeq, Illumina, USA) using a panel of DSD related genes. A compound heterozygous for a rare mutation NM_000348.4: c.485A>C (NP_000339.2:p.His162Pro) and one well-known mutation NM_000348.4:c.680G>A (NP_000339.2: p.Arg227Gln) which located on exon 3 and exon 4 of *SRD5A2* gene, respectively, were found. These two mutations were further confirmed by Sanger sequencing (Figures 2(b) and 2(c)). We submitted the NM_000348.4: c.485A>C (NP_000339.2:p.His162Pro) mutation to ClinVar database on July 14, 2020. The accession number of this mutation is VCV000973099.1 (SCV001422495.1). Further evaluation demonstrated that the mutant c.485A>C was maternal inherited, whereas c.680G>A was paternal inherited. The patient's sister was healthy. She had neither c.485A>C nor c.680G>A mutations.

Written informed consent was obtained from the parents of the patient in accordance with the Institutional Review Board of University of Medicine and Pharmacy, Hue University, Vietnam.

3. Discussion

The patient presented bilateral testes inside the hyperpigmented labia-majora-like bifid scrotum, clitoris-like phallus, perineoscrotal hypospadias, and blind-ending vagina. The primary genetic analysis revealed the 46, XY karyotype and the presence of *SRY* gene. As a result of these findings, the patient was classified as 46,XY DSD. Although patient's symptoms have been reported frequently in 5αRD2 deficiency, this phenotype in a newborn has a high overlap with other common causes of 46,XY DSD related to androgen synthesis or function, such as partial androgen insensitivity and 17-hydroxysteroid dehydrogenase deficiency [11–13]. Hormonal analysis is a valuable diagnostic tool for patients with 46,XY DSD. In newborns, the baseline testosterone level in a blood sample can indicate the ability of the testes to secrete testosterone [14]. However, this patient has a normal testosterone level, which can be found in both androgen insensitivity syndrome and 5αRD2 deficiency.

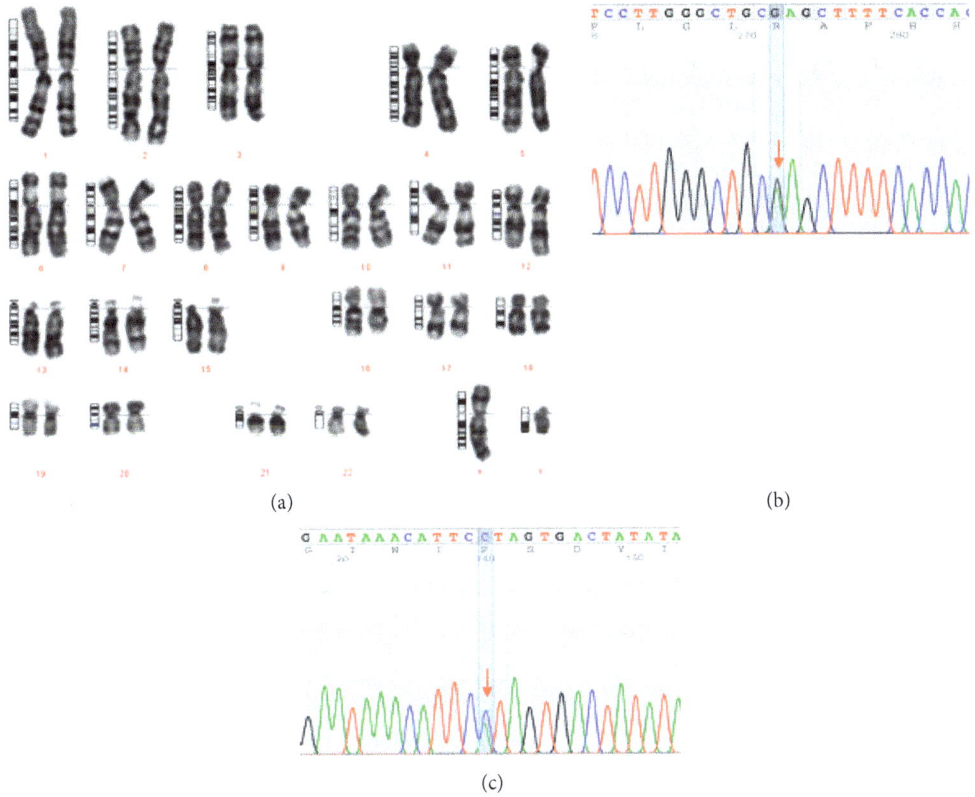

Figure 2: Genetic analysis of the patient. (a) 46,XY karyotype and (b, c) sanger sequencing results revealed c.680G>A (p.Arg227Gln) and c.485A>C (p. His162Pro) mutations.

Several genes responsible for 46,XY DSD have been identified. As a result, sequencing a panel of those candidate genes is first recommended when clinical and hormonal patterns are insufficiency to indicate a diagnosis [14]. The compound heterozygous status for c.485A>C (p.His162Pro) and c.680G>A (p.Arg227Gln) of the *SRD5A2* gene, which was identified via NGS, confirmed 5αRD2 deficiency in our patient.

To date, around 180 mutations have been described in the *SRD5A2* gene, among which missense mutations are major (Human Gene Mutation Database, HGMD, https://www.hgmd.cf.ac.uk/ac/gene.php?gene=SRD5A2). Our patient carries a rare compound heterozygous mutation of *SRD5A2* gene, including maternal inherited c.485A>C in exon 3 and paternal inherited c.680G>A in exon 4. Interestingly, exon 1 and exon 4 of the *SRD5A2* gene are known as hotspot regions, whereas the frequency of mutation happening in exon 3 is quite rare [15, 16]. This is the first report in the world of a compound heterozygous state of SRD5A2 c.485A>C and c.680G>A mutations.

The *SRD5A2* c.485A>C mutation is an extremely rare variant. In 2019, Chinese 18-year-old twin brothers with DSD (sex of rearing at birth changed from female to male) possessing a compound heterozygous state of *SRD5A2* c.485A>C (p.His162Pro) and c.16C>T (p.Glu6Ter) mutations were first reported [10]. The parental origin of these variants was not identified in Cheng et al.'s study. Our case is the second report of c.485A>C mutation in the world. We submitted the c.485A>C mutation in exon 3 of the *SRD5A2* gene to ClinVar database to enrich the variant data of this gene.

The homozygous c.680G>A (p.Arg227Gln) mutation was reported previously in three Vietnamese patients with 5αRD2 enzyme deficiency [5, 8]. However, they were all diagnosed outside of Vietnam. This mutation was also detected in a number of Asian patients with 5αRD2 deficiency, including those from China, Japan, Laos, and Mongolia [5]. In particular, Fan showed that c.680G>A (p.Arg227Gln) was the most common (39.62%) in 130 Chinese children with this disorder [9].

SRD5A2 mutations can result in either a total loss of activity, disrupting the binding domain to testosterone, or an inefficient protein assembly or a shorter half-life [4]. The c.680G>A (p.Arg227Gln) and c.485A>C (p.His162Pro) mutations have been well documented as decreasing the 5αRD2 enzyme activity by functional analysis [10, 17]. Thus, carrying these two mutations, which may result in a significant loss of enzyme activity, contributed to our patient's abnormal phenotype. According to Fan, the group with the p.Arg227Gln mutation had milder and more variable characteristics than the group without this mutation. In particular, individuals with homozygous p.Arg227Gln mutations had minor undervirilization, whereas patients with compound heterozygous p.Arg227Gln mutations had varying degrees of undervirilization depending on the combination of mutations [9]. Previously reported Vietnamese patients with the homozygous p.Arg227Gln mutation had a microphallus, bifid scrotum with testes inside;

hypospadias was recorded in two out of three [5, 8]. Our patient, who was a compound heterozygote for p.Arg227Gln and p.His162Pro, was more undervirilized than Vietnamse patients with homozygous p.Arg227Gln but less undervirilized than twin brothers with the compound heterozygous p.His162Pro and p.Glu6Ter mutations reported by Cheng et al. (female external genitalia, clitoromegaly, and gonads bilateral in inguinal position) [10].

As mentioned above, the patient's phenotypic features, such as bilateral testes in scrotum, a microphallus with clitoris-like underdeveloped glans at birth which had grown into a small penis with 1.5 cm in length at the age of 27 months, and male urethral structures and the absence of Mullerian remnants determined via ultrasound, all lean towards a male phenotype. Furthermore, the molecular diagnostics confirmed 5αRD2 deficiency in our patient. As a result, the patient was reared as a male. Psychosexuality is one of the most attentive considerations in 5αRD2 deficiency individuals. Even in the absence of dihydrotestosterone, the presence of androgens usually directs towards male psychosexuality development. This could explain the relatively high rate of gender change from female to male in 5αRD2 deficiency, estimated 56–63% [18, 19]. Because our patient was diagnosed early and was raised as a male, the conflict in identifying sex will be avoided.

Surgical repair for hypospadias is recommended, mainly focusing on chordee correction and urethral reconstruction. Orchidopexy is unnecessary as the bilateral testes are in correct position. Surgery can be performed in two or three steps due to perineoscrotal hypospadias [4]. The location of the patient's testes in the scrotum, as well as the early correction of hypospadias, will help to preserve testicular function, particularly spermatogenesis, for future fertility [20].

Hormone therapy is an important aspect of management for some types of 46,XY DSD. Most male patients with 5αRD2 deficiency do not require the testosterone replacement because of retained testicular function during puberty [4]. However, testosterone treatment may help our patient, who has a micropenis, gain a benefit in terms of growth [21].

In addition to the patient's treatment, genetic counseling is required for parents who plan to have another child. As the parents are carriers, prenatal diagnosis should be mentioned in the next pregnancy. In vitro fertilization with preimplantation genetic testing will also be an option.

In conclusion, this is the first report of the extremely rare mutation NM_000348.4:c.485A>C (NP_000339.2: p.His162Pro) of the *SRD5A2* gene in a compound heterozygous state in patients with 46,XY DSD generally as well as in Vietnamese population particularly. This finding has enriched the understanding of the spectrum of *SRD5A2* variants and phenotypic correlation in Asian patients with 46,XY DSD.

Authors' Contributions

Phan Tuong Quynh Le was involved in investigation, data collection, original draft writing. Thanh Nha Uyen Le was involved in investigation and original draft writing. Thi Thanh Binh Nguyen and Minh Thao Nguyen were involved in investigation and data collection. Thi Minh Thi Ha was responsible for investigation, data collection, data validation, supervising, reviewing, and editing. All authors read and approved the final version of this paper.

Acknowledgments

The authors sincerely thank their patient and his family for giving the consent and allowing to publish the data. The authors thank Gene Solution Company and Vietnamese Medical Genetic Institute for supporting them to conduct the genetic tests for our patients. This research was supported by a scientific grant from University of Medicine and Pharmacy Hospital, Hue University, Hue, Vietnam (Grant number: 48BV/21).

References

[1] J. Imperato-McGinley, L. Guerrero, and T. P. R. E. Gautier, "Steroid 5α-reductase deficiency in man: an inhertited form of male pseudohermaphroditism," *American Association for the Advancement of Science*, vol. 186, pp. 1213–1215, 1974.

[2] P. C. Walsh, J. D. Madden, and M. J. Harrod, "Familial incomplete male pseudohermaphroditism, type 2," *New England Journal of Medicine*, vol. 291, pp. 944–949, 1974.

[3] G. H. G. Sinnecker, O. Hiort, and L. Dibbelt, "Phenotypic classification of male pseudohermaphroditism due to steroid 5α-reductase 2 deficiency," *American Journal of Medical Genetics*, vol. 63, pp. 223–230, 1996.

[4] A. Avendaño, I. Paradisi, F. Cammarata-Scalisi, and M. Callea, "5-α-reductase type 2 deficiency: is there a genotype-phenotype correlation? a review," *Hormones*, vol. 17, pp. 197–204, 2018.

[5] L. Maimoun, P. Philibert, B. Cammas et al., "Phenotypical, biological, and molecular heterogeneity of 5α-reductase deficiency: an extensive international experience of 55 patients," *Journal of Clinical Endocrinology & Metabolism*, vol. 96, pp. 296–307, 2011.

[6] S. Andersson and D. W. Russell, "Structural and biochemical properties of cloned and expressed human and rat steroid 5α-reductases," *Proceedings of the National Academy of Sciences of the United States of America*, vol. 87, pp. 3640–3644, 1990.

[7] J. D. Wilson, J. E. Griffin, and D. W. Russell, "Steroid 5α-reductase 2 deficiency," *Endocrine Reviews*, vol. 14, pp. 577–593, 1993.

[8] O. Hiort, H. Willenbring, N. Alberts et al., *Molecular Genetic Analysis and Human Chorionic Gonadotropin Stimulation Tests in the Diagnosis of Prepubertal Patients with Partial 5-Reductase Deficiency*, Springer-Verlag, Berlin, Germany, 1996.

[9] L. Fan, Y. Song, M. Polak et al., "Clinical characteristics and genotype-phenotype correlations of 130 Chinese children in a high-homogeneity single-center cohort with 5α-reductase 2 deficiency," *Molecular Genetics and Genomic Medicine*, vol. 8, 2020.

[10] T. Cheng, H. Wang, B. Han et al., "Identification of three novel SRD5A2 mutations in Chinese patients with 5α-reductase 2 deficiency," *Asian Journal of Andrology*, vol. 21, pp. 577–581, 2019.

[11] M. Berra, E. L. Williams, B. Muroni et al., "Recognition of 5α-reductase-2 deficiency in an adult female 46XY DSD clinic," *European Journal of Endocrinology*, vol. 164, pp. 1019–1025, 2011.

[12] E. F. Costa, S. Domenice, and M. Sircili, "DSD due to 5α-reductase 2 deficiency—from diagnosis to long term outcome," *Seminars in Reproductive Medicine*, vol. 30, pp. 427–431, 2012.

[13] P. A. Lee, C. P. Houk, S. Ahmed, and I. A. Hughes, "Consensus statement on management of intersex disorders," *Pediatrics*, vol. 118, pp. e488–e500, 2006.

[14] A. B. Wisniewski, R. L. Batista, E. M. F. Costa et al., "Management of 46, XY differences/disorders of sex development (DSD) throughout life," *Endocrine Reviews*, vol. 40, pp. 1547–1572, 2019.

[15] M. Ahmadifard, A. Kajbafzadeh, and S. Panjeh-Shahi, "Molecular investigation of mutations in androgen receptor and 5-alpha-reductase-2 genes in 46, XY disorders of sex development with normal testicular development," *Andrologia*, vol. 51, pp. 1–9, 2019.

[16] B. Gui, Y. Song, and Z. Su, "New insights into 5α-reductase type 2 deficiency based on a multi-centre study: regional distribution and genotype-phenotype profiling of SRD5A2 in 190 Chinese patients," *Journal of Medical Genetics*, vol. 56, pp. 685–692, 2019.

[17] N. M. Makridakis, E. di Salle, and J. K. Reichardt, "Biochemical and pharmacogenetic dissection of human steroid 5 alpha-reductase type II," *Pharmacogenetics*, vol. 10, pp. 407–413, 2000.

[18] R. L. Batista and B. Bilharinho Mendonca, "Integrative and analytical review of the 5-alpha-reductase type 2 deficiency worldwide," *The Application of Clinical Genetics*, vol. 13, pp. 83–96, 2020.

[19] P. T. Cohen-Kettenis, "Gender change in 46, XY persons with 5α-reductase-2 deficiency and 17β-hydroxysteroid dehydrogenase-3 deficiency," *Archives of Sexual Behavior*, vol. 34, pp. 399–410, 2005.

[20] A. Nordenskjöld and S.-A. Ivarsson, "Molecular characterization of 5-reductase type 2 deficiency and fertility in a Swedish family," *The Journal of Clinical Endocrinology and Metabolism*, vol. 83, 1998.

[21] X. Zhao, Y. Song, S. Chen et al., "Growth pattern in Chinese children with 5α-reductase type 2 deficiency: a retrospective multicenter study," *Frontiers in Pharmacology*, vol. 10, 2019.

21

Acute Hyperglycemia Due to Topical Corticosteroid Administration

Laura Y. Sue[1] **and Anna Milanesi**[2]

[1] *VA Greater Los Angeles Healthcare System and Division of Endocrinology, Diabetes and Hypertension, Department of Medicine, UCLA David Geffen School of Medicine, 900 Veteran Avenue, 24-130 Warren Hall, Los Angeles, CA 90095, USA*
[2] *Department of Medicine, Veterans Affairs Greater Los Angeles Healthcare System and Division of Endocrinology, Departments of Medicine and Physiology, UCLA David Geffen School of Medicine, 11301 Wilshire Boulevard, Los Angeles, CA 90073, USA*

Correspondence should be addressed to Laura Y. Sue; lsue@mednet.ucla.edu

Academic Editor: J. Paul Frindik

We present the case of a 71-year-old man with longstanding, previously well-controlled type 1 diabetes who developed acute hyperglycemia. His insulin requirements, via his insulin pump, increased to nearly five times his typical daily dose. The patient was admitted for evaluation and treatment and started on an insulin infusion. He had minimal insulin requirements with the insulin infusion. History revealed recent use of a super potent topical corticosteroid for a psoriasis flare. The patient was transitioned back to his insulin pump, using his prior to admission settings. He was advised to discontinue using his topical corticosteroid. He had no further hyperglycemic episodes. The clinical presentation is suggestive of corticosteroid-induced hyperglycemia, suggesting that clinically significant changes can occur even with short duration use, particularly with high potency steroids used. This is to our knowledge the first case reported in which the patient required a very significant amount of extra insulin (nearly five times his typical total daily dose) after using high potency topical steroid cream. This case highlights the potentially detrimental effect of topical corticosteroid use in patients with diabetes.

1. Introduction

Systemic/oral administration of corticosteroids can induce or worsen hyperglycemia; however, there are limited reports about topical formulations of corticosteroids causing hyperglycemia. Here we report a case of acute hyperglycemia related to topical corticosteroid use in a patient with longstanding, well-controlled diabetes.

2. Case Presentation

We cared for a 71-year-old man with a 45-year history of type 1 diabetes. He had used an insulin pump for years with a current daily dose of 73 units of insulin. His hemoglobin A1C values had ranged from 5.9 to 7.4% in the last ten years.

The day prior to admission, the patient developed sudden persistent hyperglycemia. He required 326 units of insulin injections within 24 hours, in addition to the 30 units of basal insulin via his pump. His glucose finally decreased to 85 mg/dl six hours before presentation to the emergency department (see Figure 1). He had normal vitals on presentation. Evaluation, including complete blood count, chemistry panel, blood cultures, and chest radiograph, was normal. Cortisol was not measured.

Upon obtaining further history, the patient reported being in his usual state of health except for a psoriasis flare for which he had used fluocinonide 0.1% cream in the two days prior to presentation. Although he had used a small amount of cream on his hands before, this time he applied the cream to a larger area, including his abdomen, twice a day, using occlusive techniques to increase effectiveness. While hospitalized, the patient was kept on an insulin infusion, requiring 0.25-3 units/hour. On hospital day 2, he was transitioned to his insulin pump using his prior-to-admission settings. He was discharged home and advised to discontinue using the fluocinonide cream. On outpatient follow-up, he did not report further hyperglycemia.

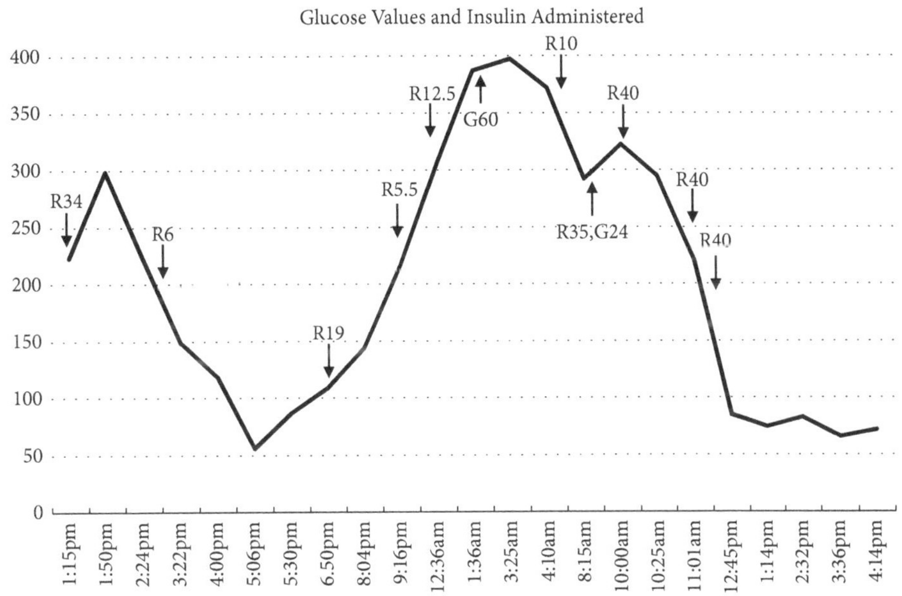

FIGURE 1: Glucose values (solid line) and insulin administered by the patient (R: regular insulin; G: glargine insulin; number denotes the number of units given) over time on the day prior to and the day of presentation.

TABLE 1: Comparison of the current case with other cases of hyperglycemia related to topical corticosteroid use.

	Patient Information	Duration of Diabetes	Details of Topical Corticosteroid Use	Glycemic Control	Diabetes Regimen Prior	Diabetes Medications During Hyperglycemic Period
Current case	71 year old Caucasian man with type 1 diabetes	45 years	Psoriasis treated in the preceding 2 days with fluocinonide 0.1% cream (class I steroid)	A1C 5.9-7.4% in the prior 10 years	Insulin pump: 73 units total daily dose	Insulin via pump and subcutaneous injections: 356 units in 24 hours
Hongo et al 2017	80 year old Japanese man with type 2 diabetes	16 years	Psoriasis treated with class III-class V steroids over a 7-8 week period	First admission: A1C 8-9%; second admission 10 days later: A1C 7.6%	Lispro insulin 42 units per day, voglibose 0.9 mg per day	First admission: insulin increased to a maximum of 36 units of neutral protamine Hagedorn (NPH) insulin and 38 units of lispro insulin per day; second admission: insulin 32 units per day (dosing by insulin type not specified)
Kahara et al 2016	68 year old Japanese man with no history of diabetes	-----	Oral lichen planus treated with class VII steroid on the oral mucosa over a 6 month period	A1C 10.8% on admission after developing thirst and polyuria	-----	Alogliptin 25 mg daily started 2 months after diagnosis of diabetes and continued for 2 months

3. Discussion

The clinical presentation is suggestive of corticosteroid-induced hyperglycemia. We know that systemic/oral administration of corticosteroids can induce or worsen hyperglycemia; however, there are limited reports about topical use causing hyperglycemia. Topical corticosteroids are classified by potency from class I (super potent) to class VII (least potent) [1]. The fluocinonide 0.1% cream that our patient used is in class I. It has been hypothesized that topical corticosteroids cause hyperglycemia through increasing alanine transport, thereby facilitating hepatic gluconeogenesis, increasing enzymatic activity, and causing a relative insulin resistance [2].

Gomez and Frost reported two patients with abnormal glucose tolerance tests who developed postprandial hyperglycemia with topical administration of high potency corticosteroid creams [3]. Two other patients, despite also having abnormal pretreatment glucose tolerance tests, had no changes in postprandial glucose values. All patients had decreased levels of measured cortisol, suggesting clinically significant systemic effects of the topical corticosteroids. Hongo et al. described an elderly man with longstanding diabetes who was diagnosed with psoriasis [1] and switched from oral to topical corticosteroid therapy. His glycemic control worsened and he required a 76% increase in total daily insulin dose (Table 1). Kahara et al. reported the case of a patient treated for oral lichen planus with a class VII (lowest potency) steroid on his oral mucosa. The patient developed new onset diabetes that required initiation of an oral anti-diabetes medication for several months (Table 1) [4]. A nested case-control study of over 192,000 patients in the Netherlands found a 1.24-fold increased risk of developing diabetes among those currently using topical corticosteroids. Risk was even higher among patients with more than 180 days of topical corticosteroid use [odds ratio (OR) 1.32, 95% confidence interval 1.14-1.54)] and among those with higher cumulative exposure (ORs ranging from 1.29 to 1.44; statistically significant) [5]. In addition to hyperglycemia, there have also been reported cases of Cushing syndrome and adrenal crisis due to topical corticosteroid use [2].

Although there are limited data about topical corticosteroid therapy causing alterations in glucose metabolism, it appears that clinically significant changes can occur even with short duration use, particularly with high potency steroids used with occlusive techniques for increased effect. This is to our knowledge the first case reported in which the patient required a very significant amount of extra insulin (nearly five times his typical total daily dose) after using high potency topical steroid cream. Hence, clinicians need to be aware of the potentially detrimental effect of topical corticosteroid use in patients with diabetes.

Acknowledgments

Anna Milanesi received support from Veterans Affairs MERIT, grant no. I01BX003665.

References

[1] E. C. Gomez and P. Frost, "Induction of Glycosuria and Hyperglycemia by Topical Corticosteroid Therapy," *Archives of Dermatology*, vol. 112, no. 11, pp. 1559–1562, 1976.

[2] U. R. Hengge, T. Ruzicka, R. A. Schwartz, and M. J. Cork, "Adverse effects of topical glucocorticosteroids," *Journal of the American Academy of Dermatology*, vol. 54, no. 1, pp. 1–15, quiz 16-8, 2006.

[3] Y. Hongo, K. Ashida, K. Ohe et al., "Change of oral to topical corticosteroid therapy exacerbated glucose tolerance in a patient with plaque psoriasis," *American Journal of Case Reports*, vol. 18, pp. 1198–1203, 2017.

[4] T. Kahara, Y. Tanaka, K. Hayashi et al., "Overt diabetes mellitus caused by the topical administration of dexamethasone ointment on the oral mucosa," *Internal Medicine*, vol. 53, no. 15, pp. 1633–1635, 2014.

[5] M. W. van der Linden, F. J. A. Penning-Van Beest, T. Nijsten, and R. M. C. Herings, "Topical corticosteroids and the risk of diabetes mellitus: A nested case-control study in the Netherlands," *Drug Safety*, vol. 32, no. 6, pp. 527–537, 2009.

22

Neonatal Cholestasis: A Rare and Unusual Presentation of Pituitary Stalk Interruption Syndrome

R. El Qadiry, A. Ouayad, H. Nassih, A. Bourrahouat, and I. Ait Sab

Pediatric B Department, Mother-Child Pole, Mohammed VI University Hospital, Marrakesh, Morocco

Correspondence should be addressed to R. El Qadiry; rabiy.elqadiry@gmail.com

Academic Editor: J. Paul Frindik

Pituitary stalk interruption syndrome (PSIS) is a very rare entity, and the clinical manifestations are nonspecific. Neonatal cholestasis due to endocrine disorders is rare and poorly recognized. Our case report describes a case of PSIS in a Moroccan infant revealed by isolated neonatal cholestasis, which is an unusual presentation in children. *Case report.* A 40-day-old girl was admitted to our department for progressive cholestatic jaundice appeared on the third day of life. She was born from a non-consanguineous marriage, and her prenatal and perinatal history went without incident. Physical examination showed icteric skin and sclera, without hepatomegaly. Analysis of pituitary hormones revealed panhypopituitarism. On brain magnetic resonance imaging (MRI), the pituitary stalk was absent, the posterior pituitary was ectopic, and the anterior pituitary was hypoplastic. The patient was diagnosed with interrupted pituitary stalk syndrome. The treatment consisted of hormone replacement with rapid improvement of her clinical condition. *Conclusion.* Panhypopituitarism, a consequence of PSIS, is a rare cause of neonatal cholestasis. However, pediatricians should keep this syndrome in mind for patients who present with neonatal cholestasis.

1. Introduction

Pituitary stalk interruption syndrome (PSIS) is a rare congenital anomaly, characterized by pituitary hormone deficiencies along with radiological features of a thin or interrupted pituitary stalk, an ectopic or absent posterior pituitary, or a hypoplastic or absent anterior pituitary [1].

Clinical signs are variable and nonspecific, which may lead to delayed diagnosis. Neonatal cholestasis due to endocrine disorders is rare and poorly recognized.

Our case report describes a case of PSIS in a Moroccan infant revealed by isolated neonatal cholestasis, which is an unusual presentation in children.

2. Case

A 40-day-old girl was admitted to our department for progressive cholestatic jaundice appeared on the third day of life. The child was born at full term from a non-consanguineous marriage with a birth weight of 3500 g (25–50th birth weight percentile). Her perinatal history went without incident; no episodes of hypoglycemia or seizures were noted. Family history did not involve hepatobiliary disease or endocrine disorder.

Physical examination showed icteric skin and sclera, with dark urine and pale stool, without hepatomegaly or splenomegaly. No obvious facial dysmorphism was observed.

Laboratory results revealed total bilirubin of 154 mg/l with 136 mg/l corresponding to conjugated bilirubin. The serum alkaline phosphatase (ALP) was elevated (719 IU/L) (N: 0–449), while gamma-glutamyl transpeptidase (γ-GTP), serum liver enzymes, and prothrombin time (PT) were within the normal range (γ-GTP: 38 UI/L, AST: 58 UI/L, ALT: 22 IU/L, and PT: 84%). Plasma glucose level was normal (85 mg/dL).

Abdominal ultrasound and magnetic resonance cholangiopancreatography showed normal liver and gallbladder anatomy and patent hepatobiliary tract, ruling out the possibility of biliary atresia. Amino acid analyses did not show any abnormalities. Test screening for hepatitis viruses (TORCH infections) was negative. Hemoglobin was 9.6 g/dl,

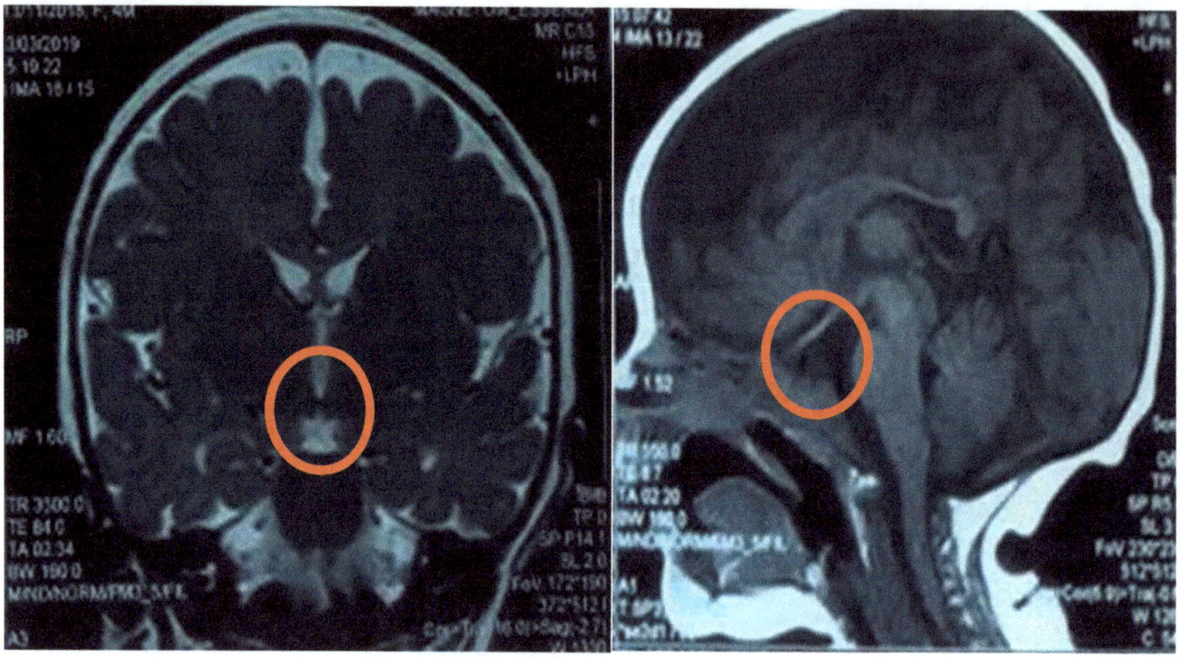

FIGURE 1: MRI of the head revealed a small anterior pituitary gland, an invisible stalk, and an ectopic posterior lobe.

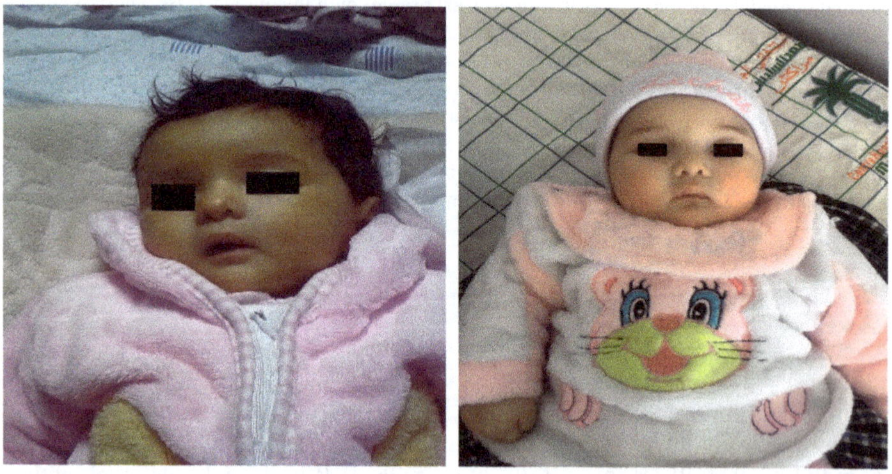

FIGURE 2: After 3 months of follow-up, the jaundice disappeared completely.

white blood cells were 12400/mm^3, CRP was 18 mg/l (<6), and urine cytobacteriological examination showed a urinary tract infection with *Klebsiella pneumoniae*, and she had been treated successfully, but jaundice persisted.

Then, pituitary hormonal profiles showed a low morning serum cortisol level at 1.30 μg/dl (reference range: 8, 7–22, 40 μg/dl) and a normal plasma adrenocorticotropic hormone (ACTH) level at 8.9 ng/l (reference range: 5–60 ng/l), indicating secondary adrenal insufficiency. Thyroid function tests showed a low free T4 level of 8.6 pmol/L (reference range: 12–22 pmol/L) and a normal TSH level of 3.61 mIU/L, suggesting central hypothyroidism. A low, insulin-like growth factor-1 (IGF-1) level <10 ng/ml (reference range: 19–104 ng/l) in combination with deficiency of more than two pituitary hormones was highly indicative of growth hormone deficiency. A magnetic resonance imaging (MRI) of the head revealed a small anterior pituitary gland, an invisible stalk, and an ectopic posterior lobe (Figure 1). The infant was diagnosed with pituitary stalk interruption syndrome.

The treatment consisted of hormone replacement with hydrocortisone (15 mg/m^2/day) and subsequently L-thyroxin (3.5 μg/kg/day). GH therapy is not yet initiated.

After 3 months of follow-up, the jaundice disappeared completely and the growth was still within the norms (Figure 2).

3. Discussion

Pituitary stalk interruption syndrome (PSIS) is a rare entity, with incidence rate of 0.5/1,000,000 per birth. The exact mechanism of this pathology is unclear. It can occur in a variety of ways. Earlier signs may include hypoglycemia, jaundice, cryptorchidism, and seizures [2].

Panhypopituitarism, a consequence of PSIS, is a rare cause of cholestasis in infants. In addition, it is generally neglected and misdiagnosed in infants with isolated cholestasis [3]. Our case underlines the importance of endocrine disorders as one of the etiologies of neonatal cholestasis. However, in the absence of physical findings suggestive of hypopituitarism, the diagnosis is less apparent.

While hormone deficiency is probably the strongest explanation for neonatal cholestasis in PSIS patients, it is not exactly known how hormone deficiencies cause cholestasis. It has been suggested that thyroid hormone and cortisol can influence the bile acid-independent bile flow and bile formation. In addition, growth hormone can modulate the biosynthesis and secretion of bile acids, and it has been shown that bleary flow recovers after hydrocortisone and GH treatment. However, cholestasis in isolated GH deficiency was never reported. For our patient, the cholestasis resolved before GH therapy instauration [3, 4].

Diagnosis can be achieved after clinical suspicion of hypopituitarism symptoms; laboratory tests and exact diagnosis can be achieved via imaging methods. MRI, with detailed hormone analysis, is the key diagnostic method for the exact diagnosis [5].

After diagnosis, hormonal therapy should be started first with cortisol and then thyroxine. This is because restoration of a euthyroid state can destabilize a patient with ACTH deficiency. GH therapy is often required later in infancy [6].

4. Conclusion

Pituitary stalk interruption syndrome is a very rare entity, and the clinical manifestations are nonspecific. Cholestasis may be the only clinical feature in the neonatal period. Consequently, many cases are exposed to extensive diagnostic tests before coming up to the suspicion of an endocrine disorder, and the treatment is delayed exposing patients to serious complications. Therefore, pediatricians should keep this syndrome in mind for patients who present with neonatal cholestasis.

Consent

Informed consent has been obtained from the patient's parents for publication of the case report.

References

[1] I. Alali, R. Saad, and Y. Kabalan, "Two cases of pituitary stalk interruption syndrome in Syrian children," *Case Reports in Endocrinology*, vol. 2020, no. 1, Article ID 2039649, 5 pages, 2020.

[2] B. Agridag Ucpinar, A. Ucar, and E. Ozmen, "Pituitary stalk interruption syndrome: presentation of a rare case," *Journal of Pediatric Neurology*, vol. 17, no. 5, pp. 176–179, 2019.

[3] U. Chan, W. T. Chan, W. H. Ting, C. S. Ho, H. C. Liu, and H. C. Lee, "Cholestasis caused by panhypopituitarism and acquired cytomegalovirus infection in a 2-month-old male infant: a case report," *Medicine (Baltimore)*, vol. 96, no. 17, Article ID e6757, 2017.

[4] D. Braslavsky, A. Keselman, M. Galoppo et al., "Neonatal cholestasis in congenital pituitary hormone deficiency and isolated hypocortisolism: characterization of liver dysfunction and follow-up," *Arquivos Brasileiros de Endocrinologia and Metabologia*, vol. 55, no. 8, pp. 622–627, 2011.

[5] A. G. Ioachimescu, A. H. Hamrahian, M. Stevens, and R. S. Zimmerman, "The pituitary stalk transection syndrome: multifaceted presentation in adulthood," *Pituitary*, vol. 15, no. 3, pp. 405–411, 2012.

[6] D. Altay, E. Eren, T. B. Ozkan, T. Ozgur, and O. Tarım, "Liver involvement in congenital hypopituitarism," *The Indian Journal of Pediatrics*, vol. 86, no. 5, pp. 412–416, 2019.

23

Triglyceride Levels Greater than 10,000 mg/dL in a 49-Year-Old Female without Evidence of Pancreatitis

Anika Toor,[1] Amit Toor,[1] Koroush Khalighi,[2] and Mahesh Krishnamurthy[1]

[1]*Department of Internal Medicine, Easton Hospital, Easton, PA 18045, USA*
[2]*Drexel University, EP Lab, Easton Hospital, Easton, PA 18045, USA*

Correspondence should be addressed to Anika Toor; anikalamba511@gmail.com

Academic Editor: Lucy Mastrandrea

We present a rare case of a 49-year-old female with very severe hypertriglyceridemia (HTG) having a total triglyceride (TG) count of > 10,000 mg/dL in the absence of pancreatitis. Based on literature review, this is one of the highest recorded TG counts in an adult without evidence of pancreatitis. HTG is a common occurrence in clinical practice, but rarely do numbers exceed 2000 mg/dl. It is crucial to evaluate and rapidly lower TG levels to prevent potentially life-threatening complications such as severe pancreatitis. Removal of potential predisposing medications, control of underlying diseases known to cause HTG, and maintenance therapies are essential to prevent reoccurrence.

1. Introduction

HTG is a common form of dyslipidemia with the potential to cause significant morbidity and mortality. In cases of severely elevated TG levels, rapid lowering to levels < 500–1000 mg/dL can be achieved with aggressive use of intravenous insulin and heparin (caution needs to be exercised when using heparin in cases of pancreatitis) and fasting.

2. Case Description

Our case is a 49-year-old Hispanic female who presented to our hospital with multiple episodes of chest pain. The onset of her pain was 5 days prior to admission. She complained of left sided pain "5 out of 10" intensity described as chest tightness. The pain was nonradiating and not precipitated by activity, inspiration, or position. The patient stated that she would have almost 5 episodes of pain daily with each episode lasting 2-5 minutes in length. This was not associated with any diaphoresis, shortness of breath, vomiting, or abdominal pain. The frequency and intensity of her pain episodes increased which led her to come to the emergency department. Her past medical history is significant for hypertension and difficult-to-control asthma requiring frequent hospital admissions. In the past she was on medication for "high cholesterol" but stopped taking it years ago as she was never told she had very high cholesterol levels. She denied any history of abnormal lipid profile, myocardial infarction or angina, congestive heart failure, or diabetes mellitus. Her medications included inhaled fluticasone and vilanterol combination, albuterol inhalation as needed, losartan, meloxicam, montelukast, verapamil, omalizumab, and intermittent short courses of prednisone for asthma exacerbations. She denied any alcohol consumption or illicit drug use. She admitted to smoking about a quarter pack a day for 15-20 years and quit 13 years ago. Family history was significant for hypertension in her mother, and a sister with stroke at the age of 44. There was no family history of dyslipidemia.

On physical examination she was found to have temperature of 97.8 degrees F, heart rate of 92 bpm, respiratory rate of 19/min with oxygen saturation of 96% on room air, and blood pressure of 152/98 mmHg. Her body mass index (BMI) was 27.7 on admission. Cardiovascular examination revealed chest wall tenderness to palpation on the upper left side. On auscultation there were no significant murmurs. Slight wheezing was audible in bilateral lung fields on auscultation. Examination of the skin did not reveal any xanthomas or xanthelasmas. Ophthalmologic examination did not reveal corneal arcus or lipemia retinalis. The examination of the nervous system and the head and neck was within normal limits.

TABLE 1: Patient's HTG trend along with therapies used and diet.

	Day 1	Day 2	Day 3	Day 4	Day 5	Day 6	Day 7	Day 8	Day 9
TG Levels (mg/dL)	>10,000	8,887	4,119	1,617	1,315	1,120	1,138	937	825
IV Drip	Insulin	Insulin	Insulin	Insulin	Insulin	Insulin	Insulin	Insulin	None
Diet	NPO	0 fat 0 carb	0 fat 0 carb	0 fat 0 carb	0 fat 0 carb	Low fat Low carb	Low fat Low carb	Low fat Low carb	Low fat Low carb
Oral Medication	G & A	G & A	G & A	G & A Niacin	G & A Niacin	G & A Niacin	G & A Niacin	G & A Niacin	F & R Niacin

G = Gemfibrozil; A = Atorvastatin; F = Fenofibrate; R = Rosuvastatin.

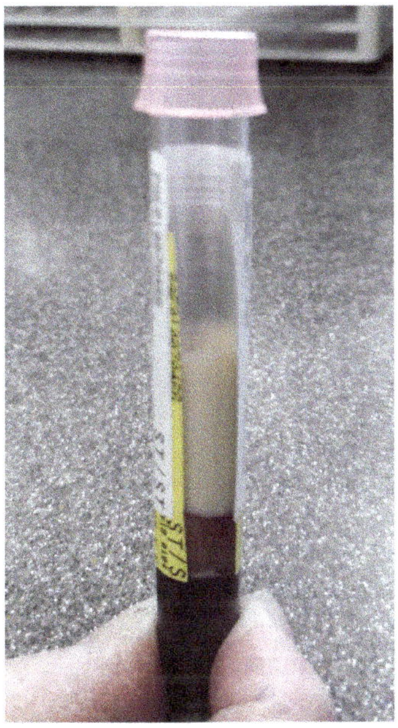

FIGURE 1

Relevant laboratory results on admission were as follows. Initial blood draw when centrifuged on gross examination was heavily lipemic (see Figure 1). Subsequent lipid panel studies were ordered which were significant for serum triglyceride (TG) of >10,000 mg/dL, serum cholesterol of 1,029 mg/dL, direct measure low density lipoprotein (LDL) of 33 mg/dL, and high-density lipoprotein (HDL) of 22 mg/dl. Other pertinent lab values included WBC count 7900/cumm, Hb of 11.6 g/dL, serum lipase of 160 units/dL, which was 46 units/dL when repeated and consistently remained within normal limits during hospitalization, serum sodium 130 mmol/L, serum magnesium of 5.2 mg/dL, and blood glucose of 111 mg/dL (random). Serum TSH was 2.39 mcIU/mL and HbA1c was of 5.3%. Initial troponin was of <0.03 ng/mL. Bicarbonate on admission was 22 mmol/L. EKG showed normal sinus rhythm with no ST-T wave changes. Chest X-ray was normal.

The patient was started on conservative management. She was kept nothing by mouth except medications for one day and started on IV regular insulin drip at a rate of 4 units/hr with IV fluids containing 5% dextrose to prevent hypoglycemia along with heparin 5000 units subcutaneously every 8 hours. Heparin drip was not initiated because PTT could not be accurately measured secondary to lipemia. She was also started on gemfibrozil, atorvastatin, and niacin at the time of admission. All of her home medications were stopped. A cardiac diet with no fats and no carbohydrates was initiated by day 2. Cardiology was consulted. Echocardiogram was done which was normal with an EF of 72%.

The patient's old medical record was reviewed to obtain previous lipid panel test results. Her lipid panel from 2016 revealed a serum triglyceride of 212 mg/dL and serum cholesterol of 182 mg/dL.

Lipid panel was repeated daily over the course of 9 days with significant decrease in patient's triglyceride and cholesterol levels. On day 9, serum triglyceride levels came down to 825 mg/dL and serum cholesterol was noted to be 360 mg/dL (see Table 1). Her diet was slowly advanced to a low fat and low carbohydrate diet which she tolerated well.

The patient also underwent treadmill myoview stress SPECT study once the serum triglyceride levels were < 2000 mg/dL in view of chest pain, which was normal. The patient's chest pain and serum triglyceride levels improved. She did not require any other interventions besides insulin drip and subcutaneous heparin. She was discharged on day 9 in medically stable condition and was closely monitored as outpatient. She was discharged on Rosuvastatin, Fenofibrate, and prescription omega-3 fatty acids. Repeat lipid panel was done in one month after discharge and the serum triglyceride levels were found to be 142 mg/dL and serum cholesterol of 117 mg/dL. Apolipoprotein B level was measured at 186 mg/dL. The patient was instructed for further genetic testing after discharge but did not follow up after this.

3. Discussion

Hypertriglyceridemia (HTG) is one of the most common lipid abnormalities and has been known to be associated with other metabolic derangements. It is estimated that the number of patients with HTG who have levels exceeding 500 mg/dL has risen to >4 million Americans and that this is more common in the Hispanic-American population [1, 2]. The presence of very severe HTG (TG levels greater than 2000 mg/dL) is estimated to be 1.8 cases per 10,000 white adults [3]. Hypertriglyceridemia is defined as TGs >150 mg/dL. The Endocrine Society 2010 guidelines further classify HTG into mild (150–199 mg/dL), moderate (200–999 mg/dL), severe (1000–1999 mg/dL), and very severe (greater than or equal to 2000 mg/dL) [4]. Severe and very severe HTG

Table 2: Fredrickson classification of primary hypertriglyceridemia [6, 8].

TYPE	ELEVATED LIPOPROTEIN	LIPID PROFILE	CLINICAL MANIFESTATIONS	RELATIVE FREQUENCY
I - Familial chylomicronemia	Chylomicron	TC + TG +++	Presents in infancy, eruptive xanthomas, recurrent pancreatitis, failure to thrive	<1%
II b - Familial Combined Hyperlipidemia	LDL, VLDL, Apo-B	TC ++ TG ++	Xanthomas less common. Risk of premature CVD	40%
III - Familial dysbetalipoproteinemia	IDL	TC ++ TG ++	Palmar xanthomas, risk of premature CVD	<1%
IV - Familial Hypertriglyceridemia	VLDL	TC + TG ++	Associated w/ DM, insulin resistance, obesity, HTN	45%
V - Primary Mixed Hyperlipidemia	Chylomicron, VLDL	TC +++ TG +++	Similar to type I but develops in adulthood	5%

TC = total cholesterol; TG = triglycerides; DM = Diabetes Mellitus; HTN = Hypertension; CVD = cardiovascular disease; LDL = low-density lipoprotein; VLDL = very low-density lipoprotein; IDL = intermediate density lipoprotein; Apo-B = apolipoprotein B.

have been shown to increase the risk for acute pancreatitis and cardiovascular disease. When levels are > 1,000 mg/dL, the risk of pancreatitis rises to approximately 5%, and, when levels are >2000 mg/dl, the risk significantly rises to 10-20% [5].

The etiologies of HTG can be further classified into primary and secondary. The Fredrickson classification scheme is commonly used to organize various primary hypertriglyceridemias into different categories (Table 2). In the United States, the most common primary HTGs include familial combined hyperlipidemia (Fredrickson type IIb) and familial hypertriglyceridemia (Type IV) [6]. Secondary causes frequently include medical conditions such as obesity, untreated diabetes mellitus, excessive alcohol intake, hypothyroidism, nephrotic syndrome, liver disease, and pregnancy [4]. Certain medications are also well known to cause elevations of TG levels such as estrogens, glucocorticoids, thiazides, beta-blockers, antipsychotics (Olanzapine), immunosuppressants, protease inhibitors, isotretinoin, and bile acid resins [4, 6].

There is a broad spectrum of clinical manifestations of HTG, the most common of which being patients who are asymptomatic. Other symptoms may include mid-epigastric abdominal pain, nausea, and vomiting in relation to acute pancreatitis. Cutaneous manifestations are usually associated with elevations of LDL levels and include eruptive cutaneous xanthomas, palmar crease xanthomas, tendinous xanthomas, tuberous xanthomas, and eyelid xanthelasmas [7]. Ophthalmologic features can include lipemia retinalis. The risk of pancreatitis increases when TG levels exceed 1000-2000 mg/dL and is the third leading cause of pancreatitis after alcohol and gallstones. There are also moderate to highly significant associations between triglyceride values and the risk of coronary heart disease. We theorize that our patient experienced chest pain possibly as a result of accumulation of chylomicrons in the coronary arteries leading to ischemia which was relieved with rapid lowering of TG levels.

Diagnosis of specific HTG disorders requires extensive and costly workup. Therefore, the most critical initial step is to exclude secondary causes. This includes medication review, evaluation of body mass index (BMI), hemoglobin A1c, TSH, and renal and liver function testing [6]. When potential secondary causes have been ruled out, patients should be evaluated for various primary HTG.

Management of severe and very severe HTG involves rapidly lowering total TG levels to prevent development of acute pancreatitis. This comprises of both immediate dietary modifications and use of TG lowering medications which may require hospitalization [4]. During acute rapid lowering of TG levels, patients are typically kept NPO, and a no-fat diet is generally introduced when TG drops to <1000 mg/dL. For chronic maintenance, patients are instructed to avoid simple carbohydrates completely as well as reducing fat intake to less than 10% of daily caloric intake [8]. This is to decrease the risk of postprandial chylomicronemia since lipoprotein lipase (LPL) levels are maximally saturated from existing severe elevations of TG levels [9]. Rapid lowering of TG levels can be achieved with administration of IV Insulin drip with glucose and IV Heparin which are potent activators of LPL to effectively remove TGs from circulation [10, 11]. The effective goal to reduce the risk of pancreatitis is to reduce TG levels to less than 500-1000 mg/dL [4, 12–14]. Concomitantly, oral TG lowering medications should be initiated. First line medical therapy of isolated HTG is fibrates [6]. The preferred fibrate is Fenofibrate of which the onset of action may take a few weeks [4]. For patients with associated elevations of low-density lipoprotein (LDL) levels, a statin medication can be given. With this combination, risk of myopathy should be assessed with baseline creatinine kinase (CK) levels, and again if patients become symptomatic [15]. Suggested prescriptions of Omega-3-fatty acids and Niacin can be added as well. For patients who develop acute pancreatitis secondary to HTG, plasmapheresis can be performed to rapidly lower TG levels [16].

We postulate that our patient had a form of familial dyslipidemia which was exacerbated by the use of estrogens and steroids. Given her elevated apolipoprotein B levels, it is more likely that she had type IIb familial combined hyperlipidemia (FCHL).

4. Conclusion

Hypertriglyceridemia is frequently encountered in clinical practice. Very severe hypertriglyceridemia above 1000-2000 mg/dL should be evaluated for primary and secondary causes. Rapidly lowering triglyceride levels is essential to prevent serious complications such as acute pancreatitis. Long term effects of elevated TG count have also been associated with coronary artery disease. Rapid lowering can be achieved with intravenous insulin drip, even in nondiabetic patients, and intravenous heparin. Maintenance therapy with dietary changes and medications such as fibrates is highly recommended.

References

[1] M. Miller, N. J. Stone, C. Ballantyne et al., "Triglycerides and cardiovascular disease: a scientific statement from the American Heart Association," *Circulation*, vol. 123, no. 20, pp. 2292–2333, 2011.

[2] J. B. Christian, N. Bourgeois, R. Snipes, and K. A. Lowe, "Prevalence of severe (500 to 2,000 mg/dl) hypertriglyceridemia in United States adults," *American Journal of Cardiology*, vol. 107, no. 6, pp. 891–897, 2011.

[3] J. Jang, "Lipid/Cardiovascular Disorders/Hypertension," *Endocrine Practice*, vol. 22, Supplement 2, pp. 115–126, 2016.

[4] L. Berglund, J. D. Brunzell, A. C. Goldberg et al., "Evaluation and treatment of hypertriglyceridemia: an endocrine society clinical practice guideline," *The Journal of Clinical Endocrinology & Metabolism*, vol. 97, no. 9, pp. 2969–2989, 2012.

[5] S. Melnick, S. Nazir, D. Gish, and M. R. Aryal, "Hypertriglyceridemic pancreatitis associated with confounding laboratory abnormalities," *Journal of Community Hospital Internal Medicine Perspectives*, vol. 6, no. 3, Article ID 31808, 2016.

[6] R. N. Pejic and D. T. Lee, "Hypertriglyceridemia," *Journal of the American Board of Family Medicine*, vol. 19, no. 3, pp. 310–316, 2006.

[7] S. S. Vangara, K. D. Klingbeil, R. M. Fertig, and J. L. Radick, "Severe hypertriglyceridemia presenting as eruptive xanthomatosis," *Journal of Family Medicine and Primary Care*, vol. 7, no. 1, pp. 267–270, 2018.

[8] A. Brahm and R. A. Hegele, "Hypertriglyceridemia," *Nutrients*, vol. 5, no. 3, pp. 981–1001, 2013.

[9] J. D. Brunzell, W. R. Hazzard, D. Porte Jr., and E. L. Bierman, "Evidence for a common, saturable, triglyceride removal mechanism for chylomicrons and very low density lipoproteins in man," *The Journal of Clinical Investigation*, vol. 52, no. 7, pp. 1578–1585, 1973.

[10] Z. Berger, R. Quera, J. Poniachik, D. Oksenberg, and J. Guerrero, "Heparin and/or insulin treatment of acute pancreatitis caused by hypertriglyceridemia," *Revista Médica de Chile*, vol. 129, pp. 1373–1378, 2001.

[11] M. A. Jabbar, M. I. Zuhri-Yafi, and J. Larrea, "Insulin therapy for a non-diabetic patient with severe hypertriglyceridemia," *Journal of the American College of Nutrition*, vol. 17, no. 5, pp. 458–461, 1998.

[12] Expert Panel on Detection, Evaluation, and Treatment of High Blood Cholesterol in Adults, "Executive summary of the third report of the National Cholesterol Education Program (NCEP) expert panel on detection, evaluation, and treatment of high blood cholesterol in adults (adult treatment panel III)," *Journal of the American Medical Association*, vol. 285, no. 19, pp. 2486–2497, 2001.

[13] V. G. Athyros, O. I. Giouleme, N. L. Nikolaidis et al., "Long-term follow-up of patients with acute hypertriglyceridemia-induced pancreatitis," *Journal of Clinical Gastroenterology*, vol. 34, no. 4, pp. 472–475, 2002.

[14] E. P. DiMagno and S. Chari, "Acute pancreatitis," in *Sleisenger & Fordtrans Gastrointestinal and Liver Disease*, M. Feldman, L. S. Friedman, and L. H. Sleisenger, Eds., pp. 913–942, W.B. Saunders, St. Louis, Mo, USA, 2002.

[15] D. Moßhammer, E. Schaeffeler, M. Schwab, and K. Mörike, "Mechanisms and assessment of statin-related muscular adverse effects," *British Journal of Clinical Pharmacology*, vol. 78, no. 3, pp. 454–466, 2014.

[16] N. Ewald and H.-U. Kloer, "Treatment options for severe hypertriglyceridemia (SHTG): the role of apheresis," *Clinical Research in Cardiology Supplements*, vol. 7, supplement 1, pp. 31–35, 2012.

24

A Case of Unresectable Papillary Thyroid Carcinoma Treated with Lenvatinib as Neoadjuvant Chemotherapy

Hiroyuki Iwasaki,[1] **Soji Toda**,[1] **Hiroyuki Ito**,[2] **Daiji Nemoto**,[2] **Daisuke Murayama**,[1] **Yoichiro Okubo**,[3] **Hiroyuki Hayashi**,[4] **and Tomoyuki Yokose**[3]

[1]*Department of Breast and Endocrine Surgery, Kanagawa Cancer Center, Yokohama, Japan*
[2]*Department of Respiratory Surgery, Kanagawa Cancer Center, Yokohama, Japan*
[3]*Department of Pathology, Kanagawa Cancer Center, Yokohama, Japan*
[4]*Department of Pathology, Yokohama City Hospital, Yokohama, Japan*

Correspondence should be addressed to Hiroyuki Iwasaki; iwasaki.h@kcch.jp

Academic Editor: Carlo Capella

A 75-year-old woman visited a nearby clinic with complaints of right clavicle discomfort, and she underwent diagnostic thoracoscopic lung biopsy, being diagnosed with lung metastasis and a right-upper mediastinal mass. The superior mediastinum mass was extrapulmonary and covered by the pleura, and it was not biopsied. Papillary thyroid carcinoma was diagnosed following biopsy of the lung metastasis. Only a small tumor, with a maximum diameter of 70 mm from the right neck to the superior mediastinum, in the thyroid gland invades the internal jugular vein and subclavian vein, forming a tumor embolus in the right brachiocephalic vein and reaching the vicinity of the superior vena cava. For life-saving purposes, we obtained approval from the Cancer Board of Kanagawa Cancer Center and used lenvatinib according to unresectable undifferentiated cancer IRB approval number 28–41. The tumor had shrunk after 4 months, and surgery was performed. The postoperative course has been good, and the patient is being followed up. The patient is alive three months after surgery, and lung metastases have disappeared on CT images. This case is reported as a successful case of neoadjuvant chemotherapy and interval debulking surgery.

1. Introduction

Lenvatinib has been recognized to be effective against radioactive iodine (RAI) refractory-differentiated thyroid carcinoma following disease progression [1]. It has also been approved for the treatment of anaplastic thyroid cancer in Japan, and clinical results have been reported [2, 3]. The neoadjuvant approach to BRAF-mutated anaplastic thyroid cancer (ATC) has been reported as clinical trials [4, 5]. Still, there are no reports for the use of neoadjuvant chemotherapy (NAC) + interval debulking surgery for patients with unresectable differentiated thyroid cancers (DTC).

2. Case Presentation

The case report involved a 75-year-old woman with no special medical history. The patient's height and weight were 147 cm and 49 kg, respectively. She visited a nearby clinic and presented with a tumor on the right clavicle and a sense of discomfort. Computed tomography (CT) revealed a large right-upper mediastinal tumor and micropulmonary metastases (Figures 1(a) and 1(b)). The large tumor extended to the neck, subclavicle, and right-upper mediastinum. Partial resection of the lung metastasis was performed under thoracoscopy to diagnose the primary tumor. We did not biopsy the superior mediastinal tumor because it was an extrapulmonary lesion with no continuity with the lung lesion, which was covered by pleura. The pathological diagnosis was lung metastasis of papillary thyroid carcinoma. Although a small mass was also found in the thyroid gland, there was no malignant finding, and treatment was prioritized without further examination. Because the tumor obstructed the right brachiocephalic vein and approached the superior vena cava (SVC) junction, there was a risk of

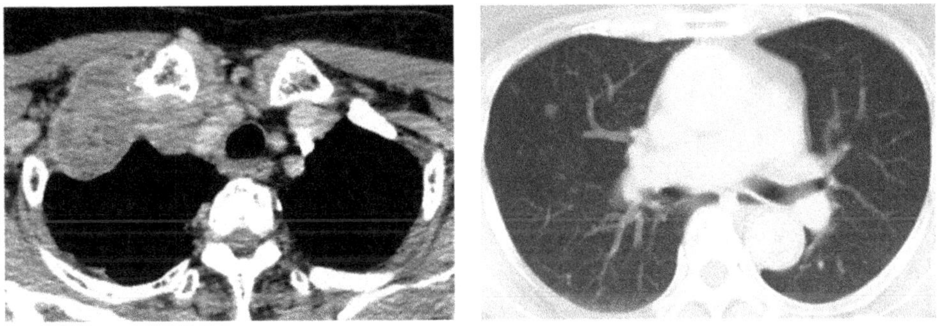

(a) (b)

FIGURE 1: Images taken during the initial visit. Computed tomography revealed a large right-upper mediastinal tumor (a) and micropulmonary metastases (b).

SVC occlusion and pulmonary embolism (Figure 2(a)). We decided to start treatment as soon as possible to avoid sudden death from pulmonary embolism. Lenvatinib treatment was started with approval from the Cancer Board of Kanagawa Cancer Center (IRB approval number 28–41). The tumor shrank upon treatment, and the major axis was reduced from 68 to 48 mm in diameter. The tumor embolus regressed from the junction of the SVC, permitting the right brachiocephalic vein to be clamped and ligated safely (Figure 2(b)).

2.1. Treatment Progress. The adverse events induced by lenvatinib included grade 2 HT, grade 2 hand-foot syndrome, and grade 2 anorexia, and thus, the dose was reduced to 10 mg after 3 weeks. After 16 weeks of treatment, her weight loss reached 10 kg, and it was clinically assessed that further continuation of lenvatinib was impossible. Then, surgery was performed 1 week after withdrawal of lenvatinib. Total thyroidectomy and resection of the first rib, right internal jugular vein, right subclavian vein, and tumor were performed, and the right brachiocephalic vein was clamped and separated from the SVC junction at the periphery. Infiltration of the subclavian artery and vagal nerve was found on the dorsal side of the tumor, and a tumor approximately 1 cm^2 in size remained at the site. The risk of SVC syndrome and pulmonary embolism was resolved, and the tumor was largely resected. Figure 3 shows the schema of the surgical procedure and CT after the operation. The sternum was incised as shown in the figure, the sternoclavicular joint and collarbone were flipped outward, and surgery was performed. We planned to conduct follow-up of the efficacy of RAI therapy and thyroid stimulating hormone (TSH) suppression for small residual tumors and lung metastases.

2.2. Pathological Findings. No primary lesion remained in the thyroid gland, and the lenvatinib had a beneficial effect on papillary carcinoma originating from the upper mediastinum. Figure 4(a) presents a histopathological image of the central region of the papillary carcinoma lesion. Figure 4(b) presents a histopathological image of the periphery of the tumor. Extensive necrosis and fibrosis caused by lenvatinib were observed. Treatment efficacy was clearly recognized. The patient's preoperative thyroglobulin and TgAb levels were 4690 ng/mL and 18 IU/mL, respectively, decreasing to 451 ng/mL and <10 IU/mL, respectively, after the operation.

3. Discussion

3.1. Choice of Treatment. In this case, if the tumor had progressed without treatment, obstruction of the SVC would have led to SVC syndrome, and once the embolus flowed to the pulmonary artery, there would have been a risk of sudden death from pulmonary embolism. In fact, micropulmonary metastasis was recognized because a small tumor embolus reached the lung and caused distant metastasis. Under these conditions, surgical resection is extremely risky, and radiotherapy cannot reduce the risk of tumor embolism. Lung metastasis is a differentiated thyroid carcinoma in the histological diagnosis; thus, a good prognosis can still be expected if the lesion can be resected, and RAI therapy can be performed after total thyroidectomy.

3.2. Selection of Dose and Timing of Interval Debulking Surgery. The initial dose of lenvatinib was set as 14 mg because of the possibility of tumor embolism due to the rapid tumor disintegration and bleeding caused by the collapse of large blood vessels. We previously reported that the antitumor effect is expected to be the same even at low doses [6]. Adverse events and treatment progress were described. As previously reported [7], surgery should be performed at the time when tumor reduction stops after 3 months of treatment because anaplastic transformation or regrowth may occur.

3.3. Withdrawal Period and Problems during and after Surgery. According to the pharmacokinetics of lenvatinib [8], the half-life is 34.5 h, which means that the half-life reached approximately five times in 7 days, meaning that the initial dose had been reduced by 32-fold. Previous experimental data indicated that a 7 day withdrawal had no therapeutic effect on VEGF inhibition, and regrowth was observed [9]. Thus, surgery was performed on day 7. At the

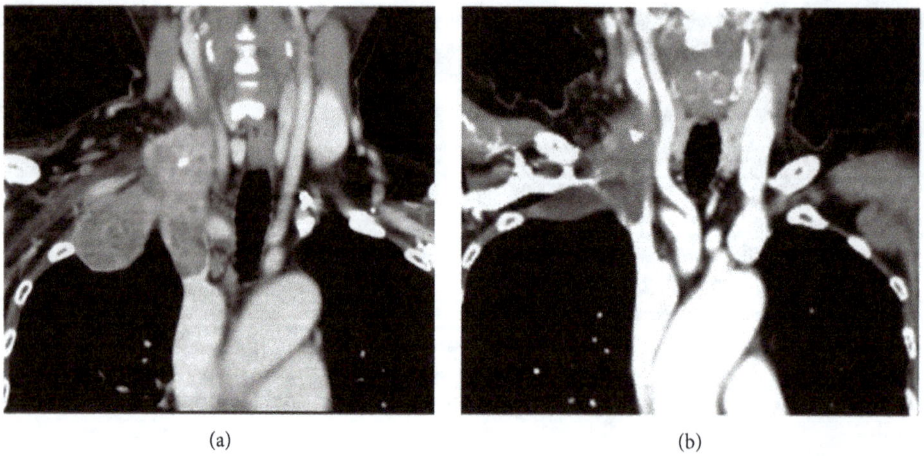

Figure 2: Images taken at baseline and 14 weeks after lenvatinib treatment. The tumor shrank upon treatment, and the major axis was reduced in diameter from 68 to 48 mm. The tumor embolus regressed from the junction of the superior vena cava.

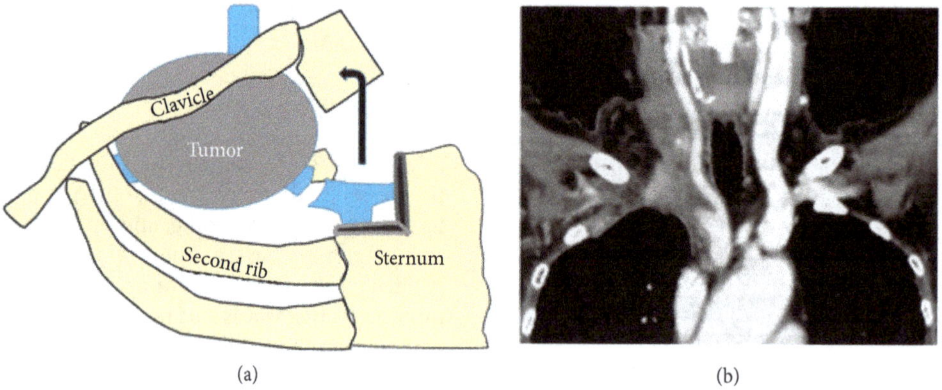

Figure 3: Surgical procedure and after surgery image ((a) and (b)). The sternum was incised as shown in the figure; the sternoclavicular joint and collarbone were flipped outward, and surgery was performed.

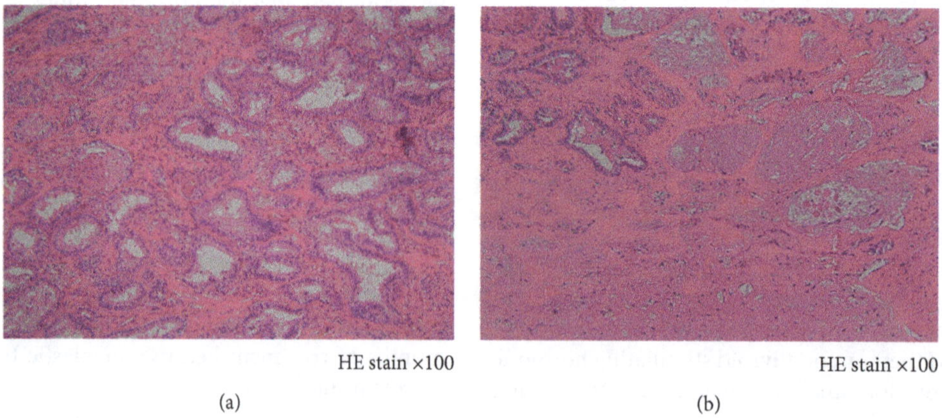

Figure 4: Histologic sections of resected tumor ((a) and (b)). (a) Histopathological image of the central part of the papillary carcinoma tumor. The tumor formed a papillary structure. Individual cancer cells had nuclear grooves, and findings suggestive of nuclear inclusions were also observed. Original magnification 100×. (b) Histopathological image of the periphery of the tumor. Extensive necrosis and fibrosis caused by lenvatinib were observed. Original magnification 100×.

time of surgery, adhesion was around the tumor only at the invaded site, and resection was performed as a normal surgical operation. Our greatest concern was delayed wound healing. Despite our concerns, healing was normal. A large tumor was removed, and the right cephalic vein, apical pleura, and first rib were also removed. Therefore, postoperative leachate retention continued for approximately 1 month, which was not sufficient for drainage. Edema of the right-upper limb was observed for approximately 1 week, after which it was resolved. No upper limb movement limitation or paresthesia was observed. The patient is alive three months after surgery, and lung metastases have disappeared on CT images so far. In the future, if NAC + surgery can be safely selected even for patients with difficult resection, it may be possible to improve the treatment results of advanced thyroid cancer.

Acknowledgments

The authors would like to thank Enago (http://www.enago.com) for the English language review.

References

[1] M. Schlumberger, M. Tahara, L. J. Wirth et al., "Lenvatinib versus placebo in radioiodine-refractory thyroid cancer," *New England Journal of Medicine*, vol. 372, no. 7, pp. 621–630, 2015.
[2] M. Tahara, N. Kiyota, T. Yamazaki et al., "Lenvatinib for anaplastic thyroid cancer," *Frontiers in Oncology*, vol. 7, p. 25, 2017.
[3] H. Iwasaki, H. Yamazaki, H. Takasaki et al., "Lenvatinib as a novel treatment for anaplastic thyroid cancer: a retrospective study," *Oncology Letters*, vol. 16, no. 6, pp. 7271–7277, 2018.
[4] M. E. Cabanillas, R. Ferrarotto, A. S. Garden et al., "Neoadjuvant BRAF- and immune-directed therapy for anaplastic thyroid carcinoma," *Thyroid*, vol. 28, no. 7, pp. 945–951, 2018.
[5] J. R. Wang, M. E. Zafereo, R. Dadu et al., "Complete surgical resection following neoadjuvant dabrafenib plus trametinib in BRAFV600E-mutated anaplastic thyroid carcinoma," *Thyroid*, vol. 29, no. 8, pp. 1036–1043, 2019.
[6] H. Yamazaki, H. Iwasaki, H. Takasaki et al., "Efficacy and tolerability of initial low-dose lenvatinib to treat differentiated thyroid cancer," *Medicine (Baltimore)*, vol. 98, no. 10, Article ID e14774, 2019.
[7] H. Yamazaki, H. Iwasaki, N. Suganuma et al., "Anaplastic thyroid carcinoma diagnosed after treatment of lenvatinib for papillary thyroid carcinoma," *Endocrinology, Diabetes & Metabolism Case Reports*, vol. 2019, no. 1, 2019.
[8] A.-C. Dubbelman, H. Rosing, C. Nijenhuis et al., "Pharmacokinetics and excretion of 14C-lenvatinib in patients with advanced solid tumors or lymphomas," *Investigational New Drugs*, vol. 33, no. 1, pp. 233–240, 2015.
[9] M. R. Mancuso, R. Davis, S. M. Norberg et al., "Rapid vascular regrowth in tumors after reversal of VEGF inhibition," *Journal of Clinical Investigation*, vol. 116, no. 10, pp. 2610–2621, 2006.

Ketogenic Diet-Induced Diabetic Ketoacidosis in a Young Adult with Unrecognized Type 1 Diabetes

Suranut Charoensri,[1] **Jin Sothornwit**,[1] **Akeatit Trirattanapikul**,[2] **and Chatlert Pongchaiyakul**[1]

[1]*Division of Endocrinology and Metabolism, Department of Medicine, Faculty of Medicine, Khon Kaen University, Khon Kaen, Thailand*
[2]*Department of Medicine, Faculty of Medicine, Khon Kaen University, Khon Kaen, Thailand*

Correspondence should be addressed to Suranut Charoensri; armsunut@hotmail.com

Academic Editor: Lucy Mastrandrea

Ketogenic diet, a very low-carbohydrate diet and high-fat diet, has emerged as a popular approach for weight reduction, particularly in young adults. However, a serious but rare complication of the ketogenic diet is ketoacidosis associated with low carbohydrate intake, which should be cautiously monitored in people with a predisposition to the condition. We report a 22-year-old Thai woman with an unremarkable past medical history who presented with an acute onset of dyspnea of 2 days' duration. Diabetic ketoacidosis was diagnosed by elevated capillary blood glucose, significant metabolic acidosis, and a high serum beta-hydroxybutyrate level. Low C-peptide level and positive islet autoantibodies confirmed the new diagnosis of type 1 diabetes in this patient. After her conditions were stabilized, the patient revealed that she began a ketogenic diet for weight reduction 4 days before her illness. Other precipitating factors were not identified. This highlights that ketogenic diet may increase diabetic ketoacidosis risk at the presentation of previously unrecognized type 1 diabetes.

1. Introduction

A number of dietary patterns have been proposed as an effective method for weight reduction [1, 2]. Guideline recommendations support several weight-loss approaches that focus on the alteration of macronutrients, including low-fat, low-carbohydrate, and high-protein diets [3]. All of these approaches have resulted in similar clinically meaningful weight loss [4, 5]. The ketogenic diet, a very low-carbohydrate diet and high-fat diet, has emerged as a popular approach, especially for young adults. This diet restricts the daily intake of carbohydrates to less than 50 grams per day, leading to reduced insulin secretion and the conversion of fatty acids to ketone bodies for energy consumption [6, 7]. However, a serious but rare complication of the ketogenic diet is ketoacidosis associated with low carbohydrate intake [8], which should be cautiously monitored in people with a predisposition to the condition, including pregnancy, chronic alcoholism, and type 1 diabetes [9]. Here, we report the case of a healthy young adult who developed diabetic ketoacidosis (DKA) as the first presentation of type 1 diabetes following the course of ketogenic diet.

2. Case Report

A 22-year-old Thai woman with an unremarkable past medical history presented to the emergency department with an acute onset of dyspnea of 2 days' duration. She was unable to tolerate any food or drink since the symptoms started. On examination, her vital signs included temperature 38°C, pulse rate 110 bpm, blood pressure 110/80 mmHg, and

Table 1: Initial laboratory investigations.

Lab	Value	Reference	Units
Hemoglobin	13.7	12.0–14.3	g/dL
Hematocrit	41	36.0–47.7	%
White blood cells	15.8	4.60–10.60	k/mm^3
Neutrophils	82	43.7–70.9	%
Platelets	294	173–383	k/mm^3
Sodium	144	136–145	mEq/L
Potassium	3.6	3.5–5.0	mEq/L
Chloride	115	98–106	mEq/L
Bicarbonate	4.8	23–30	mEq/L
Anion gap	24.2	3–11	—
BUN	3.8	6.0–20.0	mg/dL
Creatinine	0.49	0.51–0.95	mg/dL
Glucose	390	70–99	mg/dL
Hemoglobin A1C	14	4.6–6.5	%
Lactate	1.2	0.4–2.0	mmol/L
Serum ketones	6.65	0–3	mmol/L
Urine glucose	4+	Negative	—
Urine ketones	2+	Negative	—
Arterial pH	7.15	7.35–7.45	—

Table 2: The "ketogenic diet" that the patient had before her illness.

Day	Lunch	Dinner
Day 1	(i) One serving of Thai papaya salad (ii) Half serving of fried fish (iii) A coconut	(i) Eight servings of spiced duck (ii) One cup of black coffee
Day 2	(i) One serving of Thai papaya salad (ii) Half serving of fried fish (iii) One cup of black coffee (iv) One bottle of soda	(i) One serving of stir-fried pork with basil leaves (without rice) (ii) One serving of omelette (iii) A coconut (iv) One dish of fried pupa
Day 3	(i) One serving of Chinese clear soup with braised pork (ii) A coconut (iii) One cup of latte	(i) A tablespoon of avocado (ii) 30 grams of pumpkin seed
Day 4	(i) One serving of Chinese clear soup with braised pork	(i) One serving of Thai suki

respiratory rate 32/minute with a kussmaul breathing pattern. Other physical examinations were unremarkable except for severe dehydration. The initial testing revealed the results in Table 1, which included capillary blood glucose of 356 mg/dL, serum bicarbonate of 4.8 mEq/L, arterial pH of 7.15, and a serum beta-hydroxybutyrate level of 6.65 mmol/L, while the lactate level was normal. The urinalysis showed glucosuria and ketonuria. A diagnosis of new-onset diabetes and diabetic ketoacidosis (DKA) was established. However, the type of diabetes was undetermined at that time. Fasting C-peptide level and islet autoantibodies were sent to evaluate for type 1 diabetes.

She was admitted to the intensive care unit and treated with intravenous saline, intravenous insulin infusion, and electrolyte repletion. Blood glucose levels and metabolic acidosis improved. Oral intake and subcutaneous insulin were initiated two days later. Despite a BMI of 22.3 kg/m^2, the patient felt that she needed to lose weight. A week prior, she initiated an intensive weight management regimen including a ketogenic diet. She had restricted her carbohydrate intake to less than 15 grams per day 4 days. The specifics of her ketogenic meal are shown in Table 2. She denied participating in a heavy exercise which could lead to dehydration. Other precipitating factors of DKA were not identified.

After 6 days of hospital admission, she was discharged with multiple daily injection (MDI) insulin therapy without further complications. One week later, the results of special investigations for identifying the type of diabetes showed C-peptide level 0.2 ng/mL, anti-GAD 8.79 U/mL (normal <5), and anti-IA2 130.95 U/mL (normal <7.5), which confirmed the diagnosis of type 1 diabetes in this patient.

3. Discussion

This case demonstrates the development of DKA following a low-carbohydrate, ketogenic diet in a patient with unrecognized type 1 diabetes. It is important for physicians to be aware of this rare potential complication of ketogenic diet, particularly in those with increased risk for type 1 diabetes.

DKA is a life-threatening complication, usually affecting children with newly diagnosed type 1 diabetes [10, 11]. Although the mortality rate is low, DKA is associated with adverse neurological outcomes [12]. The most common precipitating factors in the development of DKA are infection and discontinuation of insulin in type 1 diabetes [13]. Factors that may lead to insulin omission in young patients include fear of weight gain, fear of hypoglycemia, rebelliousness from authority, and stress of chronic disease [14]. Theoretically, carbohydrate-restricted dietary ketosis may predispose to ketoacidosis in people with type 1 diabetes, particularly in the setting of insulin omission or in the rare situation of undiagnosed type 1 diabetes, not on insulin therapy [9].

Adolescent obesity is a global epidemic with a growing prevalence impacting all socioeconomic groups [15]. However, perceptions of overweight in late adolescence and early adulthood are much more common than being actual overweight. Up to 60% of normal weight young women consider themselves to be overweight in both Western and Asian cultures [16, 17]. These beliefs, whether true or not, are correlated with unhealthy habits, including maladaptive weight-loss strategies [18, 19]. Ketogenic diet is one of the most popular weight-reduction methods in Thailand. Ketosis status from this form of dietary pattern is predicted. However, severe ketoacidosis inducing metabolic acidosis is rare [20]. In patients with near-normal or normal insulin activity, the concentration of plasma beta-hydroxybutyrate during a ketogenic diet should be comparable to those who fasted because the rate of hepatic ketone body synthesis is balanced by ketone utilization and ketone excretion in the urine [9, 21–23]. Therefore, there will be no alteration of the acid-base balance during dieting. On the contrary, serious ketoacidosis may occur in people with lower than normal insulin activity, including type 1 diabetes, pregnant women, alcoholics, and certain diabetic patients currently using sodium-glucose cotransporter-2 inhibitors (SGLT-2i). These patients with higher risk for ketoacidosis should be monitored more closely if choosing to pursue a ketogenic diet. The patient reported in our case had an unrecognized insulin deficiency, combined with a strict ketogenic diet of less than 15 grams of carbohydrates per day, which led to a presentation of DKA. It is important to make individuals aware of this potential complication. In those at higher risk for type 1 diabetes, especially in first-degree relatives of type 1 diabetes patients or other high-risk populations, clinicians should consider screening for overt diabetes prior to patients starting a ketogenic diet, and in those with type 1 diabetes on ketogenic diets, insulin omission should be avoided.

References

[1] U.S. Department of Health and Human Services and U.S. Department of Agriculture. 2015–2020 Dietary Guidelines for Americans., http://health.gov/dietaryguidelines/2015/guidelines/.

[2] A. Makris and G. D. Foster, "Dietary approaches to the treatment of obesity," *Psychiatric Clinics of North America*, vol. 34, no. 4, pp. 813–827, 2011.

[3] M. D. Jensen, D. H. Ryan, C. M. Apovian et al., "2013 AHA/ACC/TOS guideline for the management of overweight and obesity in adults," *Circulation*, vol. 129, no. 25, pp. S102–S138, 2013.

[4] L. Schwingshackl and G. Hoffmann, "Long-term effects of low-fat diets either low or high in protein on cardiovascular and metabolic risk factors: a systematic review and meta-analysis," *Nutrition-Journal*, vol. 12, p. 48, 2013.

[5] F. M. Sacks, G. A. Bray, V. J. Carey et al., "Comparison of weight-loss diets with different compositions of fat, protein, and carbohydrates," *New England Journal of Medicine*, vol. 360, no. 9, pp. 859–873, 2009.

[6] E. A. Murphy and T. J. Jenkins, "A ketogenic diet for reducing obesity and maintaining capacity for physical activity," *Current Opinion in Clinical Nutrition & Metabolic Care*, vol. 22, no. 4, pp. 314–319, 2019.

[7] R. Ting, N. Dugré, G. M. Allan, and A. J. Lindblad, "Ketogenic diet for weight loss," *Canadian family physician Medecin de famille canadien*, vol. 64, no. 12, p. 906, 2018.

[8] P. Shah and W. L. Isley, "Ketoacidosis during a low-carbohydrate diet," *New England Journal of Medicine*, vol. 354, no. 1, pp. 97-98, 2006.

[9] J. R. Oster and M. Epstein, "Acid-base aspects of ketoacidosis," *American Journal of Nephrology*, vol. 4, no. 3, pp. 137–151, 1984.

[10] A. Rewers, F. Dong, R. H. Slover, G. J. Klingensmith, and M. Rewers, "Incidence of diabetic ketoacidosis at diagnosis of type 1 diabetes in colorado youth, 1998-2012," *The Journal of the American Medical Association*, vol. 313, no. 15, pp. 1570–1572, 2015.

[11] A. Rewers, G. Klingensmith, C. Davis et al., "Presence of diabetic ketoacidosis at diagnosis of diabetes mellitus in youth: the search for diabetes in youth study," *Pediatrics*, vol. 121, no. 5, pp. e1258–e1266, 2008.

[12] F. J. Cameron, S. E. Scratch, C. Nadebaum et al., "Neurological consequences of diabetic ketoacidosis at initial presentation of type 1 diabetes in a prospective cohort study of children," *Diabetes Care*, vol. 37, no. 6, pp. 1554–1562, 2014.

[13] W. Ahuja, N. Kumar, S. Kumar, and A. Rizwan, "Precipitating risk factors, clinical presentation, and outcome of diabetic ketoacidosis in patients with type 1 diabetes," *Cureus*, vol. 11, no. 5, Article ID e4789, 2019.

[14] W. H. Polonsky, B. J. Anderson, P. A. Lohrer, J. E. Aponte, A. M. Jacobson, and C. F. Cole, "Insulin omission in women with IDDM," *Diabetes Care*, vol. 17, no. 10, pp. 1178–1185, 1994.

[15] M. Raj and R. K. Kumar, "Obesity in children & adolescents," *Indian Journal of Medical Research*, vol. 132, pp. 598–607, 2010.

[16] F. Bellisle, M. O. Monneuse, A. Steptoe, and J. Wardle, "Weight concerns and eating patterns: a survey of university students in Europe," *International journal of obesity and related metabolic disorders: journal of the International Association for the Study of Obesity*, vol. 19, pp. 723–730, 1995.

[17] Y. Wong and Y.-C. Huang, "Obesity concerns, weight satisfaction and characteristics of female dieters: a study on female Taiwanese college students," *Journal of the American College of Nutrition*, vol. 18, no. 2, pp. 194–200, 1999.

[18] R. Isomaa, A.-L. Isomaa, M. Marttunen, R. Kaltiala-Heino, and K. Björkqvist, "Longitudinal concomitants of incorrect weight perception in female and male adolescents," *Body Image*, vol. 8, no. 1, pp. 58–63, 2011.

[19] A.-L. Winter, N. A. De Guia, R. Ferrence, and J. E. Cohen, "The relationship between body weight perceptions, weight control behaviours and smoking status among adolescents," *Canadian Journal of Public Health*, vol. 93, no. 5, pp. 362–365, 2002.

[20] D. Gomez-Arbelaez, A. B. Crujeiras, A. I. Castro et al., "Acid-base safety during the course of a very low-calorie-ketogenic diet," *Endocrine*, vol. 58, no. 1, pp. 81–90, 2017.

[21] W. S. Yancy, M. K. Olsen, T. Dudley, and E. C. Westman, "Acid-base analysis of individuals following two weight loss diets," *European Journal of Clinical Nutrition*, vol. 61, no. 12, pp. 1416–1422, 2007.

[22] G. F. Cahill, "Fuel metabolism in starvation," *Annual Review of Nutrition*, vol. 26, no. 1, pp. 1–22, 2006.

[23] O. E. Owen, P. Felig, A. P. Morgan, J. Wahren, and G. F. Cahill, "Liver and kidney metabolism during prolonged starvation," *Journal of Clinical Investigation*, vol. 48, no. 3, pp. 574–583, 1969.

26

An Adolescent with Transient Hyperthyroxinemia after Blunt Trauma to Head and Neck

Michelle Romijn,[1] **Leo M. G. Geeraedts Jr.**,[2] **Jonathan I. M. L. Verbeke**,[3] **and Martijn J. J. Finken**[1]

[1]*Department of Pediatric Endocrinology, Emma Children's Hospital, Amsterdam UMC, Amsterdam, Netherlands*
[2]*Department of Surgery, Section Trauma Surgery Amsterdam UMC, Location VUmc, Amsterdam, Netherlands*
[3]*Department of Radiology and Nuclear Medicine, Amsterdam UMC, Location VUmc, Amsterdam, Netherlands*

Correspondence should be addressed to Michelle Romijn; m.romijn1@amsterdamumc.nl

Academic Editor: J. Paul Frindik

Background. Thyroid storm is a well-known complication of surgical procedures in the lower neck, but is rare after a blunt neck trauma. The cases described previously have mainly focussed on adults with pre-existent thyroid disease. In this case report, we describe the disease course of a previously healthy adolescent who had asymptomatic hyperthyroxinemia after a blunt trauma of the jaw and neck. *Case Presentation.* A 17-year-old girl presented at our emergency department after she fell on her head while roller blading. On physical examination, among other injuries, she had a swelling in the lower neck, which appeared to involve the thyroid gland. Subsequent laboratory analysis was indicative of primary hyperthyroxinemia, with a free T4 of 59 pmol/L (reference range: 12–22) and a TSH of 0.46 mU/L (reference range: 0.5–4.3), but the patient had no symptoms fitting with this. Four weeks after the initial presentation, the patient reported only complaints regarding tenderness in the jaw and neck region. She was no longer hyperthyroidic on biochemical evaluation (with a free T4 level of 15.6 pmol/L and a TSH level of 0.33 mU/L), and antibodies against thyroid peroxidase or TSH receptor were not present. *Conclusions.* This case might indicate that hyperthyroxinemia following a neck trauma may go unnoticed if hyperthyroid symptoms are mild or absent and thyroid function tests are not performed.

1. Introduction

Thyroid storm is a well-known complication of surgical manipulation of the thyroid gland, for example, during parathyroidectomy or laryngectomy [1–5]. However, thyroid storm induced by thyroid injury after blunt trauma to the neck is a rare finding [6, 7]. This clinical entity has been described following attempted suicide by hanging [8, 9], a severe neck trauma [6, 10], and thyroid ultrasonography [11, 12]. A great majority of patients described so far were adults, of whom the majority experienced severe hyperthyroid symptomatology and were known with pre-existent thyroid disease [6, 7, 13]. Thyroid storm is a potentially life-threatening complication of thyroid injury that starts abruptly and is characterized by four main symptom clusters, including fever, supraventricular arrhythmias or tachycardia, and gastrointestinal system and central nervous system symptomatology. Early recognition and prompt treatment seem necessary [6]. In this case report, we describe the disease course of a previously healthy adolescent who had asymptomatic hyperthyroxinemia after a blunt trauma to the head and neck.

2. Case Presentation

A previously healthy, 17-year-old girl presented at the emergency department after she fell on her head while roller blading. She complained about pain in her jaw and neck. On physical examination, the patient was an alert girl with stable vital parameters, including a heart rate of 70 bpm, a blood pressure of 125/85 mmHg, a peripheral oxygen saturation of 99% on room air, and a temperature of 37.6°C. Injuries noted were a fractured mandible and a painless, mobile swelling in the lower neck at the level of the thyroid region. There was no audible stridor or other signs of upper airway obstruction.

Computed tomography (CT) scanning of the head and neck was performed, showing an enlarged and inhomogeneous thyroid gland and a fractured mandible (see Figure 1). Subsequently, contrast-enhanced CT scanning and ultrasonography of the neck showed enlargement and asymmetry of the thyroid gland, with more hypodense areas in the right lobe, suspicious of contusion or laceration, though the possibility of autoimmune thyroiditis could not be excluded (see Figure 2).

After the imaging results, thyroid function tests were performed, demonstrating a free T4 level of 59.0 pmol/L (reference range: 12–22) and a TSH level of 0.46 mU/L (reference range: 0.5–4.3). The patient did not experience symptoms of hyperthyroidism, in particular no jittery, no palpitations, no excessive sweating, and no previous weight loss. She had no history of a neck swelling. The family history was unremarkable, with no family members reporting a history of thyroid or autoimmune disease. The day after admission, the laboratory tests were repeated, showing a decline in the free T4 level (see Table 1). The patient still did not experience symptoms of hyperthyroidism, and 24 hours later, she was discharged.

At an outpatient visit 4 weeks after presentation, the patient reported to be nearly recovered, except for tenderness in her jaw and neck region. On physical examination, her vital signs were stable and her thyroid gland was no longer enlarged. Thyroid function tests showed a free T4 level of 15.6 pmol/L and TSH level that was still slightly suppressed at 0.33 mU/L and absence of antibodies against thyroid peroxidase or TSH receptor (see Table 1). The transient hyperthyroxinemia could therefore most likely be attributed to thyroid injury.

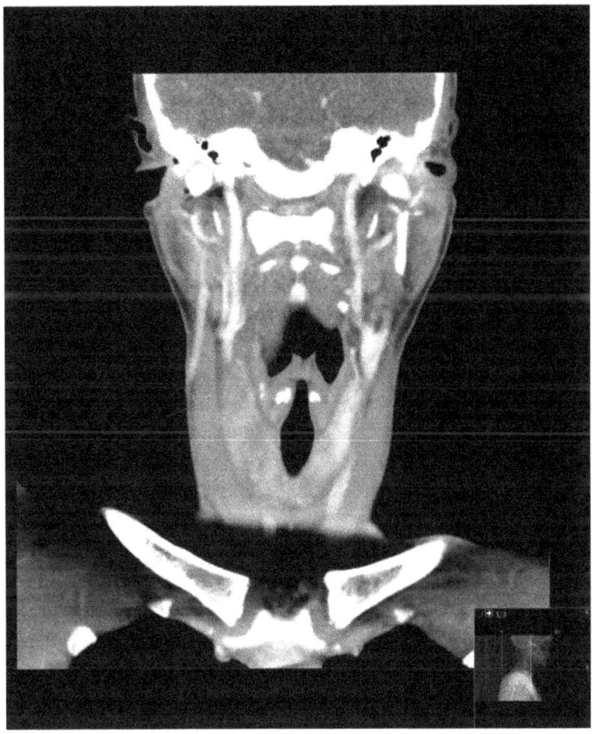

Figure 1: Contrast-enhanced CT image of head and neck, demonstrating thyroid enlargement and asymmetry. After the administration of contrast, the right lobe contained more hypodense areas without enhancement compared to the left lobe, as indicated by the arrows. There was no extravasation of the contrast medium. These findings are suspicious of contusion or laceration, though the possibility of autoimmune thyroiditis could not be excluded.

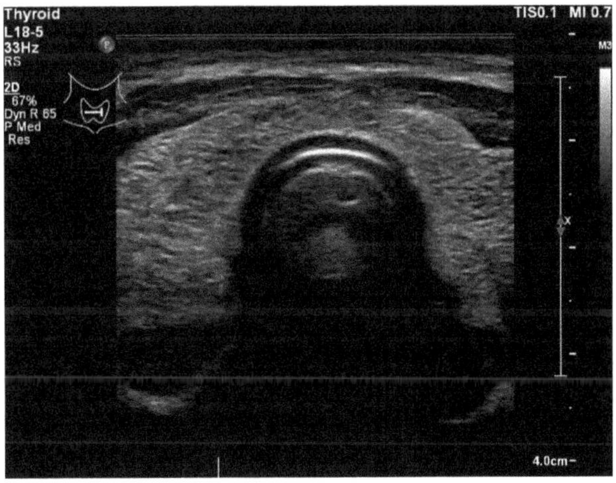

Figure 2: Thyroid ultrasonography of the patient demonstrating thyroid enlargement and inhomogeneity. The size of the left lobe was 1.5 × 1.6 × 2.8 cm, and the size of the right lobe was 1.7 × 1.5 × 3.5 cm. Anterior from both thyroid lobes was fluid accumulation.

3. Discussion

We have presented a patient with transient, asymptomatic hyperthyroxinemia after a blunt trauma of the head and neck. The pathomechanism of trauma-induced hyperthyroxinemia is thought to involve rupture of acini and liberation of thyroid hormones in the bloodstream, which may result in a potentially life-threatening condition called thyroid storm [6]. Thyroid storm is a rare finding among trauma patients that has previously been described only in those with a severe trauma to the neck, such as after hanging and strangulation [8, 9]. There are only a few reports describing thyroid injury and thyroid storm after a blunt neck trauma [6, 7, 10]. Most of the cases described before were adult females, with a median age of 44 (range: 8–89) years, and approximately half of them were known with pre-existing thyroid disease [7]. Newer theories suggest that thyroid storm represents a form of allostatic failure in situations, where severe illness would normally result in euthyroid sick syndrome, but where the patient is unable to downregulate T3 concentrations due to thyrotoxicosis [14]. However, in our patient, T3 concentrations were not measured.

Another complication of thyroid injury is a rapidly expanding hematoma that may cause airway compression

TABLE 1: Thyroid function tests of the patient.

	Day 1	Day 2	Day 28	Reference range
TSH (mU/L)	0.46	0.14	0.33	0.5–4.3
FT4 (pmol/L)	59.0	47.3	15.6	12–22
Anti-TPO antibodies (kU/L)			<30	<60
Anti-TSH receptor antibodies (U/L)			<0.1	<1.8

TSH = thyroid stimulating hormone; FT4 = Free thyroxine; TPO = thyroid peroxidase.

requiring hemithyroidectomy. It has been described that nearly half of the patients with thyroid injury required hemithyroidectomy due to a rapidly expanding hematoma of the thyroid [6, 15]. The onset of symptoms of an expanding hematoma, such as a painful pre- and paratracheal swelling and dyspnoea, may be delayed in approximately 50% of the patients [7, 13], necessitating inhospital monitoring for more than 24 hours.

Thyroid function tests of the patient were indicative of primary hyperthyroidism. During the follow-up, her free T4 level recovered, while her TSH level remained slightly suppressed, which may be attributed to a delayed pituitary response, as evidenced from Jostel's TSH Index (7.16, 4.40, and 0.99 at days 1, 2, and 28, respectively). Given the lack of antibodies directed against the thyroid gland and the absence of evidence for a pre-existing thyroid disease, it is amenable that the hyperthyroxinemia in the patient could be explained by thyroid trauma. This case is special and interesting in such a way that it concerned a 17-year-old adolescent who did not experience symptoms suggestive of hyperthyroxinemia. In addition, the patient had no own or family history of thyroid disease. Despite the absence of hyperthyroid symptoms, thyroid function tests showed hyperthyroxinemia. The lack of hyperthyroid symptoms in our patient could be explained by the fact that she was young and previously healthy. For the publication of this case report, we obtained a written informed consent from our subject.

With this case report, we add that hyperthyroxinemia following a neck trauma may go unnoticed if hyperthyroid symptoms are mild or absent and thyroid function tests are not performed. Therefore, hyperthyroxinemia may occur more frequent after a blunt trauma of the neck than previously expected.

Ethical Approval

For this case report, the ethical approval was not required.

Consent

Written informed consent was obtained from the patient for publication of the clinical details and images.

Acknowledgments

The authors would like to thank the patient for consent to publish this case as a case report.

References

[1] R. A. Calle and K. L. Cohen, "Transient thyroiditis due to surgical trauma," *The American Journal of Medicine*, vol. 95, no. 5, pp. 546–548, 1993.

[2] P. Lindblom, S. Valdemarsson, J. Westerdahl, J. Tennvall, and A. Bergenfelz, "Hyperthyroidism after surgery for primary hyperparathyroidism," *Langenbeck's Archives of Surgery*, vol. 384, no. 6, pp. 568–575, 1999.

[3] M. T. Stang, J. H. Yim, S. M. Challinor, S. Bahl, and S. E. Carty, "Hyperthyroidism after parathyroid exploration," *Surgery*, vol. 138, no. 6, pp. 1058–1065, 2005.

[4] G. Rudofsky, M. Tsioga, P. Reismann et al., "Transient hyperthyroidism after surgery for secondary hyperparathyroidism: a common problem," *European Journal of Medical Research*, vol. 16, no. 8, pp. 375–380, 20118.

[5] E. S. Thieroldt, J. B. Lama, S. M. Abad, and A. M. De La Torre, "Transient hyperthyroidism after total laryngectomy for laryngeal cancer," *Nutricion hospitalaria*, vol. 31, no. 1, pp. 380–383, 2015.

[6] S. Delikoukos and F. Mantzos, "Thyroid storm induced by blunt thyroid gland trauma," *The American Surgeon*, vol. 73, no. 12, pp. 1247–1249, 2007.

[7] J. Lemke, M. N. Schreiber, D. Henne-Bruns, G. Cammerer, and A. Hillenbrand, "Thyroid gland hemorrhage after blunt neck trauma: case report and review of the literature," *BMC Surgery*, vol. 17, no. 1, p. 115, 2017.

[8] J. I. Ramírez, P. Petrone, E. J. Kuncir, and J. A. Asensio, "Thyroid storm induced by strangulation," *Southern Medical Journal*, vol. 97, no. 6, pp. 608–610, 2004.

[9] J. M. Shrum, B. Byers, and K. Parhar, "Thyroid storm following suicide attempt by hanging," *BMJ Case Report*, vol. 2014, 2014.

[10] A. Hagiwara, A. Murata, T. Matsuda, S. Sakaki, and S. Shimazaki, "Thyroid storm after blunt thyroid injury: a case report," *Journal of Trauma: Injury, Infection & Critical Care*, vol. 63, no. 3, pp. E85–E87, 2007.

[11] K. Nakabayashi, N. Nakazawa, T. Suzuki et al., "Thyroid echography-induced thyroid storm and exacerbation of acute heart failure," *Internal Medicine*, vol. 55, no. 16, pp. 2209–2212, 2016.

[12] R. K. Yatavelli and S. N. Levine, "Transient hyperthyroidism induced by thyroid ultrasound," *Annals of Otology, Rhinology & Laryngology*, vol. 127, no. 8, pp. 558–562, 2018.

[13] E. E. Schipper, D. R. Kool, T. Wobbes, and L. M. G. Geeraedts Jr, "Management of thyroid gland hemorrhage after blunt trauma: a case report and review of the literature," *European Journal of Trauma and Emergency Surgery*, vol. 35, no. 6, pp. 587–590, 2009.

[14] A. Chatzitomaris, R. Hoermann, J. E. Midgley et al., "Thyroid allostasis-adaptive responses of thyrotropic feedback control

to conditions of strain, stress, and developmental programming," *Front Endocrinol (Lausanne)*, vol. 8, p. 163, 2017.

[15] F. Zawawi, R. Varshney, R. J. Payne, and J. J. Manoukian, "Thyroid gland rupture: a rare finding after a blunt neck trauma," *International Journal of Pediatric Otorhinolaryngology*, vol. 77, no. 5, pp. 863–865, 2013.

New-Onset Diabetes in Children during COVID-19: Clinical Case Report

M. Aabdi,[1] A. Aarab,[2] O. Es-Saad,[1] K. Malki,[1] H. Bkiyar,[1] and B. Housni[1]

[1]*Anesthesiology and Intensive Care Unit Department, MOHAMMED VI University Hospital Center, Oujda, Morocco*
[2]*Laboratory Unit Department, MOHAMMED VI University Hospital Center, Oujda, Morocco*

Correspondence should be addressed to M. Aabdi; med.aabdi@gmail.com

Academic Editor: Suat Simsek

Introduction. Data of COVID-19 in newborns and children are limited, and clinical manifestations are nonspecific and might delay the diagnosis, which might lead to severe complications. In this clinical case, we will describe new-onset diabetes with consciousness impairment as an atypical revealing way of COVID-19. *Case.* A 3-year-old child presented to the Emergency Department with loss of consciousness (without fever), lethargy, and stupor. Clinical assessment on admission found an unconscious child with a pediatric Glasgow Coma Scale of 10/15 with no localizing signs or meningeal syndrome, polypneic of 35 breaths/min, pulse oximetry of 90%, with signs of overall dehydration: skin folds, sunken eyes, tachycardia of 160 beats/minute, and recoloring time superior at 3 seconds. Laboratory findings showed hyperleukocytosis of 16000/mm^3, lymphopenia of 450/mm^3, glycemia of 5 g/L with a correct ionogram : corrected natremia of 139 mmol/L, serum potassium of 4.5 mmol/L, glycosuria of 3+, ketonuria of 2+, and HbA1c of 10%, and COVID-19 RT-PCR came back positive. *Conclusion.* COVID-19 might be revealed with atypical symptoms including new-onset diabetes and diabetic ketoacidosis; therefore, clinicians must suspect it in children with blood glucose and HbA1c at the time of admission. This will help to manage patients with hyperglycemia early.

1. Introduction

From March 2020, Anesthesiology and Intensive Care Unit Department, Mohammed VI University Hospital Center, Oujda, Morocco, has been facing an unprecedented outbreak of coronavirus disease and spread of 2019 novel coronavirus or severe acute respiratory syndrome coronavirus 2 (SARS-CoV-2), which has now become a global pandemic [1, 2]. The disease caused by SARS-CoV-2 was termed "COVID-19," and the World Health Organization declared the COVID-19 outbreak a public health emergency of international concern and officially was declared a pandemic on March 11, 2020 [2].

Data from the early months of 2020 suggest that there is a bidirectional relationship between COVID-19 and diabetes [3]. Diabetes is associated and is continuously suggested as a risk factor that contributes to the severity and mortality of COVID-19 [1]. Multiple forms of diabetes might be observed in patients with COVID-19 including new-onset diabetes and metabolic complications such as diabetic ketoacidosis and hyperosmolarity [4]. Nonetheless, data on new-onset type 1 diabetes during the COVID-19 pandemic, particularly in children, are limited [5]. In this article, we describe a clinical case of a 3-year-old child who presented to the Emergency Department (ED) in a ketoacidosis decompensation state, a recent diagnosis with COVID-19 infection, and who was retrospectively diagnosed with new-onset diabetes.

2. Clinical Case

A 3-year-old child presented to the ED with loss of consciousness (without fever), lethargy, and stupor. Clinical assessment on admission found an unconscious child with a pediatric Glasgow Coma Scale (GCS) of 10/15 with no localizing signs or meningeal syndrome, polypneic of 35 breaths/min, pulse oximetry of 90%, with signs of overall dehydration (skin folds), sunken eyes, tachycardia of 160 beats/minute, and recoloring time superior at 3 seconds.

Laboratory findings showed hyperleukocytosis of 16000 mm^3, lymphopenia of 450 mm^3, glycemia of 5 g/L with a correct ionogram : corrected natremia of 139 mmol/L, serum potassium of 4.5 mmol/L, glycosuria of 3+, ketonuria of 2+, and HbA1c of 10%.

Brain computed tomography (CT) came back normal; the search for a primary infection site led us to carry out a chest X-ray showing an alveolar-interstitial syndrome (Figure 1), supplemented by a thoracic CT revealing a bilateral ground-glass opacification consistent with viral pneumopathy, with moderate impairment with a level of suspicion scored CO-RADS 4 (Figure 2). Given the epidemiological context, a COVID-19 RT-PCR came back positive.

Diabetic ketoacidosis (DKA) is the most common hyperglycemic emergency and is associated with increased morbidity and mortality. In children and adolescents with type 1 diabetes, DKA accounts for the most common cause of death. DKA is characterized by hyperglycemia, ketosis, and metabolic acidosis [6].

Management of DKA consisted of rehydration with Ringer's lactate 20 ml/kg initially and physiological serum as well as insulin therapy with a dose of 0.05 IU/kg/h along with monitoring of blood sugar levels and any complications. The prognosis was favorable with neurological, respiratory, and metabolic improvement; the child was transferred to the pediatric endocrinology department for further assessment.

3. Discussion

Coronaviruses are positive-strand ribonucleic, large viruses. Only two genera of the viruses can infect humans: a and b types, and they are called human coronaviruses (HCoVs) [7].

HCoVs are used to be mild phenotypes in humans because of their inconsequential pathogenic effect. However, two epidemics emerging in the early 21st century (severe acute respiratory syndrome (SARS) and Middle East respiratory syndrome (MERS)) with a high rate of morbidity and mortality changed the knowledge about this [8].

COVID-19 is generally more frequent among adults more than 15 years old with less confirmed cases among children [9]. However, the number of children infected has increased due to the pathogen detection campaigns and the lack of protective measures [10].

A report of a multicenter regional data from North West London of new-onset type 1 diabetes and DKA in children has estimated an increase of 80% of new type 1 diabetes cases during the COVID-19 pandemic and postulates that COVID-19 exposure contributed to the observed increase in cases by precipitating or accelerating type 1 diabetes onset [5]. A previous paper reported that children accounted for 5% of confirmed COVID-19 cases and presented with a milder disease symptom, and they have a better prognosis compared with adults, with very low mortality rate [7, 9]. But children with newly diagnosed diabetes, either it is new--onset or previously undiagnosed, tend to have increased levels of inflammatory markers and indicators of multiorgan injury leading to severe or critical illness of COVID-19 [11]. They also present severe hyperglycemic complications such as DKA and hyperosmolar hyperglycemic syndrome requiring high doses of insulin [12]. COVID-19 patients with newly diagnosed diabetes have higher mortality rate than those with known diabetes [11].

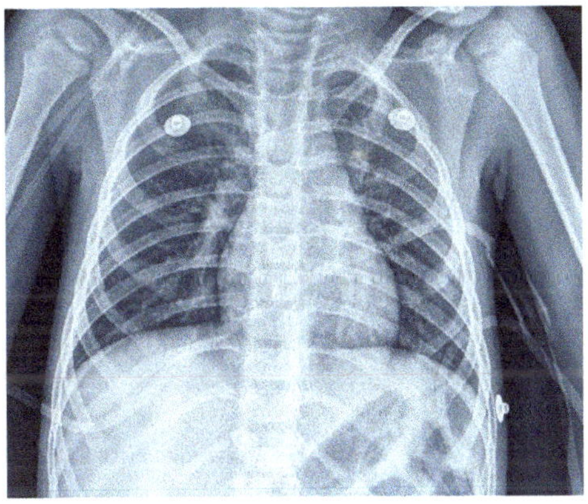

Figure 1: Chest X-ray showing an alveolar-interstitial syndrome.

The pathophysiological mechanisms implicated with the increased frequency and severity of COVID-19 in people with diabetes are not yet elucidated, and several hypotheses have been elaborated to explain the link between COVID-19 and high rate and worst outcomes in diabetic people [2].

Diabetes is associated with an increased risk of infections, including viral ones due to defects in the innate immunity affecting phagocytosis, neutrophil chemotaxis, and cell-mediated immunity [1, 13]. Besides, diabetes and insulin resistance are associated with endothelial dysfunction and increased platelet aggregation and activation leading to the hypercoagulable prothrombotic state [13]. The latter associated with the low-grade chronic inflammation might promote the cytokine storm, a severe complication of COVID-19 characterized by excessive production of inflammatory cytokines [14]. Furthermore, COVID-19 spike protein gains entry to its target cells by using the angiotensin-converting enzyme 2 (ACE2) as the receptor, which has protective effects primarily regarding inflammation [1]. COVID-19 infection reduces ACE2 expression inducing cellular damage, hyperinflammation, and respiratory failure and can lead to a direct effect on β-cell function, which not only explains that diabetes might be a risk factor for a severe form of COVID-19 disease but also explains that infection could induce new-onset diabetes [1, 9, 15–18].

New-onset diabetes must be detected in all nondiabetic patients especially those at high risk for metabolic disease who have contracted the viral infection. Besides, most patients present multiple stresses with COVID-19 including respiratory failure and sepsis requiring intravenous infusion of insulin and fluid balance to control the glycemia levels [19]. In addition, potassium balance must be carefully considered in the context of insulin treatment, as hypokalemia is a common feature of COVID-19 and may be exacerbated after the introduction of insulin [19].

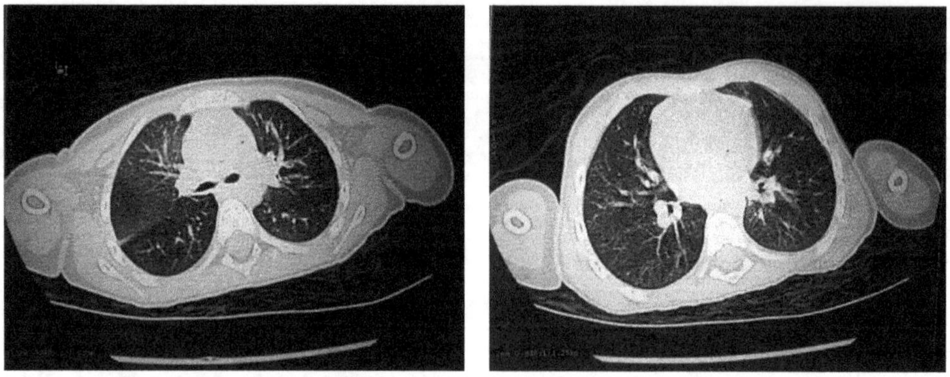

(a) (b)

FIGURE 2: Chest CT scan showing images in favor of pneumopathy COVID-19 CO-RADS 4.

4. Conclusion

This clinical case supports the strong link between COVID-19 infection and diabetes. Therefore, physicians should consider this in all nondiabetic children and screen them at their admission with blood glucose and HbA1C for appropriate and early management.

Ethical Approval

This study was exempt from ethical approval at our institution, as it was an observational finding in regular practice.

Consent

Written informed consent was obtained from the child holder for publication of this case report and accompanying images.

Authors' Contributions

Dr. Aabdi Mohammed contributed to conceptualization, methodology, validation, formal analysis, and visualization and wrote the original draft. Dr. Aarab Adnane contributed to formal analysis and visualization and reviewed and edited the manuscript. Dr. Es-Saad Ounci provided resources and developed software and was responsible for data curation. Dr. Malki Khalil, Pr. Housni Brahim, and Pr. Houssam Bkiyar were responsible for visualization. Pr. Houssam Bkiyar reviewed and edited the manuscript. Pr. Housni Brahim was responsible for project administration; provided resources; contributed to conceptualization, methodology, and validation; and reviewed and edited the manuscript. Dr. Aarab Adnane, Dr. Es-Saad Ounci, Dr. Malki Khalil, Pr. Housni Brahim, and Pr. Houssam Bkiyar approved the final version of the manuscript.

Acknowledgments

The authors acknowledge the frontline medical staff working day and night in Morocco to rescue critical cases and protect the public health. The authors know that these great efforts are now and will be in the future crucial in overcoming COVID-19.

References

[1] S. R. Bornstein, F. Rubino, K. Khunti et al., "Practical recommendations for the management of diabetes in patients with COVID-19," *The Lancet Diabetes & Endocrinology*, vol. 8, no. 6, pp. 546–550, 2020.

[2] E. Papadokostaki, N. Tentolouris, and E. Liberopoulos, "COVID-19 and diabetes: what does the clinician need to know?" *Primary Care Diabetes*, vol. 14, no. 5, pp. 558–563, 2020.

[3] Y. Chen, X. Gong, L. Wang, and J. Guo, "Effects of hypertension, diabetes and coronary heart disease on COVID-19 diseases severity: a systematic review and meta-analysis MedRxiv," p. 280, 2020.

[4] M. Paul Zimmet, M. D. George Alberti, M. D. Stefan Bornstein et al., "New-onset diabetes in COVID-19," *The New England Journal of Medicine*, vol. 383, no. 8, pp. 787–789, 2020.

[5] R. Unsworth, S. Wallace, N. S. Oliver et al., "New-onset type 1 diabetes in children during COVID-19: multicenter regional findings in the UK," *Diabetes Care*, vol. 43, no. 11, pp. e170–e171, 2020.

[6] M. Fayfman, F. J. Pasquel, and G. E. Umpierrez, "Management of hyperglycemic crises," *Medical Clinics of North America*, vol. 101, no. 3, pp. 587–606, 2017.

[7] Y. Dong, Y. Dong, X. Mo, Y. Hu, X. Qi, and F. Jiang, "Epidemiology of COVID-19 among children in China," *Pediatrics*, vol. 145, no. 6, 2020.

[8] A. H. De Wilde, J. Eric, M. K. Snijder, and M. J. Van, "Host factors in coronavirus replication," in *Assessment & Evaluation in Higher Education*, p. 435, Springer International Publishing, New York, NY, USA, 2012, Available from: http://books.google.com/books?id=_DDwCqx6wpcC&printsec=frontcover&dq=unwritten+rules+of+phd+research&hl=&cd=1&source=gbs_api%255Cnpapers2://publication/uuid/48967E01-55F9-4397-B941-310D9C5405FA%255Cnhttp://medcontent.metapress.com/index/A65RM03P4874243N.p.

[9] J. She, L. Liu, and W. Liu, "COVID-19 epidemic: disease characteristics in children," *Journal of Medical Virology*, vol. 92, no. 7, pp. 747–754, 2020.

[10] C. Jiehao, X. Jin, L. Daojiong et al., "A case series of children with 2019 novel coronavirus infection: clinical and epidemiological features," *Clinical Infectious Diseases*, vol. 71, no. 6, pp. 1547–1551, 2020.

[11] T. Sathish, Y. Cao, and N. Kapoor, "Newly diagnosed diabetes in COVID-19 patients," *Primary Care Diabetes*, vol. 15, no. 1, p. 194, 2020.

[12] Y. Jie, S. Jia, H. Ng, and E. Yeoh, "Diabetic ketoacidosis precipitated by COVID-19 in a patient with newly diagnosed diabetes mellitus," *Diabetes Research and Clinical Practice*, vol. 164, Article ID 108166, 2020.

[13] W. Abu-ashour, L. Twells, J. Valcour et al., "The association between diabetes mellitus and incident infections : a systematic review and meta-analysis of observational studies," *BMJ Open Diabetes Research and Care*, vol. 5, no. 1, 2017.

[14] W. Guo, M. Li, Y. Dong et al., "Diabetes is a risk factor for the progression and prognosis of COVID-19," *Diabetes Metabolism Research and Reviews*, vol. 36, no. 6, Article ID e3319, 2020.

[15] S. M. Bindom and E. Lazartigues, "The sweeter side of ACE2: physiological evidence for a role in diabetes," *Molecular and Cellular Endocrinology*, vol. 302, no. 2, pp. 193–202, 2020.

[16] M. Apicella, M. C. Campopiano, M. Mantuano, L. Mazoni, A. Coppelli, and S. Del Prato, "COVID-19 in people with diabetes: understanding the reasons for worse outcomes," *The Lancet Diabetes & Endocrinology*, vol. 8, no. 9, pp. 782–792, 2020.

[17] J.-K. Guo, S.-S. Lin, X.-J. Ji, and L.-M. Guo, "Binding of SARS coronavirus to its receptor damages islets and causes acute diabetes," *Acta Diabetologica*, vol. 47, no. 3, pp. 193–199, 2010.

[18] L. Fang, G. Karakiulakis, and M. Roth, "Are patients with hypertension and diabetes mellitus at increased risk for COVID-19 infection?" *The Lancet Respiratory Medicine*, vol. 8, no. 4, p. e21, 2020.

[19] R. P. Dellinger, M. M. Levy, A. Rhodes et al., "Surviving sepsis campaign : international guidelines for management of severe sepsis and septic shock ," *Critical Care Medicine*, vol. 41, no. 2, pp. 580–637, 2013.

28

An Uncommon Presentation of Adrenal Cyst with Subclinical Cushing's Syndrome: A Diagnosis Dilemma

A. Tahri,[1] W. Abdellaoui,[1] S. Benyakhlef,[1] K. Boujtat,[1] I. Mahroug,[1] I. Kamaoui,[2] A. Barki,[3] F. Kettani,[4] S. Rouf,[1] and H. Latrech[1,5]

[1]*Department of Endocrinology-Diabetology, Mohammed VIth University Hospital, Faculty of Medicine and Pharmacy of Oujda, Mohammed the First University, Oujda, Morocco*
[2]*Department of Urology, Mohammed VIth University Hospital, Faculty of Medicine and Pharmacy of Oujda, Mohammed the First University, Oujda, Morocco*
[3]*Department of Radiology, Mohammed VIth University Hospital, Faculty of Medicine and Pharmacy of Oujda, Mohammed the First University, Oujda, Morocco*
[4]*United Nations Center of Cytopathology, Rabat, Morocco*
[5]*Laboratory of Epidemiology, Clinical Research and Public Health, Faculty of Medicine and Pharmacy of Oujda, Mohammed the First University, Oujda, Morocco*

Correspondence should be addressed to H. Latrech; hlatrech@hotmail.fr

Academic Editor: Suat Simsek

Adrenal cysts are a rare entity that is usually nonfunctional and asymptomatic. Their association with adrenal neoplasms was rarely described in the literature. We report a unique case of a 40 -year-old woman who was referred for evaluation of a left adrenal incidentaloma with subclinical Cushing's syndrome. The tumor was suspicious for malignancy regarding computed tomography scan (CT scan) features. Therefore, a laparoscopic left partial adrenalectomy was performed. Pathology examination showed multilocular spaces lined by endothelial cells which are compatible with endothelial adrenal cyst, associated to an adrenocortical adenoma. We further discuss the management of adrenal cyst with review of the literature.

1. Introduction

Adrenal cysts are rare cystic masses that arise from the adrenal gland. They are usually nonfunctional and asymptomatic measuring less than 10 cm. These lesions may occur simultaneously with other adrenal tumors associated with hormonal hypersecretion. Only few papers describe the association between an adrenal cyst and adrenocortical adenoma.

We report one of the rare cases of a functioning adrenal cyst incidentally discovered.

2. Case Presentation

A 40-year-old woman was referred to our endocrinology department to evaluate a left adrenal incidentaloma discovered when a CT scan was performed because of her history of ureteral stones revealing a left adrenal mass of 34×27 mm. She had also hypertension treated with amlodipine 10 mg 2 months ago and did not complain neither of headache nor diaphoresis or palpitations.

No clinical features of Cushing's syndrome were noticed on physical examination regardless of moderate obesity with android distribution (weight: 94 kg, body mass index 30 kg/m^2, and waist size 105 cm). But, her blood pressure levels were not well controlled under amlodipine 10 mg.

Laboratory examination showed a normal value of 24-hour urine metanephrines/normetanephrine, plasma renin, and plasma aldosterone concentration (Table 1).

Her plasma levels of midnight cortisol of two different days were 5, 2–4, and 2 ug/dL (normal value: 1.8 ug/dL with the immunoassay technique), urine free cortisol values of

TABLE 1: Value of U-metanephrine, U-normetanephrine, the plasma renin, and the plasma aldosterone concentration.

U-metanephrine (mg/day), *N*: 0.04–0.20 with the liquid chromatography-mass spectrometry technique		0.07
U-normetanephrine (mg/day), *N*: 0.07–0.38 with the liquid chromatography-mass spectrometry technique		0.14
Plasma aldosterone pg/ml radioimmunoassay method	Seated position *N*: 30–146	128
	After 1 hour of upright position *N*: 75–361	345
Plasma renin mUI/ml chemiluminescence method	Seated position *N*: 2.8–39.9	6.1
	After 1 hour of upright position *N*: 4.4–46.1	20.1
Aldosterone-renin ratio (ARR)	Seated position *N*: < 64	58
	After 1 hour of upright position *N*: <64	48

three different days were 36.3, 42.8, and 3.25 ug/day (normal value: 4.3–176), and serum dehydroepiandrosterone sulfate level was 119 ug/dL (normal value: < 600 ug/dL with the chemiluminescence method). However, her plasma adrenocorticotropic hormone (ACTH) concentration was at the low limit: 10.4 ng/L (normal value: 10.3–48.2 with the electrochemiluminescence method), and the overnight 1 mg dexamethasone suppression test (2.7 μg/dL; reference range <1.8 μg/dL) besides the low-dose dexamethasone suppression test (DST) showed an absence of cortisol suppression, which was consistent with the European Society of Endocrinology criteria of autonomous cortisol secretion [1].

Laboratory tests concerning associated comorbidities showed an increased level of total cholesterol: 2.23 g/L (normal value < 2 g/L) and triglyceride: 3.21 g/l (normal value < 1,5 g/L) and decreased level of HDL cholesterol: 0.47 g/L (normal value: < 0.60 g/L). Fasting blood sugar level was 0.85 g/L (N: 0.70–1.10 g/L) and hemoglobin A1c level (HbA1c) was 5.2%. The 75 g oral glucose tolerance test noted an impaired glucose tolerance. Bone density was normal.

The CT scan revealed a rounded well-defined hypodense lesion of the left adrenal. Its size increased to 44 × 29 mm. Spontaneous density was 22 Hounsfield unit (HU) (Figure 1(a)), and absolute washout reached 50%. The wall of this lesion did not enhance after contrast injection, and calcification was detected (Figure 1(b)). The right adrenal gland was normal.

According to the clinical, laboratory, and imaging findings, the left adrenal mass was suspicious. Laparoscopic retroperitoneal cystic resection and left partial adrenalectomy were performed. It is the elective surgical procedure adopted by our urologist, for numerous advantages, especially for a shorter surgery duration and a minor intraoperative bleeding. Hydrocortisone replacement was not administered after the surgery because the patient did not have signs or symptoms of adrenal insufficiency.

At three months after surgery, her weight turned to 88 kg and her hypertension was stabilized under amlodipine 10 mg. Plasma 8 am ACTH concentration increased to 28 pg/mL, and plasma cortisol concentration decreased compared with her preoperative levels (Table 2). Moreover, plasma cortisol concentration was suppressed in reaction to the overnight 1 mg DST without impaired glucose tolerance (Table 2).

Pathological analysis of the resected tumor reported a 4 * 2.3 * 1.7 cm mass weighing 13 g with a partially yellowish cystic appearance.

Histological examination of the different specimens showed a cystic cavity with a fibrous wall and constituted of multilocular spaces lined by endothelial cells and filled with red blood cells (Figure 2(a) (star)). This morphological feature was consistent with an endothelial cyst. A proliferation of well-defined clear cells was found at the rim of this lesion (Figure 2(a) (arrow)) arranged in an alveolar pattern (Figure 2(b)) without cytonuclear atypia (Figure 2(c)). According to Weiss's criteria, these pathological features were suggestive of an adrenocortical adenoma. This finding suggested the diagnosis of adrenocortical adenoma [2].

3. Discussion

Adrenal cysts are generally rare, and around 600 cases have been documented in the literature so far [3, 4]. The incidence of adrenal cysts in autopsy series ranges from 0.06% to 0.18%. They may occur at any age, although most of them may appear in the 3rd to 4th decade of life with a female preponderance [4, 5]. Our case was in the same range of age. Cyst size varies from millimeters to exceptional giant lesions above 20 cm. They may be unilocular or multilocular, usually solitary, involving the right and left adrenal glands with equal frequency. Neri and Nance [4] reported an incidence of 7% malignant forms, classically within the pseudocyst subclassification of adrenal cysts.

Clinical symptoms are related to the position and size of these benign cysts, although abdominal pain, gastrointestinal disorders, dyspnea, and palpable mass can be noted in large cysts. Besides, intracystic hemorrhage, infection, and hypertension have been also reported [6]. Our patient was asymptomatic with poorly controlled hypertension suggesting hormone secretion.

In 1966, Foster [7] classified 115 adrenal cysts into 4 histopathological types: epithelial cysts (9%), parasitic cysts (7%), particularly echinococcal type, pseudocysts (39%), and

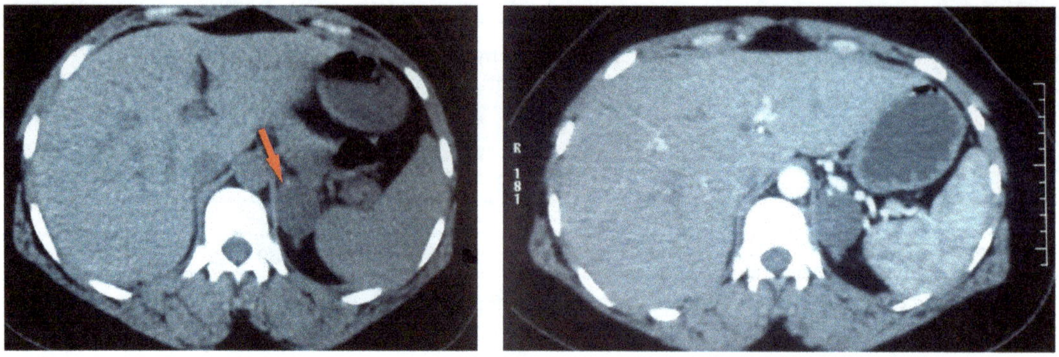

(a) (b)

Figure 1: Unenhanced computed tomography scan (a) of the abdomen showing a unilocular left adrenal cyst, without wall's enhancement after contrast injection (b).

Table 2: Comparative table of laboratory data before and after surgery.

Variable	Before surgery	3 months after surgery
Midnight cortisol* (ug/dL) Normal: < 1.8	5.2–4.2	1–1.7
u-free cortisol** (μg/day) normal: 4.3–176	36-42-3.25	23-13-9
Plasma ACTH (ng/L) 8 AM Normal: 10.30–48.30	10.7	28.5
Cortisol plasma after 1 mg DST (ug/dL) Normal <1.8	2.7	0.7
Plasma glucose at 120 min in 75 g OGTT (mg/dL) Normal <1.40	1.78	1.10

ACTH: adrenocorticotropic hormone; DST: overnight dexamethasone suppression test; DHEA-S: dehydroepiandrosterone sulfate; OGTT: oral glucose tolerance test. *In plasma examination, values of two different days are shown to view day-to-day variation. **In urine examination, values of three different days are shown to view day-to-day variation.

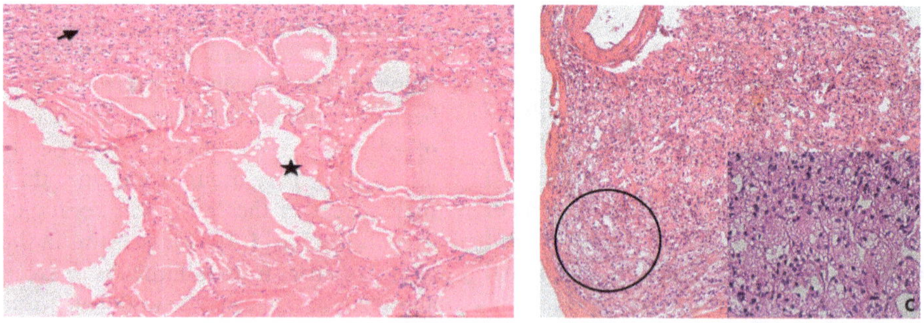

(a) (b)

Figure 2: Histological study of the lesion: (a) a cystic space lined by flattened endothelial cells filled with blood (star) associated to a proliferation of well-defined clear cells (arrow) (H&Ex100). (b) Alveolar disposition of the clear cells (circle) (H&Ex200). (c) Adrenocortical adenoma (H&Ex400).

endothelial cysts (45%). Data from this evaluation demonstrated that endothelial cysts were the most common subtype. Nevertheless, Neri and Nance [4] considered pseudocyst as the most common subtype regarding their review of 515 from a total of 613 adrenal cysts with available pathology reports.

Endothelial cysts, also known as "simple cysts," are usually thin-walled and multilocular measuring less than 2 cm. They are defined by their smooth and flattened endothelial lining, in addition to their yellow-tinged serous fluid [7]. They can be subcategorized histopathologically into angiomatous cysts and lymphangiomatous cysts which are the most common subtypes. Diagnosis can be established using the hematoxylin and eosin staining, although the immunohistochemical examination is essential to distinguish the lymphangiomatous subtype using podoplanin

(D2-40) which constitutes a marker of lymphatic endothelium, from the angiomatous subtype using the angiomatous marker (CD31 and CD34) [5]. Pathological examination of our resected tumor using hematoxylin and eosin staining lead to the diagnosis of an endothelial cyst based on the presence of a cystic cavity surrounded by a fibrous wall and composed of multilocular spaces lined by endothelial cells and filled with blood.

Endothelial cysts are typically described at CT imaging as unilateral, with different sizes, thin walls (<3.5 mm), smooth borders, and multilocular structure besides septal calcifications [8]. They have a low attenuation coefficient usually less than 20 Hounsfield units (HU) and do not enhance after contrast media injection [9]. The content of these endothelial cysts is more hemorrhagic than any other subtype which may increase the attenuation coefficient [10]. The CT scan in our case exhibits typical features of an endothelial cyst, but a malignancy cannot be neglected as the lesion's size exceeded 4 cm knowing that the spontaneous density was high at 22 HU and the absolute washout was below 50% [1].

Since functioning adrenal cysts have been described in the literature [9], all patients with this tumor (especially in the presence of arterial hypertension) should undergo adrenal functionality investigations [11, 12]. Measurements of 24-h urinary metanephrines are the most used tests for pheochromocytoma identification [1, 11, 12] and the ratio between morning plasma aldosterone and plasma renin activity (PRA) is mandatory in hypertensive patients, in order to identify aldosterone-producing tumors [1, 11, 12]. Evaluation of 24-h urinary cortisol and the overnight 1 mg dexamethasone suppression test are the most used diagnostic methods [1, 11] for the identification of hypercortisolism. Otherwise, morphological imaging (CT scan or MRI) or functional studies (MIBG scan for suspected pheochromocytoma) help with determining size, morphological features (cystic contents, density, wall thickness, and contrast enhancement), and relationship with adjacent structures, since malignancy is reported [10, 11]. Nevertheless, calcifications are not pathognomonic of malignant lesions [13].

Only a few case series and reports of endothelial cysts have been documented in the literature, and their association with other adrenal neoplasms is even uncommon. In fact, Erickson et al. reported only one case of endothelial cyst associated with pheochromocytoma [14], and Nigawara et al. were the first who described a case of adrenocortical adenoma associated with an endothelial cyst [15]. Yamada et al. also reported a case associating an endothelial cyst, an adrenocortical adenoma, and a myelolipoma. [16], and more recently, this rare entity has been delineated by Hong et al. [17]. To the best of our knowledge, this is the fourth reported case of adrenocortical adenoma associated with an endothelial cyst. Table 3 shows the three previously reported cases of endothelial cysts associated to an adrenocortical adenoma with the present case.

Our case supported what was previously described, and the gender was the same in the three cases except for the third one. The masses were incidentally discovered in the CT scan. Clinically, our patient had poorly controlled hypertension with obesity just as the case reported by Nigawara et al. [15]. Biological assessment of our case revealed an autonomous secretion of cortisol with a disturbed lipid profile and an impaired glucose tolerance, and the same findings were found in the case of Nigawara et al. The CT scan of the first case was highly suggestive of a left adrenocortical carcinoma because of the large size and the heterogeneity of the tumor (9 × 7 cm), while the second case a left adrenal myelolipoma was suspected. The CT scan of our patient was pathognomonic of an adrenal cyst, but the presence of a high spontaneous density with absolute washout below 50% was responsible of a diagnostic dilemma. On microscopic examination, the proliferation of clear cortical cells without nuclear atypia or mitotic activity was compatible with an adrenocortical adenoma, which was found in all the cases. Moreover, immunohistochemical study analysis of steroidogenic enzymes provides important information to asses the hyperfunctioning pattern of the adrenocortical adenoma [15, 16]. This includes the search for expression of the following enzymes: P450 side-chain cleavage (P450scc), 3β-hydroxysteroid dehydrogenase (3βHSD), P450c17 α-hydroxylase (P450c17) and P450 21 hydroxylase (P450c21)1, and DHEA-sulfotransferase (DHEA-ST). This exploration was carried out in case 1 and case 2; however, it was not made in our case because of economical issues.

The pathogenesis of an adrenal endothelial cyst formation within an adrenocortical adenoma is still a mysterious issue. Several theories suggested that the cyst may arise from a preexisting vascular hamartoma [5, 14] or lymphangiectasis [14] or intraparenchymal hemorrhage. In the present case, no apparent abnormal vascular channels have been identified.

Up to now, no guidelines have been established on the management and treatment of cystic adrenal lesions because of the low incidence of these lesions and the difficulty in achieving a definitive preoperative diagnosis. These particular cases require a multidisciplinary team when malignancy is suspected, a hormone secretion excess has been established, and when surgery is envisaged [1]. Indications for adrenal cystic lesions' surgery include a size exceeding 5 cm because of the risk of hemorrhage or other secondary complications, the presence of symptoms, endocrine abnormalities, and suspicion of malignancy [18–20]. All other asymptomatic, small lesions can be only followed by imaging, although no screening protocol has been described [20]. Fine-needle aspiration biopsy cytology of the cystic lesion has been suggested in case if the mass is hormonally inactive specifically excluding pheocromocytoma with nonbenign imaging in which pathology results would directly change management [1, 21]. In 1992, Assalia and Gagner [22] performed the first laparoscopic adrenalectomy which is considered as the gold standard in the treatment of adrenal tumors [11, 18].

Two procedures of laparoscopic adrenalectomy have been described in the literature. The transperitoneal approach is more appropriate to resect large tumors because it allows evaluation of the peritoneal space. However, the retroperitoneal technique provides good visualization of the

Table 3: Comparative table of the previous cases and the present case.

	Clinical presentation	Laboratory assessment	CT scan	Pathology findings	Treatment
Case 1 Nigawara et al., 2009 [15]	Incidental left adrenal mass in a 68-year-old Japanese woman, with obesity and hypertension	Subclinical Cushing's syndrome	Left adrenal tumor (9 × 7 cm) with highly heterogeneous configuration, including foci of calcification. Contrast media stained only the rim of the tumor	Vascular cyst with hyaline degeneration (lining cells were CD34 positive) within an adrenocortical adenoma. Immunohistochemical analysis of steroidogenic enzymes showed the expression of P450scc, 3βHSD, P450c17, and P450c21	Laparoscopic left adrenalectomy
Case 2 Yamada et al., 2011 [16]	Incidental right renal and left adrenal tumors discovered in a 72-year-old Japanese female, with type 2 diabetes mellitus	Normal (nonfunctioning)	Right kidney: an enhanced mass, measuring 3 cm × 3 cm. Left adrenal: a well-demarcated nodule measuring 2 cm, consisting of nonenhanced and low-density areas	Right kidney: eenal clear cell carcinoma. Left adrenal: association of myelolipoma, endothelial cyst, and adrenocortical adenoma. Immunohistochemical analysis: expression of cytochrome P450c17, 3HβSD, and DHEA-sulfotransferase	Right nephrectomy and left adrenalectomy
Case 3 Hong et al., 2020 [17]	Incidental right adrenal mass in a 53-year-old Chinese man with type 2 diabetes	Nonfunctioning adrenal mass	A right circular low-density mass measuring (6 × 7 cm), with a multiroom separation inside the mass. The CT value is 17 HU with no significant enhancement on contrast-enhanced CT	Cystic mass composed of fibrous wall tissues with local calcification. Another mass with a fibrous capsule outside the cystic wall composed of bright and dark cells, which are arranged in acinar and flaky shapes, and a large, deformed nucleus was present in the foci. Immunohistochemistry shows that the cells stained positive for CD34, D2-40, desmin, and SMA	Laparoscopic right adrenalectomy
Case 4 The present case	Incidental left adrenal lesion discovered in a 40-year-old woman, with hypertension and obesity	Subclinical Cushing's syndrome	A rounded well-defined nonenhancing hypodense lesion of the left adrenal measuring 44 × 29 mm in size, with high spontaneous density, and the absolute washout reached 50% with calcification in the wall which did not enhance after contrast injection	Endothelial cyst within an adrenocortical adenoma	Laparoscopic cystic resection and left partial adrenalectomy

retroperitonal anatomy, direct access to the adrenal tumor, and short duration of surgery and minimizes operative bleeding. Several studies have shown that the outcomes of the retroperitonal approach were superior to those of transperitoneal approches regarding adrenal tumors resection. Nevertheless, there is a lack of evidence regarding the effectiveness of the two approaches' comparison in patients [23].

Different methods have been suggested, and complete adrenalectomy was recommended by most authors [11, 24]. According to other papers, adrenal-sparing surgery may be performed after excluding hormone secretion, when the risk of malignancy is considered to be low or when the cyst is found to be large [18]. Furthermore, other centers perform adrenal-sparing resections even in the setting of functioning active tumors such as pheochromocytomas [25]. Moreover, during the last years, partial adrenalectomy has become an accepted alternative in the treatment of adrenal tumors [25, 26], especially for small ones [25]. He et al. [27] performed laparoscopic partial adrenalectomy in 87 Cushing's adenomas and showed that this procedure had extremely low morbidity and achieved an excellent outcome.

In our case, a small cystic tumor discovered at the time of the surgical exploration allowed for partial adrenalectomy.

Open surgery should be advocated either in complicated cases, larger cyst size, or preoperative evidence of massive compression or infiltration of adjacent structures to avoid mini-invasive approaches' complication [19].

To sum up, this is a case of adrenal cyst presenting with subclinical Cushing's syndrome. Preoperative diagnosis was made by CT scan, and laparoscopic partial adrenalectomy was performed without complications. The pathology was consistent with an adrenal endothelial cyst associated with adrenocortical adenoma. As far as we know, this is the fourth reported case of adrenal endothelial cyst associated with adrenocortical adenoma. Although it was regarded as a benign tumor in our particular case, the potential risk of malignancy when managing adrenal cyst should be taken into consideration before any surgery.

Disclosure

Abir Tahri and Wahiba Abdellaoui are the co-first authors.

References

[1] M. Fassnacht, W. Arlt, I. Bancos et al., "Management of adrenal incidentalomas: European society of Endocrinology clinical practice guideline in collaboration with the European network for the study of adrenal tumors," *European Journal of Endocrinology*, vol. 175, no. 2, pp. G1–G34, 2016.

[2] L. M. Weiss, L. J. Medeiros, and A. L. Vickery, "Pathologic features of prognostic significance in adrenocortical carcinoma," *The American Journal of Surgical Pathology*, vol. 13, no. 3, pp. 202–206, 1989.

[3] R. Bellantone, A. Ferrante, M. Raffaelli, M. Boscherini, C. P. Lombardi, and F. Crucitti, "Adrenal cystic lesions: report of 12 surgically treated cases and review of the literature," *Journal of Endocrinological Investigation*, vol. 21, no. 2, pp. 109–114, 1998.

[4] L. M. Neri and F. C. Nance, "Management of adrenal cysts," *The American Surgeon*, vol. 65, pp. 151–163, 1999.

[5] E. Carvounis, A. Marinis, N. Arkadopoulos, T. Theodosopoulos, and V. Smyrniotis, "Vascular adrenal cysts," *Archives of Pathology & Laboratory Medicine*, vol. 130, pp. 1733–1824, 2006.

[6] Y.-C. Chou, C.-W. Lin, C.-K. Wei, J.-E. Tseng, and K.-C. Tseng, "Laparoscopic management of a giant adrenal cyst," *Tzu Chi Medical Journal*, vol. 25, no. 3, pp. 179–181, 2013.

[7] D. G. Foster, "Adrenal cysts," *Archives of Surgery*, vol. 92, no. 1, pp. 131–143, 1966.

[8] C. Torres, J. Y. Ro, M. A. Batt, Y. W. Park, N. G. Ordonez, and A. G. Ayala, "Vascular adrenal cysts: a clinicopathologic and immunohistochemical study of six cases and a review of the literature," *Modern Pathology: An Official Journal of the United States and Canadian Academy of Pathology, Inc*, vol. 10, pp. 530–536, 1997.

[9] A. Wedmid and M. Palese, "Diagnosis and treatment of the adrenal cyst," *Current Urology Reports*, vol. 11, no. 1, pp. 44–50, 2010.

[10] Y. Erbil, A. Salmaslıoğlu, U. Barbaros et al., "Clinical and radiological features of adrenal cysts," *Urologia Internationalis*, vol. 80, no. 1, pp. 31–36, 2008.

[11] G. Cavallaro, D. Crocetti, A. Paliotta et al., "Cystic adrenal lesions: clinical and surgical management. The experience of a referral centre," *International Journal of Surgery*, vol. 13, pp. 23–26, 2015.

[12] M. Terzolo, A. Stigliano, I. Chiodini et al., "AME position statement on adrenal incidentaloma," *European Journal of Endocrinology*, vol. 164, no. 6, pp. 851–870, 2011.

[13] P. J. Kenney and R. J. Stanley, "Calcified adrenal masses," *Urologic Radiology*, vol. 9, no. 1, pp. 9–15, 1988.

[14] L. A. Erickson, R. V. Lloyd, R. Hartman, and G. Thompson, "Cystic adrenal neoplasms," *Cancer*, vol. 101, no. 7, pp. 1537–1544, 2004.

[15] T. Nigawara, S. Sakihara, K. Kageyama et al., "Endothelial cyst of the adrenal gland associated with adrenocortical adenoma: preoperative images simulate carcinoma," *Internal Medicine*, vol. 48, no. 4, pp. 235–240, 2009.

[16] S. Yamada, A. Tanimoto, K.-Y. Wang et al., "Non-functional adrenocortical adenoma: a unique case of combination with myelolipoma and endothelial cysts," *Pathology, Research & Practice*, vol. 207, no. 3, pp. 192–196, 2011.

[17] Y. Hong, Q. Yang, J. Zheng, and G. Hou, "Adrenal endothelial cyst associated with adrenocortical adenoma: a case report and literature review," *Oncology and Translational Medicine February*, vol. 6, no. 1, pp. P43–P45, 2020.

[18] R. Pogorzelski, S. Toutounchi, E. Krajewska et al., "Adrenal cysts - optimal laparoscopic treatment," *Videosurgery and Other Miniinvasive Techniques*, vol. 13, no. 3, pp. 288–291, 2018.

[19] C. Sebastiano, X. Zhao, F.-M. Deng, and K. Das, "Cystic lesions of the adrenal gland: our experience over the last 20 years," *Human Pathology*, vol. 44, no. 9, pp. 1797–1803, 2013.

[20] P. V. Pradeep, A. K. Mishra, V. Aggarwal, P. R. K. Bhargav, S. K. Gupta, and A. Agarwal, "Adrenal cysts: an institutional experience," *World Journal of Surgery*, vol. 30, no. 10, pp. 1817–1820, 2006.

[21] G. A. Tung, R. C. Pfister, N. Papanicolaou, and I. C. Yoder, "Adrenal cysts: imaging and percutaneous aspiration," *Radiology*, vol. 173, no. 1, pp. 107–110, 1989.

[22] A. Assalia and M. Gagner, "Laparoscopic adrenalectomy," *British Journal of Surgery*, vol. 91, no. 10, pp. 1259–1274, 2004.

[23] A. Arezzo, A. Bullano, G. Cochetti et al., "Transperitoneal versus retroperitoneal laparoscopic adrenalectomy for adrenal tumours in adults," *Cochrane Database of Systematic Reviews*, vol. 12, no. 12, p. 2018, 2018.

[24] P. Sadai, S. Arora, and A. J. Greenstein, "The pathological features of surgically managed adrenal cysts: a 15-year retrospective review," *The American Surgeon*, vol. 79, pp. 1159–1162, 2013.

[25] A. Miron, C. Giulea, M. Nădrăgea, and O. Enciu, "Laparoscopic partial adrenalectomy," *Chirurgia*, vol. 112, no. 1, pp. 77–81, 2017.

[26] D. Colleselli and G. Janetschek, "Current trends in partial adrenalectomy," *Current Opinion in Urology*, vol. 25, no. 2, pp. 89–94, 2015.

[27] H.-c. He, J. Dai, Z.-j. Shen et al., "Retroperitoneal adrenal-sparing surgery for the treatment of cushing's syndrome caused by adrenocortical adenoma: 8-year experience with 87 patients," *World Journal of Surgery*, vol. 36, no. 5, pp. 1182–1188, 2012.

29

Homozygous Mutation in the FANCD2 Gene Observed in a Saudi Male Infant with Severe Ambiguous Genitalia

Aida Al Jabri,[1] **Nusaybah Al Naim,**[2] **and Abeer Al Dossari**[2]

[1]*Department of Pediatrics, King Abdulaziz Hospital, Ministry of the National Guard-Health Affairs, King Abdullah International Medical Research Center, King Saud Bin Abdulaziz University for Health Sciences, Al-Ahasa, Saudi Arabia*
[2]*Department of Pediatrics, King Abdulaziz Hospital, Ministry of National Guard-Health Affairs, Al-Ahasa, Saudi Arabia*

Correspondence should be addressed to Aida Al Jabri; dr_aida_s@hotmail.com

Academic Editor: Lucy Mastrandrea

Fanconi anemia (FA) is a rare autosomal recessive inherited disease caused by gene mutations that are primarily involved in the response to or repair of DNA damage. FA characterizes by multiple congenital abnormalities and malformations including growth retardation, renal agenesis, absence of radial bones and thumbs as well, progressive bone marrow failure, irregular skin pigmentation patterns, and increased susceptibility to cancer. FANCD2 gene mutation is believed to be one of the causative mutations in Fanconi anemia, and despite many case reports that link the FANC gene mutation to multiple congenital anomalies and disease, there is no case report found to link it with genitalia abnormalities. In our paper, we report a male Saudi infant who presented to the endocrine clinic at the age of 9 months with severe ambiguous genitalia and found that he carries a homozygous variant mutation in the FANCD2 gene and we face a challenge to treat this patient since there was no previous similar case.

1. Introduction

Fanconi anemia (FA) is a rare autosomal recessive inherited disease caused by gene mutations that are primarily involved in response to or repair of DNA damage. Congenital malformations, progressive bone marrow failure, irregular skin pigmentation patterns, and cancer susceptibility also characterize the disorder [1].

With the exception of FANCB, which is located on the X chromosome, there are more than 15 FANC gene mutations associated with Fanconi anemia. All other FANC genes are autosomal recessive inheritance [2].

There are multiple congenital abnormalities such as growth retardation, renal agenesis, absence of radial bones and thumbs, and radial deviation of the hands that are also correlated with the FANCD2 gene mutation, which is believed to be one of the causative mutations in Fanconi anemia [3], nasopharyngeal carcinoma [4], hepatocellular carcinoma [5], and interstitial nephritis [6].

Although there were many case reports that link the FANC gene mutation to multiple congenital anomalies and diseases, no case report was found to link it with genitalia abnormalities.

There is some evidence in an animal study that FANCB is essential in the male germline and regulates H3K9 methylation on the sex chromosomes during meiosis [7]; also, it was found in one case report that FANCM mutation was linked to primary ovarian insufficiency [8].

In our case, we found that FANCD2 gene mutation was linked to ambiguous genitalia in males. Genital ambiguity considers one of the most important medical emergencies in pediatrics, not only because it is linked to salt wasting and electrolyte imbalance but also because it has long-term psychosocial effects for patients and their families.

The incidence of disorders of sex development (DSD) is not fully known. In 2000, Fausto-Sterling suggested that it corresponds to 1.7% of live births [9].

In one small study conducted in our region (ALHAFOUF) that included 41 newborn infants, it has been found that, in 46, XX karyotype patients, congenital adrenal hyperplasia followed by general malformation disorder was the most common cause of ambiguous genitalia in more than two-thirds of patients while in XY karyotype patients, testosterone pathway biosynthetic defects were the most common cause even in conjunction with a generalized malformation disorder [10].

2. Case Presentation

The case of a 30-month-old Saudi boy from Al-Ahsa is presented. He was born at term with ambiguous genitalia and intrauterine growth restriction (IUGR) with a birth weight of 1.6 kg by normal delivery at a local hospital. He was the fourth child in the family, and his parents are first cousins. There was no family history of ambiguous genitalia, neonatal death, or skeletal abnormalities, and the pregnancy was unremarkable.

After birth, the patient was admitted to the intermediate care nursery (ICN) for 18 days as a neonate with ambiguous genitalia for investigation. He was seen by an endocrinologist at that time, and he found that the baby was not dysmorphic with no midline defect, both gonads were palpated in the well-developed scrotum with severe hypospadias, the Stretched Penile Length (SPL) of 2 cm, and the anus was sited normally; otherwise, the examination was normal. Pelvic ultrasound (US) showed small testes with no female internal genitalia, and karyotype revealed a 46 XY. The impression at that time was a male neonate with severe hypospadias and no disorder of sex development (DSD) and to be seen by the urology team for hypospadias correction.

At the age of 9 months, he was seen by a urologist and his impression was clear ambiguous, so he was referred to another endocrinologist for further investigation and management.

In our clinic, when we saw him and on physical examination (at the age of 9 months), he was pale, with failure to thrive (FTT) and both height and weight below the −2 SD. He was not dysmorphic with no organomegaly. Genitalia exam was ambiguous with severe penile chordee, small phallus with a stretched penile length (SPL) of 2 cm, perineal hypospadias, bifid scrotum, and bilateral small testes. Laboratory investigation performed includes an HCG stimulation test. The injection of 500 international units (IUs) was given over 3 days. Testosterone, dihydrotestosterone, and androstenedione were collected before the first injection and 24 hours after the last one. The results were normal with a testosterone-to-dihydrotestosterone ratio of 10.1 and testosterone-to-androstenedione ratio of 23.

So, we sent a gene to clarify the causes of the ambiguous genitalia which showed homozygous variant (c.2605 + 1G>A p.) mutation in the FANCD2 gene (OMIM: 613984), which was considered as the first homozygous mutation of this gene.

To complete our investigation, electrolytes were normal, and complete blood count (CBC) revealed an iron deficiency anemia (IDA) with hemoglobin of 8.3 mg/dL and a low mean corpuscular volume (MCV) and mean corpuscular hemoglobin (MCH) of 56.8 fL and 18.2 fL, respectively. The red cell distribution width (RDW) was 16%, and the platelet level was normal. A skeletal survey was performed, and it was normal.

So, since this is the first case with such variant and abnormal genitalia and with no previous similar case, we planned to challenge him with testosterone injection; he received a total of 4 doses of 50 mg intramuscular (IM) injection every 4 weeks; in Figure 1, his genitalia before treatment is shown, and Figure 2 shows his genitalia after the last dose.

Genitalia examination after the last dose showed much improvement in the length of his penis with an SPL of 3.5 cm and palpable testes in the scrotum with severe hypospadias. Also, he was treated for the FTT and IDA.

One month after his last injection, he showed further improvement with an SPL of 4.5 cm, and surgical correction for the hypospadias was performed over stages.

3. Discussion and Conclusions

Fanconi anemia (FA) is an autosomal recessive genetic disorder characterized by progressive bone marrow failure, multiple congenital anomalies, and an increased risk of cancer, particularly acute myeloid leukemia [11].

The cellular phenotype is characterized by chromosomal instability and hypersensitivity to DNA interstrand cross-linking (ICL) agents such as mitomycin C (MMC), diepoxybutane, and cisplatin. There are considered to be at least eight complementation groups (FA-A, B, C, D1, D2, E, F, and G) [11].

FANCD2 is an evolutionary gene of Fanconi anemia (FA), and it is considered one of the most important genes that play a key role in reactions to DNA double-strand type damage [12].

Congenital malformations are common, and hematological symptoms occur faster and rapidly progressive in those patients with FANCD2 gene mutation rather than the other patients [12].

Although there were many case reports linking the FANC gene mutation to multiple congenital anomalies and diseases, no case report was found to link this disease with genitalia ambiguity. The phenotype of FA in children has been extensively described before including endocrine and nonendocrine manifestations; male genitalia abnormalities have a high incidence in those patients with FA, and it is around 20% of the FA clinical manifestations. It includes hypoplastic gonads, hypogenitalia, undescended testes, micropenis, cryptorchidism, hypospadias, and hypo-/azoospermia with infertility. Females may also have underdeveloped genitalia and malpositioned uterus with small ovaries [13–16].

There is some evidence in an animal study that FANCB is essential in the male germline and regulates H3K9 methylation on the sex chromosomes during meiosis [7]; also, it was found in one case report that FANCM mutation was linked to primary ovarian insufficiency [8].

In our case, we found that FANCD2 gene mutation was linked to ambiguous genitalia in Saudi male infants.

There are a lot of varieties of disorders under the term ambiguous genitalia which are labeled as DSDs or disorders of sex development. DSDs are categorized as congenital disorders in which chromosomal, gonadal, or anatomical sex

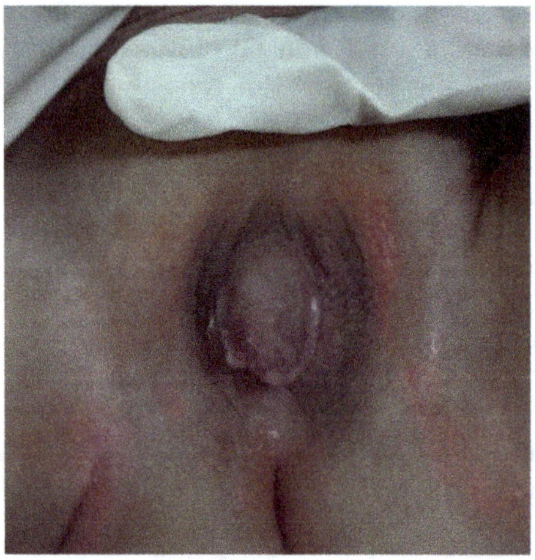

Figure 1: The genitalia before treatment.

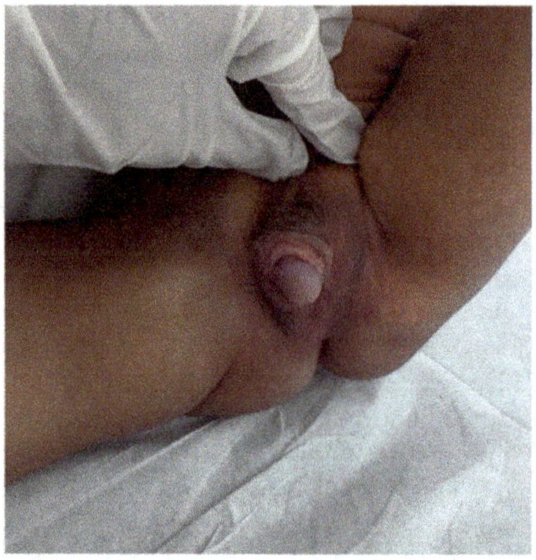

Figure 2: The genitalia after 3 doses of testosterone injection.

development is abnormal, and they include a comprehensive variety of metabolic and anatomical deficiencies and variations which can cause atypical genital appearance, and if left untreated, they can cause distress that is emotional and psychological [17].

Through a well-choreographed, well-coordinated, and localized expression of gene products, a normal sex differentiation and development progress can be developed; furthermore, the gonads, as well as internal and external genital structures all, originating from the same bipotential embryologic tissues are important to be understood or realized [17].

The first migration of bipotential primordial germ cells from the yolk sac endoderm to the urogenital ridges leads to the undifferentiated gonad beginning at 4–6 weeks [17].

Even though, histologically, changes are well underway, the male and female fetuses could not be distinguished in the first 7 weeks of pregnancy which is considered as an indifferent stage. Later on, a switch could occur that signals the determination of the sex and leads to the initiation of testicular or ovarian gonadal differentiation [17].

In normal sexual differentiation, several genes are involved. The molecular events of testis formation are triggered by the sex-determining region on the Y chromosome (SRY) [18]. Congenital adrenal hyperplasia (CAH) is one of the most causes of ambiguous genitalia. Wide-ranging phenotypes from a salt-wasting adrenal crisis in the infant to virilization in young females delayed puberty in adolescents, and even polycystic ovary syndrome- (PCOS-) like symptoms (i.e., acne, irregular menses, hirsutism, and infertility) in young women are as a result of a collection of different adrenal steroid biosynthetic disorders. In any virilized infant with nonpalpable gonads, CAH should be the primary consideration [17].

The treatment of the abnormal genital is considered a challenge for the pediatrician and endocrinologist providing care. It is crucial to determine the cause and treat it as soon as possible to minimize the medical, psychological, and social complications. It can be a mild form that required only testosterone injection to surgical sex reverse in the severe form [19, 20].

In our case, the treatment was a challenge since no case report before describes the same manifestation; however, we succeeded in treating him with testosterone injection, although we had to follow him up for further pubertal assessment.

Consent

Written informed consent was obtained from the patient for publication of this case report and the accompanying images.

References

[1] W. Deng, M. Zhao, Y. Liu, L. Cao, and M. Yang, "Fanconi anemia in twins with neutropenia: a case report," *Oncology Letters*, vol. 16, no. 4, pp. 5325–5330, 2018.

[2] J. Soulier, "Fanconi anemia," *Hematology*, vol. 2011, no. 1, pp. 492–497, 2011.

[3] R. Vazharova, S. Vragaleva, V. Dimitrova et al., "Novel hypomorphic mutation in FANCD2 gene observed in a fetus with multiple congenital anomalies," *Case Reports in Obstetrics and Gynecology*, vol. 2016, Article ID 1462818, 4 pages, 2016.

[4] S. Xu, F. Zhao, Z. Liang et al., "Expression of FANCD2 is associated with prognosis in patients with nasopharyngeal carcinoma," *International Journal of Clinical and Experimental Pathology*, vol. 12, no. 9, p. 3465, 2019.

[5] H. Komatsu, T. Masuda, T. Lguchi et al., "Clinical significance of FANCD2 gene expression and its association with tumor progression in hepatocellular carcinoma," *Anticancer Research*, vol. 37, no. 3, pp. 1083–1090, 2017.

[6] R. Airik, M. Schueler, M. Airik et al., "A FANCD2/FANCI-associated nuclease 1-knockout model develops karyomegalic interstitial nephritis," *Journal of the American Society of Nephrology*, vol. 27, no. 12, pp. 3552–3559, 2016.

[7] Y. Kato, K. G. Alavattam, H.-S. Sin et al., "FANCB is essential in the male germline and regulates H3K9 methylation on the sex chromosomes during meiosis," *Human Molecular Genetics*, vol. 24, no. 18, pp. 5234–5249, 2015.

[8] B. Fouquet, P. Pawlikowska, S Caburet et al., "A homozygous FANCM mutation underlies a familial case of non-syndromic primary ovarian insufficiency," *Elife*, vol. 6, Article ID e30490, 2017.

[9] G. B. De Paula, B. A. Barros, S. Carpini et al., "408 cases of genital ambiguity followed by single multidisciplinary team during 23 years: etiologic diagnosis and sex of rearing," *International Journal of Endocrinology*, vol. 2016, Article ID 4963574, 9 pages, 2016.

[10] A. N. Al Mulhim and H. M. Kamal, "Ambiguous genitalia in neonates: a 4-year prospective study in a localized area," *EMHJ-eastern Mediterranean Health Journal*, vol. 16, no. 2, pp. 214–217, 2010.

[11] S. Hussain, E. Witt, P. A. Huber, A. L. Medhurst, A. Ashworth, and C. G. Mathew, "Direct interaction of the Fanconi anaemia protein FANCG with BRCA2/FANCD1," *Human Molecular Genetics*, vol. 12, no. 19, pp. 2503–2510, 2003.

[12] R. Kalb, K. Neveling, H. Hoehn et al., "Hypomorphic mutations in the gene encoding a key Fanconi anemia protein, FANCD2, sustain a significant group of FA-D2 patients with severe phenotype," *The American Journal of Human Genetics*, vol. 80, no. 5, pp. 895–910, 2007.

[13] M. Tischkowitz and I. Dokal, "Fanconi anaemia and leukaemia - clinical and molecular aspects," *British Journal of Haematology*, vol. 126, no. 2, pp. 176–191, 2004.

[14] M. Schneider, K. Chandler, M. Tischkowitz, and S. Meyer, "Fanconi anaemia: genetics, molecular biology, and cancer-implications for clinical management in children and adults," *Clinical Genetics*, vol. 88, no. 1, pp. 13–24, 2015.

[15] C. Feben, T. Wainstein, J. Kromberg, F. Essop, and A. Krause, "Fanconi anaemia in South Africa: past, present and future," *South African Medical Journal*, vol. 108, no. 5, pp. 393–398, 2018.

[16] A. D. Auerbach, "Fanconi anemia and its diagnosis," *Mutation Research*, vol. 668, no. 1-2, pp. 4–10, 2009 Jul 31.

[17] J. A. Indyk, "Disorders/differences of sex development (DSDs) for primary care: the approach to the infant with ambiguous genitalia," *Translational Pediatrics*, vol. 6, no. 4, pp. 323–334, 2017.

[18] M. El-Sherbiny, "Disorders of sexual differentiation: I. Genetics and pathology," *Arab Journal of Urology*, vol. 11, no. 1, pp. 19–26, 2013.

[19] S. Nimkarn, S. Likitmaskul, P. Sangacharoenkit et al., "Ambiguous genitalia: an overview of 22 years experience and the diagnostic approach in the Pediatric Department, Siriraj Hospital," *Journal of the Medical Association of Thailand*, vol. 85, pp. S496–S505, 2002.

[20] G. Göllü, R. V. Yıldız, M. Bingol-Kologlu et al., "Ambiguous genitalia: an overview of 17 years' experience," *Journal of Pediatric Surgery*, vol. 42, no. 5, pp. 840–844, 2007.

30

Adverse Effects of Ramadan Fasting in a Girl with Salt-Losing Congenital Adrenal Hyperplasia

Valeria Calcaterra[1,2] **Francesco Bassanese,**[3] **Andrea Martina Clemente,**[3] **Rossella Amariti,**[1,3] **Corrado Regalbuto,**[3] **Anna Sala,**[2,4] **and Gian Vincenzo Zuccotti**[2,4]

[1]*Pediatric and Adolescent Unit, Department of Internal Medicine University of Pavia, Pavia, Italy*
[2]*Department of Pediatrics, Children' Hospital "Vittore Buzzi", Milan, Italy*
[3]*Pediatric Unit, Department of the Mother and Child Health Fondazione IRCCS Policlinico San Matteo and University of Pavia, Pavia, Italy*
[4]*Department of Biomedical and Clinical Science "L. Sacco", University of Milano, Milano, Italy*

Correspondence should be addressed to Valeria Calcaterra; valeria.calcaterra@unipv.it

Academic Editor: Toshihiro Kita

Objective. Congenital adrenal hyperplasia (CAH) is the most common cause of adrenal insufficiency in pediatrics. Chronic glucocorticoid replacement is the mainstay of treatment in the classic forms of CAH, and mineralocorticoid replacement therapy is mandatory in the salt-wasting form. Fasting is a mild stressor, which can expose to dehydration, hypotension, hypoglycemia, and acute adrenal crisis in patients with adrenal insufficiency. *Case.* We report the case of an adolescent affected by the classic form with salt-losing CAH, who observed Ramadan for 30 days, without individualized therapeutic management plan. After Ramadan, a dramatic increase of ACTH level (1081 pg/ml, n.v. 6–57), reduced cortisolemia, tendency to hypotension, and weight loss were recorded. She experienced insomnia, intense thirst, asthenia, and headache. The symptoms disappeared restarting the previous therapy schedule and increasing the total hydrocortisone daily dose with progressive restoring of hormonal control. *Conclusion.* Our case confirms that patients with CAH are vulnerable, especially during fasting in Ramadan, with a higher risk of acute adrenal crisis. CAH patients should reform and individualize their treatment plan and be submitted to careful monitoring.

1. Introduction

Congenital adrenal hyperplasia (CAH) is the most common cause of adrenal insufficiency in pediatrics [1]. CAH comprises a family of autosomal recessive disorders that impair adrenal steroidogenesis; the main form is due to 21-hydroxylase deficiency (21-OHD) associated with mutations in the 21-hydroxylase gene (6p21). In the case of 21-OHD, the phenotypic spectrum includes salt wasting, simple virilizing, and late onset form. The "classic form" includes salt wasting and simple virilizing forms. The "late-onset or nonclassic form" includes milder forms [1]. However, this classification system is somewhat artificial because of disease severity due to a continuum based on residual enzyme activity [2]. Chronic glucocorticoid replacement is the mainstay of treatment in the classic forms of CAH. Mineralocorticoid replacement is also necessary in salt-wasting form. Patients in glucocorticoid treatment must double or triple hydrocortisone dose during intercurrent illness (fever and gastrointestinal illness), stressful life events, surgery, or trauma in order to prevent adrenal crisis [3].

Fasting is usually considered as a mild stressor. It can expose to dehydration, hypotension, hypoglycemia, and acute adrenal crisis in patients with adrenal insufficiency. Ramadan fasting is the fourth pillar of Islam. During this holy month, Muslims must abstain from drinking, eating, and even taking oral medications, from sunrise to sunset. This practice is request to all the Muslims, beginning from adolescence, excluding pregnant women and ill subjects in which Ramadan can be dangerous [4]. Nevertheless, some people with chronic conditions still want to adhere fasting during Ramadan.

Here, we report the case of an adolescent affected by the classic form with salt-losing CAH, who observed Ramadan for 30 days, without individualized therapeutic management plan.

2. Case Report

The patient is a 13-year-old girl, third child of non-consanguineous parents, born at the end of a normal course pregnancy, by eutocic birth. Increased 17-OHP level (252 nmol/L) was found at Guthrie neonatal screening and confirmed by a second test (440 nmol/L). Classical CAH form with salt losing was diagnosed, and replacement therapy with hydrocortisone, acetate fludrocortisone, and NaCl oral supplementation was therefore started. During infancy and childhood, there were no remarkable events in her medical history except for episodes of febrile convulsions; secondary enuresis at the age of 6 was treated with oxybutynin for 6 months. Growth and neuropsycomotory development were normal. Menarche occurred at 12 years. During the follow-up (10 years), therapeutic adjustment in medications was related to weight gain and stress periods (fever). Despite the adherence of the therapy was not always optimal, major complications never occurred. The data at the last checkup visit (4 months before Ramadan beginning) are reported in Table 1. Without consulting our clinic or agreeing on therapeutic plans, the girl begins Ramadan, which she completes after a total of 30 days. During Ramadan, the girl observed fasting from sunrise to sunset, having dinner at 9 pm, snacks at midnight, and abundant breakfast at 4 am. Consequently, the patient modified therapy schedule as reported in Table 1. At the periodic endocrinological evaluation, which almost coincided with the end of Ramadan, we found a dramatic increase of ACTH level (1081 pg/ml, n.v. 6–57), reduced cortisolemia (5 mcg/dl, n.v. 4.3–22.2), tendency to hypotension, and important weight loss (−12.5% of body weight) (Table 1).

From the anamnestic collection, it emerged that, during the fasting period, the girl presented some difficulty falling asleep in the first days of Ramadan. She complained intense thirst and strong predilection for salty foods, mainly due to the fast and the saline loss, compensated only during the night. She also reported onset of asthenia and episodes of daytime headache. During this control visit, we prescribed restoring the previous therapy schedule and increasing the total hydrocortisone daily dose to 30 mg. One month after this therapeutic change, the ACTH level was diminished, still indicative of poor control of the CAH, but the symptoms had disappeared, and body weight increased by 2 kg. Four months later, at the end of Ramadan, ACTH hematic level further reduced, and the cortisolemia was within normal ranges. Progressive restoring of hormonal control was reached (Table 1).

Finally, the patient and the family discussed on the seriousness of the decision taken and on the risks that the girl could have faced.

3. Discussion

Fasting during Ramadan is a stressful period, in which food and fluid ingestion are restricted from sunrise to sunset for a complete month, each year. As in our patient, during Ramadan, the disruption of feeding and sleep schedules in lack of an adequate adaptation in therapeutic management influences the stress system response and leads to the disruption of the cortisol circadian pattern, with lower levels in the morning and higher in the evening.

The dysregulation of the cortisol circadian rhythm, which acts as a regulator between central and peripheral clocks in different tissues, can have metabolic adverse effects. In patients with adrenal insufficiency, particularly in subjects with classic CAH, Ramadan fasting exposes to the risk of hypoglycemia and dehydration, and this practice could be fatal [5]. Fatigue and asthenia, as noted in this case, can occur as symptoms of the hypoglycemic events. The pathogenic mechanism underlying hypoglycemia is accounted to low levels of cortisolemia, reduction of hepatic gluconeogenesis, and increased sensitivity to insulin, due to relationship between the cortisol rhythm and the insulin resistance rhythm [5]. Fasting shifts from carbohydrates to fatty acid metabolism, using ketones as a major cellular fuel source for the body. In lack of exogenous glucose, counterregulatory hormones, such as glucagon, epinephrine, cortisol, and growth hormone, stimulate hepatic glycogenolysis and gluconeogenesis to maintain glycemic homeostasis. A prevalent use of fatty acids from adipose tissue may also induce body weight loss. Although this reduction may seem beneficial, an exacerbation of this mechanism could lead to an acute adrenal crisis [5].

The distortion of adrenal hormones during Ramadan fasting is also attributed to changes in sleep and activity timing. Sleep rhythm and changes in metabolic status are closely and reciprocally bound: sleeping rhythm alteration can cause distortion of adrenal hormone excretion, and alteration of these later can affect the circadian rhythm, leading to sleep alteration. In our case, sleeplessness could be related to higher levels of cortisol in the evening, due to the assumption of two doses of hydrocortisone close to bedtime, when maximal glucocorticoid sensitivity of peripheral tissues is reported [4, 6]. The observed metabolic impairments during Ramadan practice highlight the need of an individualized therapeutic management plan; intramuscular hydrocortisone [7], subcutaneous glucocorticoids pumps [8], and use of long acting steroids such as dexamethasone and prednisone instead of hydrocortisone [6] could be considered as therapeutic options to adhere Ramadan.

Furthermore, they might adequate their diet habits (avoiding sugars, processed starches, caffeine, and other stimulant drugs, supplementing salt, and drinking nonsugar-laden liquids) and physical activity (increasing resting in fasting and hotter hours). Education of these patients and caregivers is mandatory to recognize warning symptoms of adrenal insufficiency, such as asthenia, nausea, and/or vomiting [9].

Table 1: Hormonal panel (8 am), blood pressure, body weight, and therapy of our patient before, during, and after Ramadan.

	Before Ramadan	During Ramadan	3 days after Ramadan	1 month after Ramadan	8 months after Ramadan
ACTH (pg/ml, n.v. 6–57)	236	na	1081	875	16.3
17-OHP (ng/ml, n.v. 0.1–1)	3.7	na	2.4	na	0.7
Cortisol (mcg/dl, n.v. 4.3–22.2)	20.6	na	5	13.2	11.6
Blood pressure (mmHg)	125/80	na	90/60	120/80	110/60
Weight (kg)	62	na	54	56	59
Hydrocortisone	8 am: 10 mg 1 pm: 10 mg 8 pm: 5 mg	4 am: 10 mg 9 pm: 10 mg Midnight: 5 mg	8 am: 10 mg 1 pm: 10 mg 8 pm: 10 mg	8 am: 10 mg 1 pm: 10 mg 8 pm: 10 mg	8 am: 10 mg 1 pm: 10 mg 8 pm: 10 mg
Fludrocortisone	1 pm: 0.1 mg	9 pm: 0.1 mg	1 pm: 0.1 mg	1 pm: 0.1 mg	1 pm: 0.1 mg

na = not available.

In conclusion, our case confirms that patients with CAH are vulnerable, especially during fasting in Ramadan, with a higher risk of acute adrenal crisis. CAH patients should reform and individualize their treatment plan and be submitted to careful monitoring.

Authors' Contributions

VC conceptualized, investigated, wrote, reviewed, and edited the study; AMC, FB, RA, CR, GVZ, and AS prepared the original draft, reviewed, and edited the article; and GVZ and VC supervised the study. All authors read and approved the submitted version.

References

[1] M. Auron and N. Raissouni, "Adrenal insufficiency," *Pediatrics in Review*, vol. 36, no. 3, pp. 92–103, 2015.

[2] S. F. Witchel, "Congenital adrenal hyperplasia," *Journal of Pediatric and Adolescent Gynecology*, vol. 30, no. 5, pp. 520–534, 2017.

[3] D. El-Maouche, W. Arlt, and D. P. Merke, "Congenital adrenal hyperplasia," *The Lancet*, vol. 390, no. 10108, pp. 2194–2210, 2017.

[4] S. O. Qasrawi, S. R. Pandi-Perumal, and A. S. Bahammam, "The effect of intermittent fasting during Ramadan on sleep, sleepiness, cognitive function, and circadian rhythm," *Sleep and Breathing*, vol. 21, no. 3, pp. 577–586, 2017.

[5] M. Debono, "Fasting during the Ramadan: a challenge for patients with adrenal insufficiency," *Endocrine*, vol. 57, pp. 196–198, 2017.

[6] N. C. Nicolaides, E. Charmandari, G. P. Chrousos, and T. Kino, "Recent advances in the molecular mechanisms determining tissue sensitivity to glucocorticoids: novel mutations, circadian rhythm and ligand-induced repression of the human glucocorticoid receptor," *BMC Endocrine Disorders*, vol. 14, p. 71, 2014.

[7] G. L. Chrisp, A. M. Maguire, M. Quartararo et al., "Variations in the management of acute illness in children with congenital adrenal hyperplasia: an audit of three paediatric hospitals," *Clinical Endocrinology*, vol. 89, no. 5, pp. 577–585, 2018.

[8] A. Khanna, R. Khurana, A. Kyriacou, R. Davies, and D. W. Ray, "Management of adrenocortical insufficiency with continuous subcutaneous hydrocortisone infusion: long-term experience in three patients," *Endocrinology, Diabetes & Metabolism Case Reports*, vol. 2015, Article ID 150005, 2015.

[9] S. Siddiqi, S. Khan, M. F. Pathan et al., "Guidelines regarding management of adrenal insufficiency in the Holy month of Ramadan," *Indian Journal of Endocrinology and Metabolism*, vol. 16, no. 4, pp. 519–521, 2012.

31

Dapagliflozin-Induced Acute Pancreatitis: A Case Report and Review of Literature

Sunam M. Sujanani, Mohanad M. Elfishawi, Paria Zarghamravanbaksh, Francisco J. Cuevas Castillo, and David M. Reich

Department of Medicine, Icahn School of Medicine at Mount Sinai, NYC Health and Hospitals/Queens, Jamaica, NY 11432, USA

Correspondence should be addressed to Sunam M. Sujanani; sunam.m.sujanani@gmail.com

Academic Editor: J. Paul Frindik

Sodium-glucose cotransporter 2 (SGLT2) inhibitors are increasingly used as add-on therapy in patients with poorly controlled type 2 diabetes mellitus (T2DM). Although pancreatitis is not a known side effect of SGLT-2 inhibitors, there have been case reports of SGLT-2 inhibitor use being associated with pancreatitis. *Case Presentation*. A 51-year-old male with a history of type 2 diabetes, dyslipidemia, and status-post cholecystectomy presented to the emergency room with a four-day history of periumbilical pain radiating to the back. He denied any history of recent alcohol intake or prior episodes of pancreatitis. On physical examination, his abdomen was diffusely tender to palpation without guarding or rebound. Initial labs were notable for a leukocyte count of 9.3×10^9/L, creatinine level of 0.72 mg/dL, calcium level of 9.5 mg/dL, lipase level of 262 U/L, and triglyceride level of 203 mg/dL. His last HbA1c was 8.5%. CT scan of his abdomen and pelvis showed findings consistent with acute pancreatitis with no biliary ductal dilatation. Careful review of his medications revealed the patient was recently started on dapagliflozin five days prior to admission in addition to his longstanding regimen of insulin detemir, sitagliptin, metformin, and rosuvastatin. His symptoms resolved after discontinuation of sitagliptin and dapagliflozin. A year later, due to increasing HbA1c levels, a decision was made to rechallenge the patient with dapagliflozin, after which he developed another episode of acute pancreatitis. His symptoms resolved upon cessation of dapagliflozin. *Conclusion*. This case highlights the possible association of SGLT-2 inhibitors and pancreatitis. Patients should be informed about the symptoms of acute pancreatitis and advised to discontinue SGLT-2 inhibitors in case such symptoms occur.

1. Introduction

Type 2 diabetes mellitus (T2DM) is the most common cause of end-stage renal failure requiring hemodialysis and is the seventh leading cause of mortality in the United States [1]. Several treatment options are used in the management of T2DM including insulin, metformin, glucagon like peptide-1 (GLP-1) receptor agonists, dipeptidyl peptidase-4 (DPP-4) inhibitors, and sodium-glucose cotransporter-2 (SGLT-2) inhibitors [2].

SGLT-2 inhibitors are a novel class of diabetes medications that work by decreasing glucose reabsorption in the kidney, thereby increasing renal glucose elimination and reducing blood glucose levels [3].

Empagliflozin, dapagliflozin, canagliflozin, and ertugliflozin are members of the SGLT-2 inhibitor class that have been approved by the Food and Drug Administration (FDA) [4]. SGLT-2 inhibitors are increasingly being used as add-on therapy in patients with inadequately controlled T2DM [2, 5]. In addition, empagliflozin and canagliflozin have also been shown to improve cardiovascular and renal outcomes in patients with T2DM [6–9]. Interestingly, dapagliflozin was shown to reduce the risk for congestive heart failure exacerbation [10, 11]. Adverse effects reported with this class of medications include genitourinary tract infections, urinary frequency, and rarely euglycemic diabetic ketoacidosis (DKA) [12, 13].

Table 1: Published case reports for SGLT-2 inhibitor-induced pancreatitis in the literature.

Author	SGLT-2 inhibitor	Age/sex	Ethnicity	Other reported medications	Time from medication administration until pancreatitis	Severity (description) and outcome
Patel et al. [14]	Canagliflozin	71/F	Not specified	Metformin, sitagliptin	84 days	Necrotizing pancreatitis, resolved
Chowdhary et al. [15]	Canagliflozin	33/F	African-American	Metformin, levothyroxine	14 days	Severe acute pancreatitis, resolved
Srivali et al. [16]	Canagliflozin	50/M	White	Metformin, glyburide	10 days	Acute pancreatitis precipitating DKA, resolved
Verma [17]	Canagliflozin	46/F	White	Metformin, insulin, lisinopril, lovastatin, citalopram, estradiol, oxybutynin	21 days	Moderately severe acute pancreatitis, resolved
Gutch et al. [18]	Dapagliflozin	48/M	Indian	Metformin	7 days	Acute pancreatitis precipitating DKA, resolved
McIntire and Bayne [19]	Empagliflozin	70/M	African-American	Insulin, HCTZ, lisinopril, atenolol, ibuprofen, ranitidine, simvastatin, simethicone	104 days	Mild pancreatitis, resolved
Lightbourne et al. [20]	Empagliflozin	52/F	Not specified	Metformin, insulin, furosemide	30 days	Acute pancreatitis, resolved

This report illustrates a case of acute pancreatitis precipitated by the addition of dapagliflozin to long-standing sitagliptin-metformin therapy and highlights the possible association between SGLT-2 inhibitors and pancreatitis.

2. Case Report

A 51-year-old Hispanic male with a past medical history significant for T2DM, dyslipidemia, and cholecystitis status-post cholecystectomy seven years ago presented to the emergency room with a four-day history of periumbilical pain radiating to the back along with nausea and decreased appetite. He denied any history of recent alcohol intake, autoimmune disorders, or prior episodes of acute pancreatitis. He is an active smoker (five cigarettes per day since thirty years).

On presentation, vital signs included a temperature of 36.4°C (97.5°F), pulse of 77 beats per minute, blood pressure of 155/96 mm Hg, respiratory rate of 18, and oxygen saturation of 100% on room air. Physical examination was remarkable for tenderness to light palpation diffusely in his abdomen with no guarding or rebound. Initial labs were notable for a leukocyte count of 9.3×10^9/L, serum creatinine level of 0.72 mg/dL, serum calcium level of 9.5 mg/dL, serum lipase level of 262 U/L, and serum triglyceride level of 203 mg/dL. His last hemoglobin A1c one month prior to presentation was 8.5%. CT scan of his abdomen and pelvis showed status-post cholecystectomy with no biliary ductal dilatation, along with findings consistent with acute pancreatitis. Patient was placed nil per os (NPO), and outpatient oral medications were held. He was managed with IV fluids, antiemetics, and insulin.

Careful review of his medications revealed that the patient was started on dapagliflozin 10 mg daily five days prior to admission in addition to his long-standing regimen of insulin detemir 20 units twice daily, sitagliptin-metformin 50–1000 mg twice daily, and rosuvastatin 20 mg daily. The patient's symptoms improved within two days, and his diet was advanced. Upon discharge, insulin, metformin, and rosuvastatin were resumed. Dapagliflozin and sitagliptin were discontinued in light of the episode of pancreatitis. One month after discharge, glimepiride was added to his regimen by his endocrinologist.

Three-month, six-month, and nine-month follow-up visits revealed no further episodes of pancreatitis, but due to increasing hemoglobin A1c levels and lack of ample evidence of dapagliflozin precipitating pancreatitis, a decision was made to rechallenge the patient with dapagliflozin 10 mg in addition to continuing the concurrent regimen of insulin detemir, metformin, and glimepiride. The patient presented to the emergency room seven days after initiation of dapagliflozin with complaints of three-day history of nausea and epigastric pain radiating to the back. Laboratory findings were notable for a leukocyte count of 8.9×10^9/L and serum lipase level of 138 U/L. CT scan of his abdomen and pelvis revealed findings suggestive of acute pancreatitis. Dapagliflozin was subsequently discontinued with resolution of symptoms. There has been no recurrence of pancreatitis since discontinuation of dapagliflozin.

3. Discussion

SGLT-2 inhibitors are being considered as possible causes of pancreatitis. Review of literature shows seven published case reports of acute pancreatitis attributed to SGLT-2 inhibitors. Four of them were associated with canagliflozin, two with empagliflozin, and one with dapagliflozin (Table 1).

Among these seven studies, the mean age of patients is 52.8 (range from 33–71), three were males, and four were females. The time interval between the initiation of SGLT-2 inhibitors and pancreatitis was 7 days with dapagliflozin,

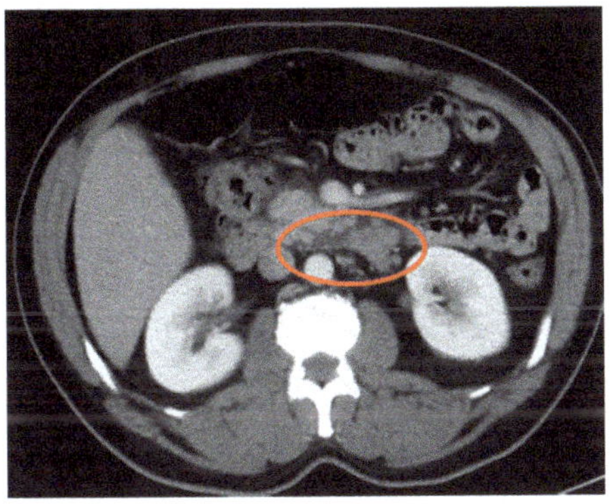

Figure 1: CT scan after initial presentation of acute pancreatitis.

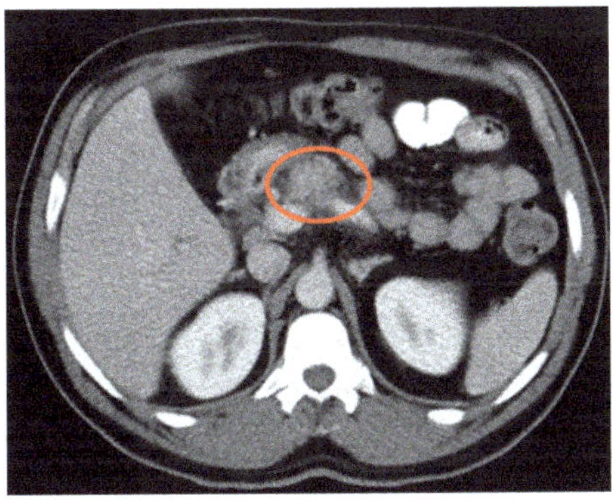

Figure 2: CT scan after subsequent episode of acute pancreatitis.

10–84 days with canagliflozin, and 30–104 days with empagliflozin. In our case report, the time interval was around 5 days after initiation of dapagliflozin in the initial presentation and subsequent presentation of pancreatitis upon rechallenge with dapagliflozin.

Metformin was listed as a concomitant diabetes medication in all published case reports with canagliflozin and dapagliflozin and one with empagliflozin. One possible mechanism could involve dehydration and lactic acidosis, leading to pancreatitis [21].

In this report, the patient presented with a picture of acute pancreatitis in the setting of newly introduced dapagliflozin in the absence of a known cause of pancreatitis such as alcohol or gallstones. Furthermore, the recurrence of pancreatitis upon rechallenge with dapagliflozin and the resolution of symptoms after dapagliflozin cessation make it a likely cause of pancreatitis.

The underlying mechanism of dapagliflozin-induced pancreatitis is unclear. It is likely to be an idiosyncratic reaction similar to other cases of drug-induced pancreatitis, occurring as a result of immunological or cytotoxic effects of the drug or its metabolites on the body [22, 23].

In conclusion, this report highlights the possible association of SGLT-2 inhibitors and pancreatitis. Patients should be informed about the symptoms of acute pancreatitis and advised to discontinue SGLT-2 inhibitors in case such symptoms occur.

SGLT-2 inhibitors, although approved for the management of T2DM, should be prescribed with caution particularly in patients with increased risk for pancreatitis. Regulatory entities such as the FDA and Health Canada have identified a potential safety issue and possible link between SGLT-2 inhibitors and acute pancreatitis [24, 25]. Further studies are required to investigate the exact etiology of the reported adverse reaction to the medication.

Figures 1 and 2 depict the patient's abnormal CT scan revealing findings of acute pancreatitis.

Disclosure

Portions of this study have been presented in abstract form at the Medical Society of the State of New York Resident, Fellow and Medical Student Poster Symposium in April 2019.

References

[1] U. S. Department of Health and Human Services, Centers for Disease Control and PreventionPrevention *C for DC and National Diabetes Fact Sheet: National Estimates and General Information on Diabetes and Prediabetes in the United States, 2011*, U.S. Department of Health and. Human Services, Centers for Disease Control and Prevention, Atlanta, GA, USA, 2011.

[2] A. J. Garber, M. J. Abrahamson, J. I. Barzilay et al., "Consensus statement by the American association of clinical endocrinologists and American college of endocrinology on the comprehensive type 2 diabetes management algorithm -2018 executive summary," *Endocrine Practice*, vol. 24, no. 1, pp. 91–120, 2018.

[3] A. J. Scheen, "Pharmacodynamics, efficacy and safety of sodium-glucose Co-transporter type 2 (SGLT2) inhibitors for the treatment of type 2 diabetes mellitus," *Drugs*, vol. 75, no. 1, pp. 33–59, 2015.

[4] M. Busko, "FDA approves SGLT2 inhibitor ertugliflozin for type 2 diabetes," 2018, http://www.medscape.com/viewarticle/890446.

[5] J. Bolinder, Ö. Ljunggren, J. Kullberg et al., "Effects of dapagliflozin on body weight, total fat mass, and regional adipose tissue distribution in patients with type 2 diabetes mellitus with inadequate glycemic control on metformin," *The Journal of Clinical Endocrinology & Metabolism*, vol. 97, no. 3, pp. 1020–1031, 2012.

[6] B. Zinman, C. Wanner, J. M. Lachin et al., "Empagliflozin, cardiovascular outcomes, and mortality in type 2 diabetes," *New England Journal of Medicine*, vol. 373, no. 22, pp. 2117–2128, 2015.

[7] C. Wanner, S. E. Inzucchi, J. M. Lachin et al., "Empagliflozin and progression of kidney disease in type 2 diabetes," *New England Journal of Medicine*, vol. 375, no. 4, pp. 323–334, 2016.

[8] V. Perkovic, M. J. Jardine, B. Neal et al., "Canagliflozin and renal outcomes in type 2 diabetes and nephropathy," *New England Journal of Medicine*, vol. 380, no. 24, pp. 2295–2306, 2019.

[9] K. I. Birkeland, M. E. Jørgensen, B. Carstensen et al., "Cardiovascular mortality and morbidity in patients with type 2 diabetes following initiation of sodium-glucose co-transporter-2 inhibitors versus other glucose-lowering drugs (CVD-REAL Nordic): a multinational observational analysis," *The Lancet Diabetes & Endocrinology*, vol. 5, no. 9, pp. 709–717, 2017.

inhibitors versus other glucose-lowering drugs (CVD-REAL Nordic): a multinational observational analysis," *The Lancet Diabetes & Endocrinology*, vol. 5, no. 9, pp. 709–717, 2017.

[10] S. D. Wiviott, I. Raz, M. P. Bonaca et al., "Dapagliflozin and cardiovascular outcomes in type 2 diabetes," *New England Journal of Medicine*, vol. 380, no. 4, pp. 347–357, 2019.

[11] J. J. V. McMurray, S. D. Solomon, S. E. Inzucchi et al., "Dapagliflozin in patients with heart failure and reduced ejection fraction," *New England Journal of Medicine*, vol. 381, no. 21, pp. 1995–2008, 2019.

[12] G. Musso, R. Gambino, M. Cassader, and G. Pagano, "A novel approach to control hyperglycemia in type 2 diabetes: sodium glucose co-transport (SGLT) inhibitors. Systematic review and meta-analysis of randomized trials," *Annals of Medicine*, vol. 44, no. 4, pp. 375–393, 2012.

[13] J. Rosenstock and E. Ferrannini, "Euglycemic diabetic ketoacidosis: a predictable, detectable, and preventable safety concern with SGLT2 inhibitors," *Diabetes Care*, vol. 38, no. 9, pp. 1638–1642, 2015.

[14] K. M. Patel, E. Pikas, and T. George, "Drug-induced necrotizing pancreatitis with a focus on canagliflozin," *American Journal of Therapeutics*, vol. 24, no. 4, p. e496, 2017.

[15] M. Chowdhary, A. Kabbani, and A. Chhabra, "Canagliflozin-induced pancreatitis: a rare side effect of a new drug," *Therapeutics and Clinical Risk Management*, vol. 11, pp. 991–994, 2015.

[16] N. Srivali, C. Thongprayoon, W. Cheungpasitporn, and P. Ungprasert, "Acute pancreatitis in the use of canagliflozin: a rare side-effect of the novel therapy for type 2 diabetes mellitus," *Journal of Basic and Clinical Pharmacy*, vol. 6, no. 3, pp. 101-102, 2015.

[17] R. Verma, "Canagliflozin-associated acute pancreatitis," *American Journal of Therapeutics*, vol. 23, no. 3, pp. e972–e973, 2016.

[18] M. Gutch, A. Bhattacharya, S. Kumar, R. K. Pahan, and R. S. Singh, "Dapagliflozin induced pancreatitis," *International Journal of Medicine and Public Health*, vol. 8, no. 1, pp. 45–47, 2018.

[19] D. R. McIntire and D. B. Bayne, "Empagliflozin-induced pancreatitis," *Annals of Pharmacotherapy*, vol. 52, no. 11, pp. 1158-1159, 2018.

[20] T. Lightbourne, N. Najafian, T. R. McCarty, and McCarty, "Consideration for empagliflozin-associated pancreatitis," *American Journal of Gastroenterology*, vol. 112, p. S710, 2017.

[21] R. S. Hundal and S. E. Inzucchi, "Metformin," *Drugs*, vol. 63, no. 18, pp. 1879–1894, 2003.

[22] W. Y. Hung and O. Abreu Lanfranco, "Contemporary review of drug-induced pancreatitis: a different perspective," *World Journal of Gastrointestinal Pathophysiology*, vol. 5, no. 4, pp. 405–415, 2014.

[23] N. Badalov, R. Baradarian, K. Iswara, J. Li, W. Steinberg, and S. Tenner, "Drug-induced acute pancreatitis: an evidence-based review," *Clinical Gastroenterology and Hepatology*, vol. 5, no. 6, pp. 648–661, 2017.

[24] Summary Safety Review-Health Canada, *SGLT2 Inhibitors (Canagliflozin, Dapagliflozin and Empagliflozin)-Health*, Government of Canada, Ottawa, Canada, 2016, https://hpr-rps.hres.ca/reg-content/summary-safety-review-detail.php?lang=en&linkID=SSR00204.

[25] M. Llamas, *FDA Investigates Link to Acute Pancreatitis in SGLT2 Diabetes Drugs*, Drugwatch, Orlando, FL, USA, 2019, https://www.drugwatch.com/news/2016/12/02/sglt2-invokana-pancreatitis-link/.

32

Case Report: Homozygous C677T MTHFR Gene Mutation in Male with Hypogonadism

Rami Salameh, Mumtaheena Miah, and Catherine Anastasopoulou

Endocrinology Department, Albert Einstein Medical Center-Philadelphia, Philadelphia, PA, USA

Correspondence should be addressed to Rami Salameh; rami_salameh@hotmail.com

Academic Editor: Hyunsik Kang

We report a 44-year-old male, who was diagnosed with hypogonadotropic hypogonadism after complaining of erectile dysfunction, depression, and fatigue. He was started on testosterone replacement therapy. He persistently complained of fatigue despite increasing the dose of testosterone over two years and having therapeutic testosterone levels. He was found to have homozygous C677T methylenetetrahydrofolate reductase (MTHFR) gene mutation. After treatment with folate and B12, his symptoms resolve completely. MTHFR is a key enzyme in the folate pathway, and it plays an essential role in homocysteine metabolism. Homozygous C677T individuals have decreased activity of MTHFR enzyme with increased homocysteine levels, which is associated with increased risk of thrombosis. An association has been reported between C677T variant and male infertility. Patients identified to have hyperhomocysteinemia should be treated with B-complex vitamin supplements. Our case emphasizes other possible etiologies for fatigue and erectile dysfunction in a male with hypogonadism on testosterone therapy. Also, it shows possible association between MTHFR gene mutation and male hypogonadism.

1. Introduction

MTHFR is a key enzyme in the folate pathway, and it plays an essential role in homocysteine metabolism. Homozygous C677T individuals have decreased activity of MTHFR enzyme with potentially increased homocysteine levels that are associated with increased risk of venous thrombosis, stroke, coronary artery disease, and recurrent pregnancy loss in females. There have also been reports of association between C677T variant and male infertility.

2. Case Report

We report a case of a 44-year-old male, who was a semi-professional football player in late teenage years, with a history of multiple head concussion between age 15 and 25.

He was diagnosed with hypogonadotropic hypogonadism in 2013, when he complained of erectile dysfunction, depression, generalized fatigue. He was started on testosterone replacement therapy. He persistently complained of fatigue despite increasing the dose of testosterone over two years and having therapeutic testosterone levels on labs while on therapy.

At that point, he underwent genetic testing, as per patient personal request, which showed homozygous C677T MTHFR gene mutation.

Other relevant labs included folate: 3.1 ng/mL (normal range: 4.2–19.9) and B12: 333 pg/mL (normal range: 210–934).

His hemoglobin was at normal levels, but interestingly, it did not increase as expected with the use of testosterone.

The patient was treated with folate and B12 supplements, which made his symptoms resolve completely (Table 1).

3. Discussion

MTHFR is a key enzyme in the folate pathway, and it plays an essential role in homocysteine metabolism, as shown in Figure 1.

Homozygous C677T individuals have decreased activity of MTHFR enzyme, thus having an increased risk for hyperhomocysteinemia when deficient in folate, vitamin

Table 1: Social history.

Smoking	Current smoker, 10 pack-year
Alcohol use	Occasional; a glass of beer or wine on occasions
Recreational drug use	None/never
Physical activity	Exercises for 1 hour 3 days a week; walking or weightlifting
BMI	28

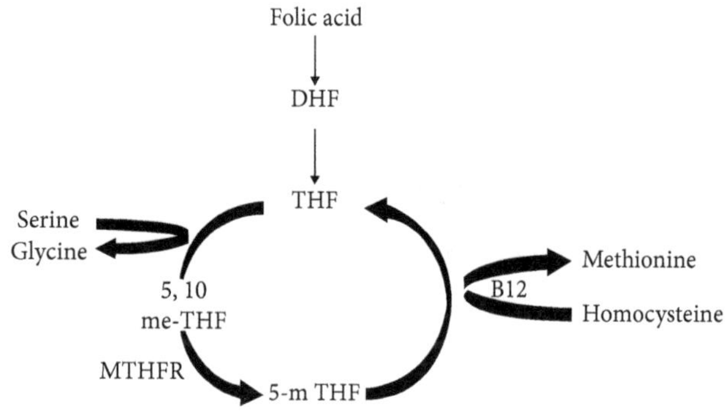

Figure 1: Folic acid is reduced to dihydrofolate (DHF) then to tetrahydrofolate (THF). THF is converted to 5,10-methylenetetrahydrofolate (5, 10-me-THF), which is then reduced to 5-methyltetrahydrofolate (5-mTHF) by MTHFR. 5-mTHF is demethylated to complete the folate cycle by donating a carbon into the methionine cycle through the methylation of homocysteine to methionine by methionine synthase and its cofactor vitamin B12.

B12, or pyridoxine [1]. Elevated homocysteine levels are associated with increased risk of venous thromboembolism, strokes, coronary artery disease, and recurrent pregnancy loss [2]. The exact cause of accelerated vascular disease is unclear, but several mechanisms have been suggested, including endothelial cell damage, lipid peroxidation, smooth muscle cell proliferation, downregulation of antithrombotic factors, and upregulation of prothrombotic factors.

Male hypogonadism, defined as decreased testosterone production and/or impaired ability to produce functional sperms, overlaps with male infertility. The association between C677T variant and male infertility has been reported in the literature.

While some studies did not find an association between C677T polymorphism and male infertility [3, 4], Bezold et al. [5] reported that the prevalence of the homozygous C677T mutation was 18.8% in infertile males as compared with 9.5% in normal fertile males. Thus, it was concluded that MTHFR products may play a role in the pathogenesis of male infertility

Mfady et al. [6] showed that in Jordanians, *MTHFR* C677T polymorphism was associated with male infertility, while *MTHFR* A1298C was not. Similar results were reported by Park et al. [7] in the South Korean population.

Gong et al. [8] conducted a meta-analysis on 26 studies involving 5,575 cases and 5,447 controls. *MTHFR* C677T polymorphism was significantly associated with male infertility in Asians as well as in Caucasians.

Other studies, on the other hand, concluded that there is an association between C677T variant and male infertility in Indian, African, and Southeast Asian populations. Data from Europe regarding this association are conflicting. The lack of similar association in Western populations could be due to the overall dietary enrichment with folates [9].

Lombardo et al. [10] studied the role of C677T MTHFR mutation with subsequent hyperhomocysteinemia in erectile dysfunction. He concluded that hyperhomocysteinemia in homozygous C677T patients may interfere with erection mechanisms and thus cause erectile dysfunction.

Patients identified to have hyperhomocysteinemia should be treated with B-complex vitamin supplements. Initiation of therapy with folic acid, B12, and B6 vitamins tends to normalize homocysteine in 1-2 months. It is unclear whether normalization of homocysteine would improve male infertility or not.

4. Conclusion

Our case emphasizes other important etiologies for fatigue and erectile dysfunction in a male with hypogonadism on testosterone therapy as well as shows the possible association between MTHFR gene mutation and male hypogonadism.

Disclosure

This abstract was presented as a poster in AACE 2019 Meeting in Los Angeles.

References

[1] P. F. Jacques, A. G. Bostom, R. R. Williams et al., "Relation between folate status, a common mutation in methylenetetrahydrofolate reductase, and plasma homocysteine concentrations," *Circulation*, vol. 93, no. 1, pp. 7–9, 1996.

[2] S.-C. Liew and E. D. Gupta, "Methylenetetrahydrofolate reductase (MTHFR) C677T polymorphism: epidemiology, metabolism and the associated diseases," *European Journal of Medical Genetics*, vol. 58, no. 1, pp. 1–10, 2015.

[3] I. M. W. Ebisch, W. L. van Heerde, C. M. G. Thomas, N. van der Put, W. Y. Wong, and R. P. M. Steegers-Theunissen, "C677T methylenetetrahydrofolate reductase polymorphism interferes with the effects of folic acid and zinc sulfate on sperm concentration," *Fertility and Sterility*, vol. 80, no. 5, pp. 1190–1194, 2003.

[4] L. Stuppia, V. Gatta, O. Scarciolla et al., "The methylenetethrahydrofolate reductase (MTHFR) C677T polymorphism and male infertility in Italy," *Journal of Endocrinological Investigation*, vol. 26, no. 7, pp. 620–622, 2003.

[5] G. Bezold, M. Lange, and R. U. Peter, "Homozygous methylenetetrahydrofolate reductase C677T mutation and male infertility," *New England Journal of Medicine*, vol. 344, no. 15, pp. 1172-1173, 2001.

[6] D. S. Mfady, M. F. Sadiq, O. F. Khabour, A. S. Fararjeh, A. Abu-Awad, and Y. Khader, "Associations of variants in

MTHFR and MTRR genes with male infertility in the Jordanian population," *Gene*, vol. 536, no. 1, pp. 40–44, 2014.

[7] J. H. Park, H. C. Lee, Yu-Mi Jeong et al., "MTHFR C677T polymorphism associates with unexplained infertile male factors," *Journal of Assisted Reproduction and Genetics*, vol. 22, no. 9-10, pp. 361–368, 2005.

[8] M. Gong, W. Dong, T. He et al., "MTHFR 677C> T polymorphism increases the male infertility risk: a meta-analysis involving 26 studies," *PLoS One*, vol. 10, no. 3, 2015.

[9] K. Singh, S. K. Singh, R. Sah, I. Singh, and R. Raman, "Mutation C677T in the methylenetetrahydrofolate reductase gene is associated with male infertility in an Indian population1," *International Journal of Andrology*, vol. 28, no. 2, pp. 115–119, 2005.

[10] F. Lombardo, P. Tsamatropoulos, E. Piroli et al., "Treatment of erectile dysfunction due to C677T mutation of the MTHFR gene with vitamin B6 and folic acid in patients non responders to PDE5i," *The Journal of Sexual Medicine*, vol. 7, no. 1, pp. 216–223, 2010.

33

The Closed-Loop System Improved the Control of a Pregnant Patient with Type 1 Diabetes Mellitus

Guillermo E. Guzmán Gómez,[1] **Julian A. Viggiano**,[2] **A. Silva-De Las Salas**,[3] **Veline Martínez**,[4] **and María A. Urbano Bonilla**[5]

[1]*Fundación Clínica Valle del Lili, Department of Endocrinology, Universidad Icesi, Cali, Colombia*
[2]*PGY3 Internal Medicine Resident, Fundación Clínica Valle del Lili, Universidad Icesi, Cali, Colombia*
[3]*Universidad Icesi, Cali, Colombia*
[4]*Fundación Clínica Valle del Lili, Department of Internal Medicine, Universidad Icesi, Cali, Colombia*
[5]*Fundación Clínica Valle del Lili, Clinical Investigations Center, Cali, Colombia*

Correspondence should be addressed to Guillermo E. Guzmán Gómez; guillermoeguzman@gmail.com

Academic Editor: Osamu Isozaki

Objective. Closed-loop insulin systems represent a technological advance in diabetes management but have rarely been studied in pregnancy. We report a case of a patient with type 1 diabetes mellitus who was previously a user of the Paradigm VEO pump and then migrated to Medtronic 670G. *Research Design and Methods.* We reviewed the case of a G1P0 patient with type 1 diabetes, treated with the Medtronic 670G system during pregnancy; a comparison with current literature was done. *Results.* The patient achieved improved glycemic control as measured by time spent in different ranges as follows: <70 mg/dL, 8–4% and 70–180 mg/dL, 83–94%. Secondary outcomes included reduction of stress, anxiety, fear of hypoglycemia, and the psychological burden related to the disease. There were no obstetric or neonatal complications. *Conclusion.* The Medtronic 670G closed-loop system was used safely in a pregnant woman; nevertheless, further research is needed to validate this system in this patient population.

1. Introduction

Type 1 diabetes mellitus (DM1) increases the risk of obstetric and neonatal complications [1]. During gestation, hormonal changes cause a diabetogenic physiological state which can lead to volatile glycemic control in diabetic patients [2]. Previous studies have shown that DM1 women are up to five times more likely to experience severe hypoglycemia during early pregnancy compared to the preconception period [3]; the management of these patients can be challenging, and there is a need for new therapies. Advances in biotechnology seek to achieve glycemic control and minimize the burden of hypoglycemia.

The Medtronic MiniMed 670G is a closed-loop hybrid insulin infusion system approved for patients with diabetes [4, 5]; however, safety in pregnancy has not been established through clinical trials. One of the challenges with this pump is that its algorithm targets fasting glucose of 120 mg/dL, higher than the standard target of <95 mg/dL during pregnancy [6–10]. Herein, we present the case of a female patient with DM1 who achieved satisfactory glycemic control using the MiniMed 670G pump.

2. Methods

A 33-year-old woman with a history of DM1 since 16 years, user of an insulin pump (Paradigm® Veo system) due to high glycemic variability and recurrent hypoglycemia, presented to the outpatient clinic seeking preconception counseling. She reported no hypoglycemic episodes since 2015 and no macrovascular or microvascular complications.

She subsequently reported her pregnancy status at week 10. At the beginning of pregnancy, her weight was 57 Kg,

Table 1: Glycemic control monitoring.

Follow-up week	Pump	Mode	Time in range (TIR)				TDD (UI)	Basal/bolus ratio (%)
			<54 mg/dl (%)	54–63 mg/dl (%)	63–140 mg/dl (%)	>140 mg/dl		
30*	VEO	N/A	1	4	87	8	40	38/62
32*	670G	Manual	1	2	80	17	45	33/67
34*	670G	Automatic	0	1	84	15	46	28/72
38*	670G	Automatic	0	2	96	2	34	24/76
1**	670G	Manual	1	2	94	3	29	21/79
4**	670G	Manual	0	1	92	7	22	45/55
6**	670G	Automatic	0	1	87	12	23	35/66

*Follow-up during pregnancy. **Postpartum follow-up. TDD, total daily dose.

body mass index (BMI) 23 Kg/m^2, and glycated hemoglobin (HbA1c) 6.7%. At week 24, laboratories showed HbA1c of 6.3%; however, she developed high glycemic variability and inadvertent hypoglycemias. Enlite Sensor® continuous glucose monitoring (CGM) dysfunction was discovered, and a switch to a MiniMed 670G pump technology was decided.

During the following four weeks, the Paradigm® Veo pump was kept without the use of a sensor, precipitating hypoglycemia with self-reported anxiety and fear of a drop in glucose levels. At week 28, maternal weight was 63 Kg, and the estimated fetal weight was 1230 g for a 67th percentile (P67). At week 30, the training process on MiniMed 670 G began, a protocol that started with two weeks in the manual mode and was then switched to the automatic mode as an off-label indication. This optimized the times in range and reduced the hypoglycemic episodes and hence the related anxiety in the patient.

By week 33, the estimated fetal weight was 2291 g (P88) and at week 35 was 2832 g (P95) with a maternal weight of 65 Kg. The glycemic control ranges remained within goal until the end of the pregnancy, which took place at week 38 via cesarean section, during which the automatic mode and dextrose infusion were maintained (Table 1). The glycemic variability was higher in weeks 30–34 with higher time in range in hyperglycemia and hypoglycemia.

There were no obstetric complications, and a healthy female newborn weighting 3635 g, suitable for gestational age (P80), was born. In the immediate postpartum period, the automatic mode was suspended due to recurrent hypoglycemic episodes and the periodic suspension of the system by the patient. The manual mode was continued for four weeks, requiring weekly adjustments due to hypoglycemia and a significant decrease in the total required daily insulin dose. At the end of the fourth postpartum week, the automatic mode was restarted, and good glycemic control was maintained.

3. Discussion

DM1 increases the risk of obstetric and neonatal complications associated with maternal hyperglycemia in pregnancy such as macrosomia, congenital anomalies, shoulder dystocia, stillbirth, and neonatal death [1, 2, 11–13]. The glucose goals of pregnant patients are stricter: fasting and preprandial target glucose is <90 mg/dL. Therefore, various pharmacological management options have been developed with less variable insulin regimens that promote better glycemic control in pregnant women [14]. The insulin infusion pump (IIP) is a treatment strategy used when insulin regimens have not been able to achieve adequate control. This syste m has proven to be effective in reducing HbA1c in the nonpregnant population [15]. Along with the development of IIP systems, continuous glucose monitoring has emerged, and in combination, they improve clinical outcomes related to glycemic control. In pregnancy, the use of an insulin pump over multiple-dose injection therapy has not shown greater benefit [16–19]. However, the CONCEPTT trial demonstrated that the use of CGM helps improve neonatal outcomes and reduce maternal hyperglycemia [20].

Research has focused on the development of an artificial pancreas, which, through prediction algorithms, can increase or decrease the supply of insulin according to glucose levels obtained with CGM [21–24]. Stewart et al. compared a closed-loop system from a DANA Diabecare R insulin pump (SOOIL) and a CGM supported by FreeStyle Navigator II vs. an open-loop system in DM1 patients. Their findings reported that women under the closed-loop system achieved better glycemic control, evidenced by fewer obstetric and neonatal complications [25].

In 2016, the FDA approved the first hybrid system, the MiniMed 670G. This system differs from others since it has an automatic glycemic control algorithm that targets a nonmodifiable glucose goal of 120 mg/dL which is higher than the standard target for pregnant patients. The TIR International Consensus established that the target range for pregnant patients is 63–140 mg/dL and to stay below this range less than 5% of the time and above of it less than 25% of the time [26].

Given the short time, this system has been on the market, and there are few reports of its use during gestation. In the case of our patient, migrating from the VEO system to 670 G reduced hypoglycemia and increased time in the target glucose range at rates higher than what is reported in literature [27].

Additionally, the control of stress, anxiety, fear of hypoglycemia, and the psychological burden of the disease play an important role in the management of the diabetic patient. The use of CGM in the CONCEPTT trial showed a reduction in anxiety related to fear of hypoglycemia [20], improving the quality of life of patients using IIP systems coupled with CGM [28].

4. Conclusion

We report an adequate glycemic control in a pregnant patient with DM1 who was transitioned to a closed-loop system at 30 weeks of gestation. The patient had no macrovascular or microvascular complications. Patient showed decreased episodes of severe hypoglycemia and hyperglycemia with better glycemic control than previously reported cases. Our findings are encouraging and open the door for further clinical studies on the use of closed-loop systems in pregnancy.

Consent

The patient has provided consent to the publication of this case.

References

[1] J. P. Vandorsten, W. C. Dodson, M. A. Espeland et al., "NIH consensus development conference: diagnosing gestational diabetes mellitus," *NIH Cconsensus and Sate-of-the-Science Statements*, vol. 29, no. 1, pp. 1–31, 2013.

[2] T. A. Buchanan and A. H. Xiang, "Gestational diabetes mellitus," *Journal of Clinical Investigation*, vol. 115, no. 3, pp. 485–491, 2005.

[3] L. R. Nielsen, U. Pedersen-Bjergaard, B. Thorsteinsson, M. Johansen, P. Damm, and E. R. Mathiesen, "Hypoglycemia in pregnant women with type 1 diabetes: predictors and role of metabolic control," *Diabetes Care*, vol. 31, no. 1, pp. 9–14, 2008.

[4] S. K. Garg, S. A. Weinzimer, W. V. Tamborlane et al., "Glucose outcomes with the in-home use of a hybrid closed-loop insulin delivery system in adolescents and adults with type 1 diabetes," *Diabetes Technology & Therapeutics*, vol. 19, no. 3, pp. 155–163, 2017.

[5] M. de Bock, J. Dart, A. Roy et al., "Exploration of the performance of a hybrid closed loop insulin delivery algorithm that includes insulin delivery limits designed to protect against hypoglycemia," *Journal of Diabetes Science and Technology*, vol. 11, no. 1, pp. 68–73, 2016.

[6] J. L. Ruiz, J. L. Sherr, E. Cengiz et al., "Effect of insulin feedback on closed-loop glucose control: a crossover study," *Journal of Diabetes Science and Technology*, vol. 6, no. 5, pp. 1123–1130, 2012.

[7] G. M. Steil, "Algorithms for a closed-loop artificial pancreas: the case for proportional-integral-derivative control," *Journal of Diabetes Science and Technology*, vol. 7, no. 6, pp. 1621–1631, 2013.

[8] S. A. Weinzimer, G. M. Steil, K. L. Swan, J. Dziura, N. Kurtz, and W. V. Tamborlane, "Fully automated closed-loop insulin delivery versus semiautomated hybrid control in pediatric patients with type 1 diabetes using an artificial pancreas," *Diabetes Care*, vol. 31, no. 5, pp. 934–939, 2008.

[9] Panel, IA of D and PSGC, International association of diabetes and pregnancy study groups recommendations on the diagnosis and classification of hyperglycemia in pregnancy," *Diabetes Care*, vol. 33, no. 3, pp. 676–682, 2010.

[10] A. D. Association, "Management of diabetes in pregnancy: standards of medical care in diabetes—2020," *Diabetes Care*, vol. 43, no. Supplement 1, pp. S183–S192, 2020.

[11] S. Handwerger and M. Freemark, "The roles of placental growth hormone and placental lactogen in the regulation of human fetal growth and development," *Journal of Pediatric Endocrinology and Metabolism*, vol. 13, no. 4, pp. 343–356, 2000.

[12] L. Barbour, "New concepts in insulin resistance of pregnancy and gestational diabetes: long-term implications for mother and offspring," *Journal of Obstetrics and Gynaecology*, vol. 23, no. 5, pp. 545–549, 2003.

[13] H. Yamashita, J. Shao, and J. E. Friedman, "Physiologic and molecular alterations in carbohydrate metabolism during pregnancy and gestational diabetes mellitus," *Clinical Obstetrics and Gynecology*, vol. 43, no. 1, pp. 87–98, 2000.

[14] L. R. Mack and P. G. Tomich, "Gestational diabetes: diagnosis, classification, and clinical care gestational diabetes," *Obstetrics and Gynecology Clinics of North America*, vol. 44, no. 2, pp. 207–217, 2017.

[15] G. Guzmán, V. Martínez, J. D. Yara et al., "Glycemic control and hypoglycemia in patients treated with insulin pump therapy: an observational study," *Journal of Diabetes Research*, vol. 2020, Article ID 1581726, 2020.

[16] O. Cohen, N. Keidar, M. Simchen, B. Weisz, M. Dolitsky, and E. Sivan, "Macrosomia in well controlled CSII treated type I diabetic pregnancy," *Gynecological Endocrinology*, vol. 24, no. 11, pp. 611–613, 2008.

[17] D. Bruttomesso, M. Bonomo, S. Costa et al., "Type 1 diabetes control and pregnancy outcomes in women treated with continuous subcutaneous insulin infusion (CSII) or with insulin glargine and multiple daily injections of rapid-acting insulin analogues (glargine-MDI)," *Diabetes and Metabolism*, vol. 37, no. 5, pp. 426–431, 2011.

[18] D. Farrar, D. J. Tuffnell, J. West, and H. M. West, "Continuous subcutaneous insulin infusion versus multiple daily injections of insulin for pregnant women with diabetes," *Cochrane Database of Systematic Reviews*, vol. 6, Article ID CD005542, 2016.

[19] G. Petrovski, C. Dimitrovski, M. Bogoev, T. Milenkovic, I. Ahmeti, and I. Bitovska, "Is there a difference in pregnancy and glycemic outcome in patients with type 1 diabetes on insulin pump with constant or intermittent glucose monitoring? A pilot study," *Diabetes Technology & Therapeutics*, vol. 13, no. 11, pp. 1109–1113, 2011.

[20] D. S. Feig, L. E. Donovan, R. Corcoy et al., "Continuous glucose monitoring in pregnant women with type 1 diabetes (CONCEPTT): a multicentre international randomised controlled trial," *Lancet (London, England)*, vol. 390, no. 10110, pp. 2347–2359, 2017.

[21] C. A. Combs, "Continuous glucose monitoring and insulin pump therapy for diabetes in pregnancy," *Journal of Maternal-Fetal and Neonatal Medicine*, vol. 25, no. 10, pp. 2025–2027, 2012.

[22] J. Kropff and J. H. DeVries, "Continuous glucose monitoring, future products, and update on worldwide artificial pancreas projects," *Diabetes Technology & Therapeutics*, vol. 18, no. Suppl 2, pp. S253–S263, 2016.

[23] M. Breton, A. Farret, D. Bruttomesso et al., "Fully integrated artificial pancreas in type 1 diabetes: modular closed-loop glucose control maintains near normoglycemia," *Diabetes*, vol. 61, no. 9, pp. 2230–2237, 2012.

[24] R. Hovorka, K. Kumareswaran, J. Harris et al., "Overnight closed loop insulin delivery (artificial pancreas) in adults with type 1 diabetes: crossover randomised controlled studies," *BMJ*, vol. 342, 2011.

[25] Z. A. Stewart, M. E. Wilinska, S. Hartnell et al., "Closed-loop insulin delivery during pregnancy in women with type 1

diabetes," *New England Journal of Medicine*, vol. 375, no. 7, pp. 644–654, 2016.

[26] M. Kalligeros, F. Shehadeh, E. K. Mylona et al., "Association of obesity with disease severity among patients with coronavirus disease 2019," *Obesity (Silver Spring)*, vol. 28, no. 7, pp. 1200–1204, 2020.

[27] S. Polsky and H. K. Akturk, "Case series of a hybrid closed-loop system used in pregnancies in clinical practice," *Diabetes/Metabolism Research and Reviews*, vol. 36, no. 3, Article ID e3248, 2020.

[28] H. Ghazanfar, S. Rizvi, A. Khurram, F. Orooj, and I. Qaiser, "Impact of insulin pump on quality of life of diabetic patients," *Indian Journal of Endocrinology and Metabolism*, vol. 20, no. 4, p. 506, 2016.

34

A BRAF V600E Mutation in RET-Negative Medullary Thyroid Cancer

Richard J. Robbins,[1] **Jessica S. Thomas**,[1,2] **Patricia Mejia Osuna**,[1] **and Jawairia Shakil**[3]

[1]*Weill Cornell Medicine, New York, NY, USA*
[2]*Department of Pathology and Genomic Medicine, Houston Methodist Hospital, Houston, TX, USA*
[3]*Division of Endocrinology, Diabetes, and Metabolism, Department of Medicine, Houston Methodist Hospital, Houston, TX, USA*

Correspondence should be addressed to Richard J. Robbins; rjrobbins@houstonmethodist.org

Academic Editor: Wayne V. Moore

We report the case of a woman with a sporadic medullary thyroid carcinoma. Genomic analysis found that her tumor did not contain any common *RET* mutations but did harbor a *BRAF* V600E mutation. Only one other well-confirmed example of the BRAF V600E mutation has been reported in an MTC patient. We conclude that this common *BRAF* mutation may independently drive neoplastic transformation of human parafollicular C cells.

1. Introduction

Medullary thyroid cancer (MTC) accounts for 1–2% of all new thyroid cancers in the US [1]. Approximately, 20% of MTC presents with a hereditary pattern, usually caused by germline mutations in the *RET* gene. The remaining MTCs are nonfamilial, and 50% of these have a somatic *RET* mutation. Patients with somatic *RET* mutations (most commonly p.M918T) have shorter overall survival compared with MTC without a *RET* mutation [2]. Less commonly sporadic MTC does not harbor a *RET* mutation, but is associated with *RAS* or *ALK* gene rearrangements. In general, *BRAF* point mutations have been found to be absent in non-*RET*-mutated MTC specimens [3].

2. Case Presentation

We report a 66 y/o African American female who was found incidentally to have a 1.3 cm thyroid nodule. A fine needle aspiration biopsy demonstrated cytological features of MTC with positive staining for calcitonin (CT). There was no family history of thyroid cancer or any other endocrine neoplasia. Serum CT was elevated at 75 pmol/L, and the serum CEA was within normal limits. Blood DNA analysis was negative for *RET* germline mutations in exons 5, 8, 10, 11, and 13–16. Pathological analysis after a total thyroidectomy and central neck lymph node dissection revealed a 1.8 cm MTC (Figure 1(a)) with multifocality, extrathyroidal extension, and MTC in 6 out of 10 lymph nodes. The tumor was microdissected out and analyzed for 50 of the most common oncogene mutations by next-generation sequencing, including *RET* and *RAS* genes. The only abnormality detected was a *BRAF* p.V600E mutation (Figure 1(b)). The presence of a *BRAF* p.V600E mutation was then confirmed by an alternate testing platform (Figure 1(c)). The *BRAF* p.V600E was detected in this patient's tumor at a low allele frequency (5–10%) on both testing platforms, likely reflecting the tumor heterogeneity and low tumor burden of the tissue sample. Imaging studies with neck and chest CT scan and MRI of the liver were negative for metastatic disease. One month following thyroidectomy, her serum calcitonin was 70.1 pmol/L. At a 2 year follow-up, she remained asymptomatic with a serum CT level of 26.3 pmol/L, a CEA of 2 mcg/L, and no clinical evidence of disease on exam or by imaging.

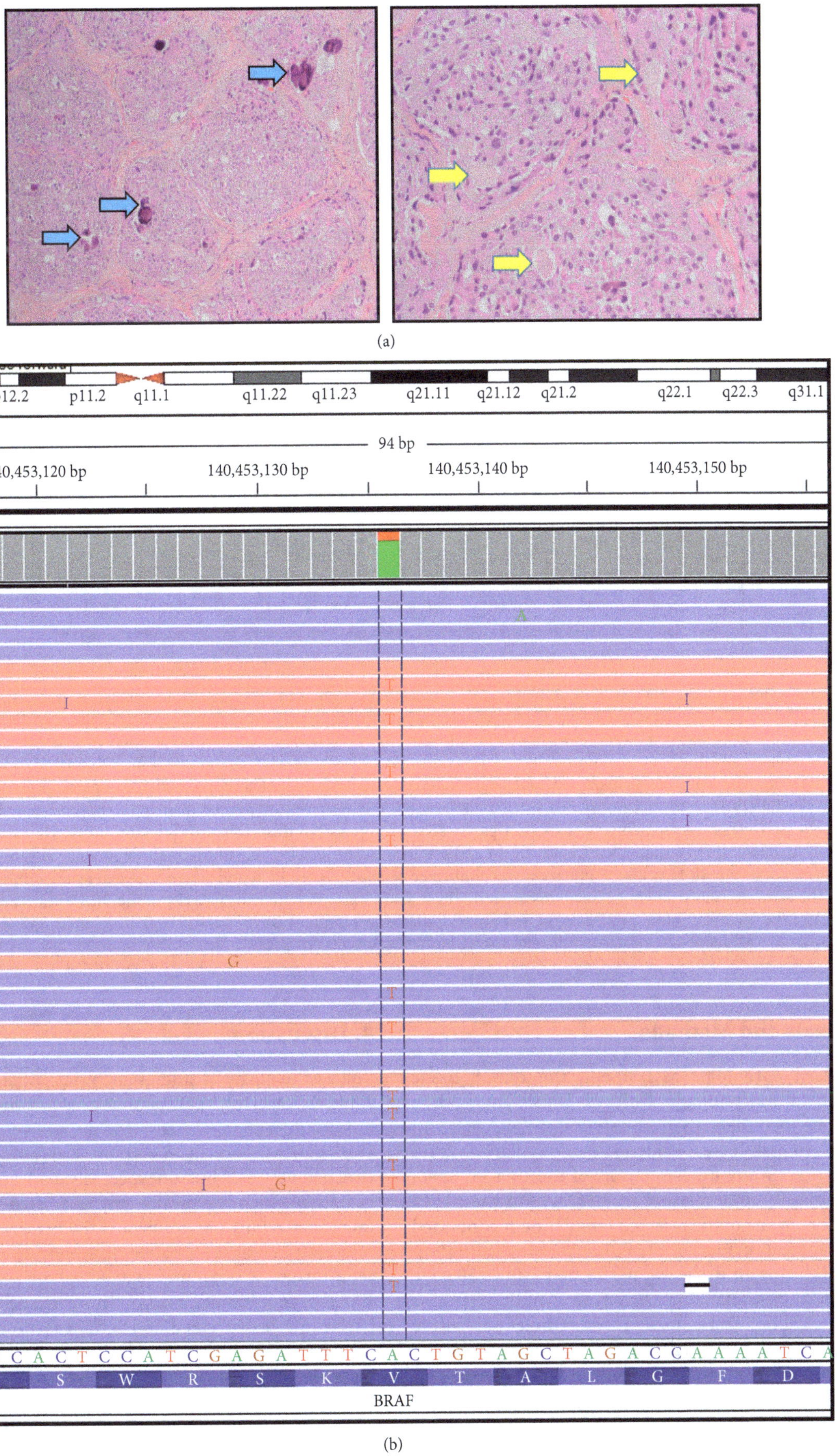

FIGURE 1: Continued.

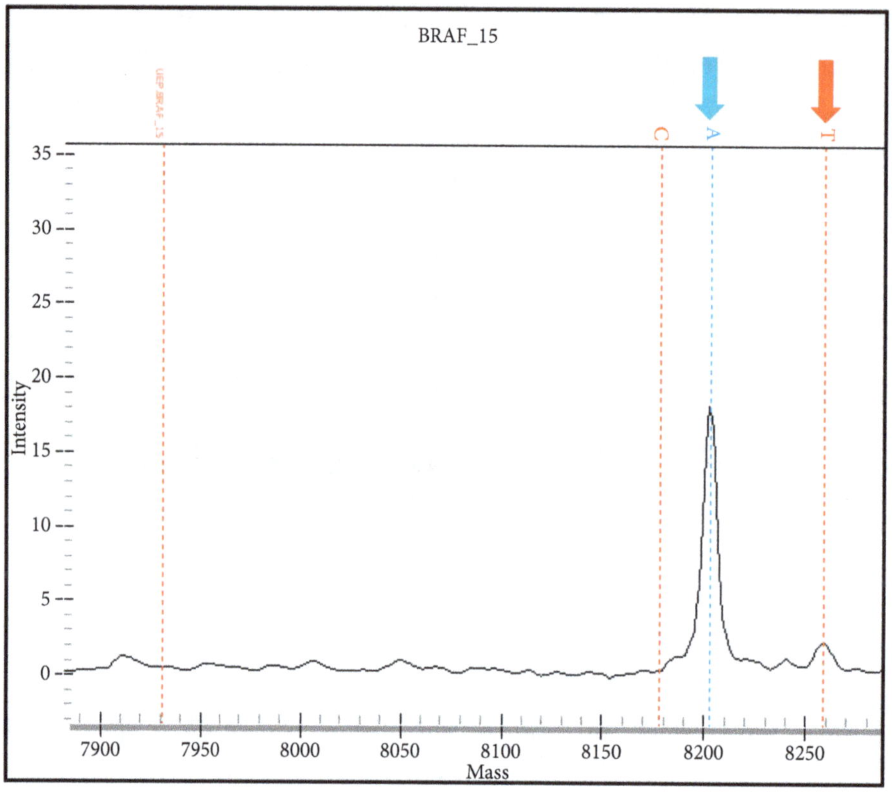

(c)

FIGURE 1: (a) An H&E-stained tissue section of the thyroid tumor at 100x (left) and 200x (right) magnification is shown. The tissue shows solid sheets and nests of cells separated by hyalinized fibrovascular stroma. Interspersed between the cells is a homogeneous, acellular, eosinophilic, extracellular matrix material, consistent with amyloid (solid yellow arrow). There are numerous scattered calcifications (solid blue arrow). Cytologically, the tumor cells are spindled, plasmacytoid, or polyhedral in shape with round to oval nuclei showing stippled, fine, uniform salt and pepper nuclear chromatin, and a moderate amount of pink granular cytoplasm. These findings are consistent with the diagnosis of medullary thyroid carcinoma. (b) Integrated Genomics Viewer representative display of the mutated sequence in *BRAF* detected by the next-generation sequencing analysis. Separate sequencing reads at this nucleotide position (1799) are shown. A (green) to T (red) nucleotide substitution (variant allele frequency, 10.3%) results in an amino acid substitution (glutamic acid for valine) at codon 600 of *BRAF*. (c) Presence of the *BRAF* p.V600E mutation was confirmed by multiplexed PCR and single-base extension with mass spectrometry analysis on the Sequenom instrument (Agena Biosciences). The mass (x-axis) and intensity (y-axis) of the *BRAF* peaks are shown. The blue arrow indicates the wildtype *BRAF* peak, and the red arrow indicates the mutant *BRAF* peak. The T to A nucleotide substitution shows results in an amino acid substitution (glutamic acid for valine) at codon 600 of *BRAF*.

3. Materials and Methods

On standard pathologic assessment, the tumor tissue demonstrated morphologic features consistent with a diagnosis of medullary thyroid carcinoma (Figure 1(a)). There was no histological evidence of a papillary thyroid cancer (PTC) in any other sections of the thyroid specimen, including no admixture of PTC within the MTC. Furthermore, none of the resected lymph nodes contained any histological evidence of PTC. Somatic mutation analysis of the tumor tissue was performed using a 50 gene next-generation sequencing assay (Ion AmpliSeq Tumor Hotspot v2, Life Technologies) and single nucleotide variant genotyping by single-base extension followed by mass spectroscopy analysis (Oncocarta Panel and Sequenom, Agena Biosciences). The report of this case was approved by the Houston Methodist Institutional Review Board (IRB #1014–0216).

4. Discussion

The vast majority of studies analyzing somatic mutations in sporadic cases of MTC continue to demonstrate that mutations other than *RET* and *RAS* are still very rare or absent. Our patient had histologically classical MTC, without concurrent PTC, but unexpectedly had a *BRAF* p.V600E mutation which is typically only associated with PTC. Only one other report has confirmed the presence of the V600E mutation in one MTC patient in Korea [4]. One remarkable report from Greece found that 68% of their MTC cases had a *BRAF* p.V600E mutation [5]. This extremely atypical result has not been confirmed and certain methodological details may have led to false positive results [4]. However, numerous other investigators [6–8] have not found any *BRAF* point mutations in hundreds of *RET* and non-*RET*-mutated MTC cases. One MTC case was found to have a unique fusion between *PARP12* (exons 1–9) and *BRAF* (exons

11–18), creating a putative oncogene [9]. B-Raf is a serine/threonine-protein kinase which is the key element in the RET/Raf/MEK/ERK pathway that is often activated in MTC. Our rare finding suggests that a gain of function *BRAF* point mutation may be able to drive malignant transformation of human parafollicular C cells, through the MEK/ERK pathway in the absence of a *RET* mutation. However, the possibility exists that this *BRAF* point mutation, which was present at a low allelic frequency, might not be the causative or "driver" mutation in this case.

Acknowledgments

This work was supported by the U.S. Centers for Medicare & Medicaid Services; Houston Methodist Hospital; the Cullen Foundation Scholars Fund; and the Occidental Petroleum Scholars Fund.

References

[1] D. W. Ball and L. Wartofsky, "Clinical aspects of medullary thyroid carcinoma," in *Thyroid Cancer: A Comprehensive Guide to Clinical Management*, L. Wartofsky and D. Van Nostrand, Eds., pp. 853–864, Springer Science + Business Media, LLC, New York, NY, USA, 3rd edition, 2016.

[2] H. G. Vuong, T. Odate, H. T. T. Ngo et al., "Clinical significance of RET and RAS mutations in sporadic medullary thyroid carcinoma: a meta-analysis," *Endocrine-Related Cancer*, vol. 25, no. 6, pp. 633–641, 2018.

[3] M. Xing, V. Vasko, G. Tallini et al., "BRAFT1796A transversion mutation in various thyroid neoplasms," *The Journal of Clinical Endocrinology & Metabolism*, vol. 89, no. 3, pp. 1365–1368, 2004.

[4] U. Cho, W. J. Oh, J. S. Bae et al., "Clinicopathological features of rare BRAF mutations in Korean thyroid cancer patients," *Journal of Korean Medical Science*, vol. 29, no. 8, pp. 1054–1060, 2014.

[5] N. Goutas, D. Vlachodimitropoulos, M. Bouka, A. C. Lazaris, G. Nasioulas, and M. Gazouli, "BRAF and K-RAS mutation in a Greek papillary and medullary thyroid carcinoma cohort," *Anticancer Research*, vol. 28, pp. 305–308, 2008.

[6] H. J. Schulten, J. Al-Maghrabi, K. Al-Ghamdi et al., "Mutational screening of RET, HRAS, KRAS, NRAS, BRAF, AKT1, and CTNNB1 in medullary thyroid carcinoma," *Anticancer Research*, vol. 31, pp. 4179–4183, 2011.

[7] F. P. Nascimento, M. G. Cardoso, S. C. Lindsey et al., "Analysis of somatic mutations in BRAF, CDKN2A/p16 and PI3KCA in patients with medullary thyroid carcinoma," *Molecular Medicine Reports*, vol. 13, no. 2, pp. 1653–1660, 2016.

[8] P. Vanden Borre, A. B. Schrock, P. M. Anderson et al., "Pediatric, adolescent, and young adult thyroid carcinoma harbors frequent and diverse targetable genomic alterations, including kinase fusions," *The Oncologist*, vol. 22, no. 3, pp. 255–263, 2017.

[9] K. Kasaian, S. M. Wiseman, B. A. Walker et al., "Putative-BRAFactivating fusion in a medullary thyroid cancer," *Molecular Case Studies*, vol. 2, no. 2, Article ID a000729, 2016.

Treatment of Growth Hormone Deficiency via Daily Intravascular Injections in a Child with Bleeding Disorder

Emir Tas[1] **Serife E. Uzun,**[2] **Vildan Tas,**[1] **and Juan D. Mejia-Otero**[1]

[1]*Department of Pediatrics, University of Arkansas for Medical Sciences, Little Rock, AR, USA*
[2]*College of Osteopathic Medicine, New York Institute of Technology, Glen Head, Long Island, NY, USA*

Correspondence should be addressed to Emir Tas; etas@uams.edu

Academic Editor: Wayne V. Moore

Objectives. The standard of treatment for pediatric growth hormone deficiency (GHD) is daily subcutaneous recombinant human growth hormone (rhGH) injections. The efficacy of rhGH treatment given as daily intravenous (IV) boluses is not known. *Case Presentation.* A female with protein C deficiency, a severe bleeding disorder characterized by thrombosis formation, was diagnosed with GHD at age four years. She has been receiving daily protein C infusion through a permanent port since the newborn period. GHD was treated with daily IV rhGH boluses given through the port following protein C infusion. She has reached a growth rate of 12 cm/year and had no side effects. Surprisingly, serum insulin-like growth factor-1 (IGF1) levels did not rise despite an excellent clinical response. *Conclusions.* IV administration may be an alternative route for GHD treatment in eligible patients with permanent vascular access. A rise in serum IGF1 levels may not be needed to achieve the growth-promoting effect of rhGH.

1. Introduction

Short stature is one of the most common referral reasons to pediatric endocrinology clinics. Among the various etiologies of short stature, growth hormone (GH) deficiency is the most common endocrine cause. Growth hormone deficiency (GHD) is estimated to have a prevalence of 1 in 4,000 to 10,000 and can be due to genetic defects, acquired causes, or idiopathic. Untreated GHD may have a profound impact on the overall health of the affected children with lasting consequences beyond childhood. Presenting symptoms and signs vary depending on the age of onset, but children with GHD usually come to medical attention with decelerated or stunted linear growth, delayed bone development, and delayed puberty. Screening tests for suspected GHD include measurement of serum growth factors, particularly insulin-like growth factor (IGF)-1, which is also used to assess adherence and monitor safety and as a guide to titrate GH dose during treatment. IGF1 is the primary mediator of GH-stimulated bone growth. Currently, the standard treatment of GHD involves daily subcutaneous injections of recombinant human growth hormone (rhGH). However, this administration route may be a source of stress in parents of children with severe underlying bleeding pathologies because of cutaneous bleeding risk. Although the likelihood of hitting a large vein in subcutaneous fat is practically zero, the parental anxiety associated with this may lead to non-adherence to GH treatment in such patients. There is a lack of knowledge regarding the efficacy and safety of daily intravenous (IV) administration of rhGH to treat GHD. We report the case of a patient with protein C deficiency who was diagnosed with GHD and successfully treated via daily IV rhGH boluses through an established port. To our knowledge, the IV route has not been previously used for long-term rhGH replacement therapy.

2. Case Presentation

A 2-year 5-month-old female was referred to for evaluation of short stature. She was born at term with a birth weight of 3845 grams and a length of 51 cm. Her history was notable for prolonged Neonatal Intensive-Care Unit (NICU) stay due to disseminated intravascular coagulation (DIC) characterized by multiple skin bruises and respiratory distress.

She required a chest tube and G-tube placement to treat chylothorax and feeding problems, respectively, and transfusion of multiple blood products to manage DIC. After an extensive workup, she was diagnosed with protein C deficiency and has begun daily IV protein C concentrate (Ceprotin®) treatment. She had no pulmonary or cardiac comorbidities upon discharge from the NICU around four months of age. The brain magnetic resonance imaging (MRI) showed nonspecific white matter injury with multiple small subdural bleeds with no known neurological sequela. She also developed right-sided blindness due to retinal detachment.

On presentation to the endocrinology clinic, she plotted below one percentile in the height-for-age and at the third percentile in the weight-for-age charts (Figure 1).

She was in no acute distress and had normal vital signs. She was developmentally at par for age. Physical examination was notable for the presence of a subcutaneous port-a-cath on the left upper chest for daily protein C concentrate infusion and well-healed small scar tissues on her chest and abdomen. She had no red reflex on the right eye and self-amputated toes on the left foot. There were no organomegaly or any other dysmorphic features. Laboratory showed undetectable insulin-like growth factor-1 (IGF-1) (<15 ng/mL) and low IGF-binding protein-3 (BP-3) (0.65 mg/L, reference range 0.8–3.9) levels, but normal thyroid studies (Table 1).

Over the next two years, she did not show catch-up growth despite improved nutritional status (Figure 1). She failed to demonstrate a normal response to the arginine-clonidine provocation test with a peak GH level of only 4.4 ng/mL and was diagnosed with GHD. Repeat brain MRI showed hypoplastic anterior pituitary without any evidence of residual white matter damage. Recombinant hGH therapy was recommended. Due to concerns of extensive bruising with daily rhGH subcutaneous injections, parents requested a trial of IV administration of rhGH therapy via her port-a-cath. They agreed to switch to subcutaneous administration if there were poor response. Parents were made aware of the off-label use of IV rhGH therapy and signed informed consent after obtaining clearance from the hematologist. The patient started standard rhGH therapy at a standard subcutaneous dose (0.3 mg/kg/week) at age 4 years and 9 months via daily IV boluses through her port-a-cath following daily protein C infusions. She had an excellent response with a growth velocity of 12 cm/year in the first year of treatment without any adverse effects. Surveillance tests for thyroid and glucose tolerance were normal. Linear growth was accompanied by a modest increase in serum IGF-1 levels a few months after starting rhGH therapy with a slight further rise in serum IGF-1 levels after 16 months of rhGH therapy (Table 1).

3. Discussion

Herein, we describe a child with congenital protein C deficiency who was later diagnosed with GHD. Congenital protein C deficiency is a rare and severe bleeding disorder, characterized by a hypercoagulable state as a result of homozygous or compound heterozygous mutation of the PROC gene [1]. Affected infants may present with purpura fulminans, disseminated intravascular coagulation (DIC), or intracranial hemorrhage due to venous thrombosis [2]. Prompt recognition of this condition is important as a delay in treatment initiation may result in irreversible consequences. Our patient presented with DIC in the newborn period with extensive skin bruising and has then suffered blindness, self-amputated toes, and white matter changes in the brain. She has had no further bleeding after protein C treatment has begun. However, she was found to have a small anterior pituitary gland while being worked up for GHD. Schmitt et al. described a case with suspected protein C deficiency who later developed hypothalamic failure manifesting with combined pituitary hormone deficiencies, including GHD [3]. Cerebrovascular occlusion due to protein C deficiency was hypothesized to be the etiology of panhypopituitarism. To our knowledge, isolated GHD has not been described previously in a patient with protein C deficiency.

Growth hormone has multiple effects on various tissues and organs in the body. Besides playing a crucial role in linear growth, it also has vital functions in metabolism and cardiovascular physiology [4]. GH regulates the endothelial function and hepatic synthesis of some coagulation factors. Studies in adults linked GHD and adverse cardiovascular outcomes, including increased thromboembolic events, but pediatric data are lacking [5]. Therefore, diagnosis and treatment of GHD in a child with an underlying bleeding disorder maybe even more important than simply focusing on the effect of GH on linear growth.

The somatomedin hypothesis suggests that GH mediates its functions, including bone growth, mainly through the induction of hepatic IGF1, which activates transmembranous receptors in chondrocytes [6]. However, Wu et al., in their animal studies, demonstrated that GH could independently promote linear bone growth even when the local IGF1 action is prevented [7]. Although the serum IGF1 level of our patient has fairly increased following over one year of GH replacement, it has remained below two standard deviations for age and sex. Our observation supports the notion that GH may promote linear growth independent of a significant increase in serum IGF1 levels even in humans.

The current standard approach for the treatment of GHD is daily subcutaneous injection of recombinant rhGH. However, this route of administration presented a challenge in our patient due to the risk of extensive bruising. Per parent's request and after clearance from her hematologist, we agreed to attempt a trial of intravenous administration of rhGH via her port-a-cath with an option to switch to subcutaneous administration if clinical responses were suboptimal. The half-life of exogenous rhGH is estimated to be around 10–15 minutes [8]. Jørgensen et al. showed that a single IV rhGH bolus in healthy adult men increased mRNA expression of IGF1 in adipose, but not in muscle tissue [9]. In a previous study conducted by the same group, the researchers compared the effects of three different IV rhGH administration schedules (two large boluses at 2000 and 0200 hours. vs. eight small boluses separated at 3-hour intervals vs. continuous infusion between 2000 and 0200

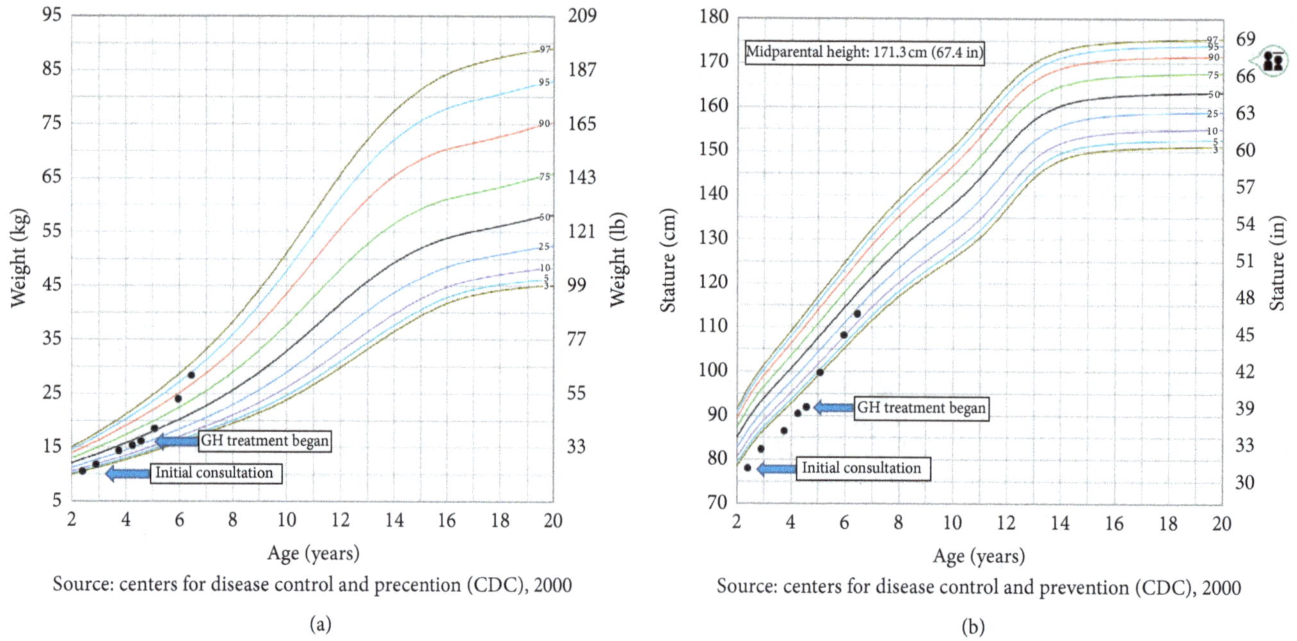

FIGURE 1: The weight (a) and height (b) data, at the time of initial consultation and when the growth hormone treatment has begun, indicated by arrows. GH, growth hormone.

TABLE 1: Laboratory results of selected biomarkers of the patient before and after growth hormone treatment.

Age (years, months)	$2^{5/12}$ years (before rhGH)	$3^{2/12}$ years (before rhGH)	$5^{2/12}$ years (5 months after rhGH)	$6^{1/12}$ years (16 months after rhGH)
IGF1 concentration (ng/mL)	<15	<15	29	41
IGF1 SDS score			−2.33	−2.17
IGFBP3 concentration (mg/L, RR: 0.8–3.9)	0.65	0.8	1.6	
TSH (mIU/L)	2.1		2.6	1.3
Free T4 (ng/dL)	1.1		0.9	0.9
Albumin (gr/dL)			4.3	
ALT (IU/L)			27	
AST (IU/L)			20	
HbA1c (%)			4.7	4.5
Protein C functional (%, RR: 40–92)	14	14	11	12

hours) on metabolic markers and IGF1 level. They found that the same amount of rhGH given as the two large boluses generated similar and significant metabolic responses on glucose and lipid markers than at baseline. All three schedules resulted in a considerable increase in IGF1 levels, but the two IV bolus groups had lower peaks in IGF1 and quicker return to baseline than the other two schedules [10]. The authors speculated that the serum GH level might need to be sustained above zero for prolonged periods to achieve its growth-promoting effects. In our patient, daily IV rhGH boluses markedly improved linear growth despite a modest increase of serum IGF1 levels.

Growth hormone stimulates hepatic IGF1 production via the activation of transmembranous receptors. Whether the expression of liver GH receptors is altered in patients with protein C deficiency or the administration of protein C concentrate immediately before the rhGH boluses had suppressed the normal hepatic response is not known. There is no standard dose for IV rhGH replacement. Moreover, we did not assess this treatment's direct effects on lipid metabolism, body composition, or cardiovascular markers. These would have provided direct evidence on the metabolic benefits of rhGH treatment on this patient.

4. Conclusions

IV administration may be an alternative route for treating GHD in eligible patients with permanent vascular access if there are challenges or potential side effects of subcutaneous administration. A significant rise in serum IGF1 levels may not be needed to achieve the growth-promoting effect of IV rhGH therapy.

Disclosure

The abstract of this manuscript was presented as a virtual poster at the annual Pediatric Endocrine Society meeting held online from April 30 to May 3, 2021.

References

[1] S. Ohga, A. Ishiguro, Y. Takahashi et al., "Protein C deficiency as the major cause of thrombophilias in childhood," *Pediatrics International*, vol. 55, no. 3, pp. 267–271, 2013.

[2] P. N. Knoebl, "Severe congenital protein C deficiency: the use of protein C concentrates (human) as replacement therapy for life-threatening blood-clotting complications," *Biologics: Targets & Therapy*, vol. 2, pp. 285–296, 2008.

[3] S. Schmitt, K. Auberger, T. Fendel, and W. Kiess, "Hypothalamic failure as a sequela of heterozygous protein C deficiency?" *European Journal of Pediatrics*, vol. 151, no. 6, pp. 428–431, 1992.

[4] J. Devesa, C. Almengló, and P. Devesa, "Multiple effects of growth hormone in the body: is it really the hormone for growth?" *Clinical Medicine Insights: Endocrinology and Diabetes*, vol. 9, Article ID CMED.S38201, 2016.

[5] C. Gazzaruso, M. Gola, I. Karamouzis, R. Giubbini, and A. Giustina, "Cardiovascular risk in adult patients with growth hormone (GH) deficiency and following substitution with GH—an update," *The Journal of Clinical Endocrinology & Metabolism*, vol. 99, no. 1, pp. 18–29, 2014.

[6] D. Le Roith, C. Bondy, S. Yakar, J.-L. Liu, and A. Butler, "The somatomedin hypothesis: 2001," *Endocrine Reviews*, vol. 22, no. 1, pp. 53–74, 2001.

[7] S. Wu, W. Yang, and F. De Luca, "Insulin-like growth factor-independent effects of growth hormone on growth plate chondrogenesis and longitudinal bone growth," *Endocrinology*, vol. 156, no. 7, pp. 2541–2551, 2015.

[8] P. C. Hindmarsh, D. R. Matthews, C. E. Brain et al., "The half-life of exogenous growth hormone after suppression of endogenous growth hormone secretion with somatostatin," *Clinical Endocrinology*, vol. 30, no. 4, pp. 443–450, 1989.

[9] J. O. L. Jørgensen, N. Jessen, S. B. Pedersen et al., "GH receptor signaling in skeletal muscle and adipose tissue in human subjects following exposure to an intravenous GH bolus," *American Journal of Physiology-Endocrinology and Metabolism*, vol. 291, no. 5, pp. E899–E905, 2006.

[10] J. O. L. Jørgensen, N. Møller, T. Lauritzen, and J. S. Christiansen, "Pulsatile versus continuous intravenous administration of growth hormone (GH) in GH-deficient patients: effects on circulating insulin-like growth factor-i and metabolic indices," *The Journal of Clinical Endocrinology & Metabolism*, vol. 70, no. 6, pp. 1616–1623, 1990.

Interleukin-6 Producing Pheochromocytoma: A Rare Cause of Systemic Inflammatory Response Syndrome

Nelson Carvalho Cunha, Leonor Gomes, Joana Saraiva, and Isabel Paiva

Department of Endocrinology, Hospitais da Universidade de Coimbra, Centro Hospitalar e Universitário de Coimbra, 3075 Coimbra, Portugal

Correspondence should be addressed to Nelson Carvalho Cunha; nelsoncarvalhocunha@gmail.com

Academic Editor: Carlo Capella

Systemic inflammatory response syndrome (SIRS) can be a rare manifestation of pheochromocytoma, since this adrenal tumor may produce cytokines and other hormones or neuropeptides besides catecholamines. We report the case of a 53-year-old female patient with a pheochromocytoma that presented with fever and weight loss of 5% in one month along with normocytic anemia, thrombocytosis, leukocytosis, and elevated C-reactive protein. In this setting, interleukin-6 (IL-6) was requested and was elevated [26.7ng/L (<7.0)]. She also presented biochemical evidence of ACTH-independent cortisol production without overt Cushing syndrome. After adrenalectomy, the inflammatory syndrome resolved and all biochemical parameters normalized, including IL-6 and ACTH. To our knowledge, this is the first case report of IL6-producing pheochromocytoma along with autonomous cortisol production.

1. Introduction

Pheochromocytoma is a tumor that arises from chromaffin cells of adrenal medulla and usually presents with paroxysms of hypertension, palpitations, sweating, and headache due to excessive catecholamine release. However, some of these tumors may secrete other hormones or neuropeptides, resulting in unusual clinical manifestations and hindering the diagnosis. Some of these are cytokines, mainly interleukin-1 (IL-1), IL-6, tumor necrosis factor-α (TNF-α), and interferon-γ (INF- γ), resulting in systemic inflammation [1]. Fever of unknown origin is uncommon in patients with pheochromocytoma, but there are few reports of patients with systemic inflammatory response syndrome (SIRS) and elevated IL-6 plasma levels due to this adrenal tumor [1–9]. The SIRS consists in a pathophysiologic response to a nonspecific insult and is characterized by fever or hypothermia, tachycardia, tachypnea, and/or leukocytosis [10]. IL-6 is a cytokine that regulates immune responses and plays a major role in inflammatory cascade by stimulating the release of acute-phase reactants such as C-reactive protein (CRP) [11]. IL-6 also regulates hematopoiesis and stimulates hypothalamic-pituitary-adrenal axis [12]. It is produced mainly by lymphocytes and monocytes and is physiologically expressed in the adrenal cortex, but not in adrenal medulla [13]. In this report, we describe a patient with a pheochromocytoma and elevated plasma IL-6 that presented with SIRS.

2. Case Presentation

A 53-year-old woman was referenced from primary care physician to her local hospital due to fever at evening and a weight loss of 5% in one month. The patient had a previous history of total hysterectomy and atrophic gastritis and was under proton pump inhibitors. No relevant familial history was known.

At admission, she was pale, with 37.9°C of temperature, normal blood pressure (119/69mmHg) and heart rate (91/min), and 61 Kg of weight (BMI 25.5Kg/m^2), without Cushing syndrome signs or other relevant clinical findings.

Patient's laboratory tests at admission (Table 1) revealed marked thrombocytosis (platelets 743x10^9/L), normocytic anemia (Hb 10.1 g/dL), and slight leukocytosis (WBC 10.2x 10^9/L) with elevated ferritin, C-reactive protein levels [(22.74 mg/dL (<0.5)], and normal procalcitonin. No pathogenic

TABLE 1: Laboratory data before and after left adrenalectomy.

	At diagnosis	After surgery	Reference range
Interleukin-6 (ng/L)	*26.7*	*<1.5*	*<7.0*
Plasma metanephrine (pg/mL)	35.9	13.1	<60
Urinary metanephrine (ug/24h)	76.5	22.1	30-350
Plasma normetanephrine (pg/mL)	3503.4	92.5	<120
Urinary normetanephrine (ug/24h)	5505.0	105.1	50-650
Plasma 3-methoxythyramine (pg/mL)	10.4	<10.0	<14
Urinary 3-methoxythyramine (ug/24h)	749.8	87.6	30-300
ACTH (pg/mL)	<5.0	19	9-52
Plasma cortisol 8am (ug/dL)	15	8.5	(5-25)
Asleep plasma cortisol 12pm (ug/dL)	7.1	1.0	<1.8
Urinary free cortisol (ug/24h)	96		10-80
Hemoglobin (g/dL)	10.1	13.8	12.0-15.0
MCV (fL)	84.3	86.5	83.0-101.0
WBC ($x10^9$/L)	10.2	6.0	4.0-10.0
Platelets ($x10^9$/L)	743	190	150-400
C-reactive protein (mg/dL)	22.74	0.11	<0.5
Procalcitonin (ng/mL)	0.11		<0.5
Ferritin (ng/mL)	566	65	15-150
Fasting blood glucose (mg/dL)	130	88	60-109
A1C (%)	6.4	5.1	4.0-6.0
Albumin (g/dL)	3.3	3.6	3.5-5.2
Calcitonin (pg/mL)	<2.0		<10
PTH (pg/mL)	68		9-72
25-hydroxyvitamin D (ng/mL)	18		>29
Calcium (mg/dL)	8.8	9.4	8.8-10.6

ACTH, adrenocorticotropic hormone; MCV, mean corpuscular volume; WBC, white blood cells; GGT, gamma-glutamyl transferase; PTH, parathyroid hormone.

agents were found on blood, urine, and cerebrospinal fluid cultures nor alcohol-acid resistant bacilli. Viral serological markers were also negative. She also presented elevated fasting blood glucose (130mg/dL) and A1C of 6.4% as well as slight elevation of liver enzymes and decreased albumin. Brain tomography showed no alterations and echocardiogram showed slightly enlarged left atrium and normal left ventricular ejection fraction.

The patient was initially medicated with levofloxacin during 7 days but without any improvement. Then, a thoracic and abdominal tomography (CT) was performed and revealed a nodular lesion of 4.2 cm length, with heterogeneous contrast enhancement, not clear if the origin was the gastric fundus or the left adrenal (Figure 1). Upper digestive endoscopy showed a hiatus hernia and erosive antral gastritis, without any suspicious features. The abdominal magnetic resonance imaging revealed a left adrenal tumor with 4.3cm length, hyperintense in T2-weighted images and hypointense in T1, with peripheral contrast enhancement and increased washout, possibly indicating a pheochromocytoma. The patient was then referred to our department and when asked, she also referred 3 to 4 episodes per day of palpitations, sweating, headache, and limbs paresthesia, mainly related with efforts, which were not initially considered. At biochemical evaluation, she presented elevation of plasma and urinary normetanephrine [3503 pg/mL (<120) and 5505 ug/24h (50-650) resp.] with plasma and urinary metanephrine and 3-methoxythyramine within reference range (Table 1). Adrenal androgens were also normal. However, ACTH was suppressed [<5pg/mL (9-52)] with asleep plasma midnight cortisol [7.1ug/dL (<1.8)], urinary free cortisol [96ug/24h (10-80)], and cortisol after 1 mg overnight dexamethasone suppression test (3.7ug/dL) slightly

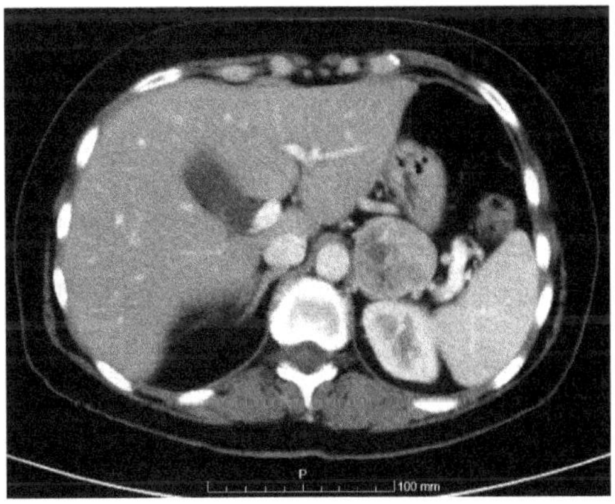

FIGURE 1: *Adrenal tumor on abdominal CT scan.* Adrenal tumor with 4.2cm length and heterogeneous iodine contrast uptake.

TABLE 2: Pheochromocytoma of the Adrenal Gland Scaled Score by Thompson.

Feature	Points assigned	Presence in patient's tumor
Large nests or diffuse growth (>10% of tumor volume)	2	Yes
Central (middle of large nests) or confluent tumor necrosis	2	Yes
High cellularity	2	Yes
Cellular monotony	2	No
Tumor cell spindling	2	No
Mitotic figures > 3/10HPF	2	No
Atypical mitotic figures	2	No
Extension into adipose tissue	2	Yes
Vascular invasion	1	No
Capsular invasion	1	Yes
Profound nuclear pleomorphism	1	Yes
Nuclear hyperchromasia	1	Yes
Total	*20*	*11*

HPF: high-power field.

elevated, consistent with autonomous cortisol production. ^{125}I-metaiodobenzyl guanidine (MIBG) scintigraphy showed an accumulation of the isotope in the left adrenal tumor. After integration of these clinical, laboratory, and imaging data, the diagnosis of pheochromocytoma was made. In the presence of a SIRS in a patient with a newly diagnosed pheochromocytoma, the measurement of plasma IL-6 was requested and it was elevated [26.7 ng/L (<7.0)], consistent with IL-6-producing pheochromocytoma. Biochemical screening of MEN2 syndrome was negative.

Patient started preoperative alpha-blockade treatment with phenoxybenzamine 10 mg id that was increased to 10 mg 2id after one week and beta-blockade treatment was added with propranolol 10 mg id. During treatment, her minimum BP was 86/53mmHg and maximum was 116/57mmHg and minimum heart rate was 73/min and maximum was 115/min. She remained without fever during this period. After 23 days of alpha-blockade single-port laparoscopy, left adrenalectomy was performed without complications. Histological examination showed a well-delimitated pheochromocytoma with 3.0x2.5x1.8cm and potential malignant biological behavior with PASS score = 11 (Table 2) (potential malignant biological behavior if PASS score ≥ 6 [14]). Immunohistochemistry revealed strong positivity to chromogranin A, synaptophysin, and neuron-specific enolase and negativity to cytokeratin AE1/AE3, calretinin, and inhibin A. Ki67 proliferation index was 1-2%. After surgery, the alpha- and beta-blockade was stopped and due to autonomous cortisol production with suppressed ACTH, hydrocortisone was initially prescribed at stress dose and then tapered to 20 mg per day.

In reevaluation two months after surgery she had no complaints. Plasma and urinary normetanephrine were within reference range and IL-6 was undetectable (Table 1). Total blood count and inflammatory parameters have all normalized. Hydrocortisone was tapered to suspension just before revaluation and a short Synacthen® test was performed, which excluded adrenal insufficiency (plasma cortisol 60 minutes after 250 μg of tetracosactide: 19 mg/dL). Abdominal CT and MIBG scintigraphy had no evidence of persistent disease. A genetic test was requested and no germline mutations were detected in the following genes: RET, VHL, SDHAF2, SDHB, SDHC, SDHD, MAX, and TMEM127.

3. Discussion

This case shows a very rare presentation of an inflammatory syndrome of unknown origin in a patient with a newly diagnosed pheochromocytoma and elevated levels of IL-6 which resolved after adrenalectomy.

Although she presented some paroxysmal events of palpitations, sweating, headache, and limbs paresthesia, the main clinical sign was the fever accompanied by the elevation of inflammatory markers, normocytic anemia, and thrombocytosis, which delayed the correct diagnosis. The lack of improvement after antibiotic therapy and the nonidentification of pathogenic agent led to the identification of an adrenal tumor on abdominal tomography and consequently to the diagnosis of a pheochromocytoma. The presence of an inflammatory syndrome in a patient with a newly diagnosed pheochromocytoma led us to measure the plasma IL-6 which was significantly elevated.

This patient also presented suppressed plasma ACTH with slightly elevated midnight plasma cortisol, urinary free cortisol, and plasma cortisol after overnight dexamethasone suppression test consistent with autonomous adrenal cortisol secretion. It is described that IL-6 can stimulate HPA axis by increasing ACTH secretion, either directly or by augmenting the effect of CRH [15], as well as adrenal cells to produce cortisol [16]. However, its mechanism is not fully understood. To the extent of our knowledge, this is the first published pheochromocytoma producing IL-6 with associated autonomous cortisol secretion.

After adrenalectomy, the inflammatory syndrome resolved as well as all blood and biochemical parameters, including normetanephrine, C-reactive protein, IL-6, and ACTH. Hydrocortisone was prescribed at stress dose during adrenalectomy and no complications were noted. The dose was tapered and stopped until the short Synacthen® test was done which excluded adrenal insufficiency.

Another major point in this case is the potential risk of malignancy, since some histological features of malignancy as well as predominant normetanephrine secretion were present. It is known that pheochromocytomas with malignant behavior are associated with a predominant secretion of normetanephrine [17]. However, all of the reported IL-6-producing pheochromocytomas were found to secrete predominantly norepinephrine and none were described as malignant. After one year of follow-up, our patient presented no clinical, biochemical, or imaging evidence of relapse or distant metastases. Germline mutations in genes associated with malignant behavior were absent, lessening the malignancy potential [18].

This case shows a very rare presentation of a pheochromocytoma with associated IL-6 production and accompanied by autonomous cortisol secretion. The clinical presentation of an inflammatory syndrome of unknown origin may hamper the correct diagnosis, being extremely important to be aware of this condition to do the prompt diagnosis and the potentially curative treatment.

Disclosure

This research received no specific grant from any funding agency in the public, commercial, or not-for-profit sectors.

References

[1] M. Minetto, A. Dovio, M. Ventura et al., "Interleukin-6 producing pheochromocytoma presenting with acute inflammatory syndrome," *Journal of Endocrinological Investigation*, vol. 26, no. 5, pp. 453–457, 2003.

[2] A. Salahuddin, T. Rohr-Kirchgraber, R. Shekar, B. West, and J. Loewenstein, "Interleukin-6 in the fever and multiorgan crisis of pheochromocytoma," *Scandinavian Journal of Infectious Diseases*, vol. 29, no. 6, pp. 640–642, 1997.

[3] S. Fukumoto, T. Matsumoto, S.-I. Harada, J. Fujisaki, M. Kawano, and E. Ogata, "Pheochromocytoma with pyrexia and marked inflammatory signs: A paraneoplastic syndrome with possible relation to interleukin-6 production," *The Journal of Clinical Endocrinology & Metabolism*, vol. 73, no. 4, pp. 877–881, 1991.

[4] K. Suzuki, A. Miyashita, Y. Inoue et al., "Interleukin-6-producing pheochromocytoma," *Acta Haematologica*, vol. 85, no. 4, pp. 217–219, 1991.

[5] C. Shimizu, M. Kubo, K. Takano et al., "Interleukin-6 (IL-6) producing phaeochromocytoma: direct IL-6 suppression by non-steroidal anti-inflammatory drugs," *Clinical Endocrinology*, vol. 54, no. 3, pp. 405–410, 2001.

[6] S. Yarman, O. Soyluk, E. Altunoglu, and R. Tanakol, "Interleukin-6-producing pheochromocytoma presenting with fever of unknown origin," *Clinics (Sa~o Paulo, Brazil)*, vol. 66, no. 10, pp. 1843–1845, 2011.

[7] H. Tokuda, T. Hosoi, K. Hayasaka, K. Okamura, N. Yoshimi, and O. Kozawa, "Overexpression of protein kinase C-delta plays a crucial role in interleukin-6-producing pheochromocytoma presenting with acute inflammatory syndrome: a case report," *Hormone and Metabolic Research*, vol. 41, no. 4, pp. 333–338, 2009.

[8] M. Takagi, T. Egawa, T. Motomura et al., "Interleukin-6 secreting phaeochromocytoma associated with clinical markers of inflammation," *Clinical Endocrinology*, vol. 46, no. 4, pp. 507–509, 1997.

[9] J. M. Kang, W. J. Lee, W. B. Kim et al., "Systemic inflammatory syndrome and hepatic inflammatory cell infiltration caused by an interleukin-6 producing pheochromocytoma," *Endocrine Journal*, vol. 52, no. 2, pp. 193–198, 2005.

[10] R. A. Balk, "Systemic inflammatory response syndrome (SIRS): where did it come from and is it still relevant today?" *Virulence*, vol. 5, no. 1, pp. 20–26, 2014.

[11] T. Tanaka, M. Narazaki, and T. Kishimoto, "IL-6 in inflammation, immunity, and disease," *Cold Spring Harbor Perspectives in Biology*, vol. 6, no. 10, Article ID a016295, 2014.

[12] D. A. Papanicolaou, "Interleukin-6: the endocrine cytokine," *The Journal of Clinical Endocrinology & Metabolism*, vol. 85, no. 3, pp. 1331–1333, 2000.

[13] G. Päth, S. R. Bornstein, M. Ehrhart-Bornstein, and W. A. Scherbaum, "Interleukin-6 and the interleukin-6 receptor in the human adrenal gland: expression and effects on steroidogenesis[1]," *The Journal of Clinical Endocrinology & Metabolism*, vol. 82, no. 7, pp. 2343–2349, 1997.

[14] V. E. Strong, T. Kennedy, H. Al-Ahmadie et al., "Prognostic indicators of malignancy in adrenal pheochromocytomas: clinical, histopathologic, and cell cycle/apoptosis gene expression analysis," *Surgery*, vol. 143, no. 6, pp. 759–768, 2008.

[15] G. P. Chrousos, "The hypothalamic-pituitary-adrenal axis and immune-mediated inflammation," *The New England Journal of Medicine*, vol. 332, no. 20, pp. 1351–1362, 1995.

[16] M. Ciacciarelli, D. Bellini, A. Laghi et al., "IL-6-producing, noncatecholamines secreting pheochromocytoma presenting as fever of unknown origin," *Case Reports in Medicine*, vol. 2016, Article ID 3489046, 5 pages, 2016.

[17] N. Kimura, K. Takekoshi, and M. Naruse, "Risk stratification on pheochromocytoma and paraganglioma from laboratory and clinical medicine," *Journal of Clinical Medicine*, vol. 7, no. 9, p. 242, 2018.

[18] J. W. M. Lenders, Q.-Y. Duh, and G. Eisenhofer, "Pheochromocytoma and paraganglioma : an endocrine society clinical practice guideline," *The Journal of Clinical Endocrinology & Metabolism*, vol. 99, no. 6, pp. 1915–1942, 2014.

37

Poorly Controlled Type 3c Diabetes due to use of Veterinarian Insulin Syringes

Francisco Barrera and Natia Murvelashvili

Amita Health Saint Francis Hospital, 355 Ridge Avenue, Evanston, IL 60202, USA

Correspondence should be addressed to Francisco Barrera; franxabae@hotmail.com

Academic Editor: Lucy Mastrandrea

Initiation of insulin therapy can be challenging for patients; proper training should be given by physicians and certified educators to ensure correct and safe use for outpatient population. Different insulin strengths are now available in the US; while U-40 insulin does not exist in the United States for humans, it is a very common strength used in animals. We are reporting a 30-year-old male that became insulin dependent after hospitalization for necrotizing pancreatitis who was using U-40 syringes to draw from the prescribed insulin U-100 and also presented with repeated hypoglycemic episodes.

1. Introduction

The proportion of patients with diabetes currently on any insulin (includes insulin only and insulin plus oral diabetes medications) was 29.1% in 2005–2012 and has been relatively stable since 1988 with 30.3% [1]. Diabetes secondary to pancreatic diseases is commonly referred to as pancreatogenic diabetes or type 3c diabetes mellitus; it is a clinically relevant condition with a prevalence of 5%-10% among all diabetic subjects in Western populations. Those with type 3c diabetes require insulin therapy more urgently than those with type 2, and most of them are discharged on insulin from the hospital [2].

2. Case Presentation

A 30-year-old male presented in December 2017 to the emergency department complaining of abdominal pain, which started around 3 am, and the pain was characterized as sharp, epigastric, nonradiating, and 9/10 in intensity. He admitted drinking alcohol, used to drink 5-6 glasses of wine/cocktails a day, but claimed he stopped a week ago, and he denied smoking or another illicit drug use.

Laboratory exams on admission were significant for lactic acid 3.7 (0.7-2.0 mmol/L), lipase >3000IU/L (11-82 IU/L), WBC 33,300 mmcu (4,000-11,000mmcu), and glucose 147mg/dl (70-99mg/dl). Patient underwent CT abdomen that showed acute pancreatitis. The next day patient glucose increased to 502mg/dl, bicarbonate was 18mg/dl (21-31mg/dl), and anion gap was 14. Patient then was transferred to Intensive Care Unit (ICU) for insulin infusion and management of diabetic ketoacidosis (DKA). His hemoglobin A1c was 5.5%.

Repeat CT abdomen with contrast (Figure 2) was concerning for necrotizing pancreatitis. After few days he was switched to subcutaneous insulin glargine/aspart and transferred back to general medical floor. Because patient developed fever and had persistent leukocytosis, and he was started on meropenem. His conditioned improved and antibiotics were changed to oral doxycycline and levofloxacin; he was discharged on insulin glargine 20U at bedtime and correctional insulin.

Patient continued to follow up as an outpatient. His blood sugars were ranging between 80 and 200 and A1c at the office visit was 4% in April 2017. Glargine was decreased to 15U nightly and sliding scale with meals was continued. In June 2017 glargine was reduced by a primary care provider to 7U due to symptomatic hypoglycemia. In July 2017 at an endocrinologist's office, A1c was 6.4%, and he allegedly reported daily fasting blood sugars ranging between 70 and 200. Glargine then was stopped and patient was advised to

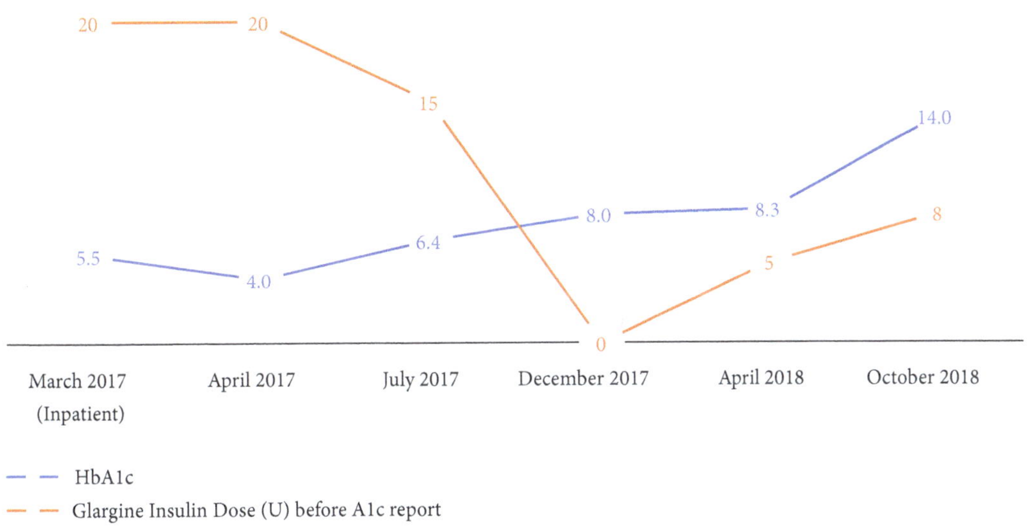

FIGURE 1: Trend of A1c and glargine insulin dose.

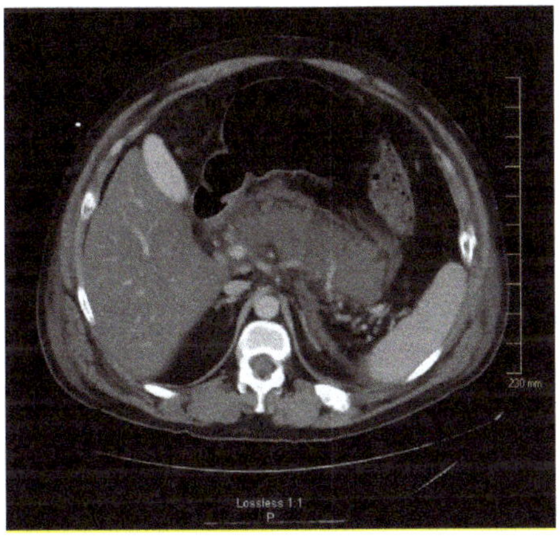

FIGURE 2: Second abdominal CT showing worsening pancreatitis.

continue taking correctional aspart insulin to administer 3U if glucose>150 (Figure 1).

In December 2017, while the patient was off glargine, A1c worsened to 8%. Patient was only using aspart as indicated and blood sugars were rarely >200s. Glargine was reinstated 5U nightly and Humalog started 4U with meals with an instruction not to take it if glucose was <110. However, in April 2018, HbA1c was 8.3% and he had episodes of symptomatic hypoglycemia. After further investigation, patient disclosed that, to avoid extra expenses, he used veterinary U-40 insulin syringes for the prescribed U100 insulin that he was getting from his wife, who herself worked in a veterinarian clinic. Unfortunately, he stopped checking his sugars regularly and on the next appointment in October 2018, HbA1c was 14%. Patient was taking glargine 8U at bedtime and Humalog 4 U if glucose was <150 and 7 U if glucose was 250-350 (Figure 1).

3. Discussion

There are different strengths of insulin. The standard and most commonly used strength in the United States is U-100. Insulin is labeled "U-100," which means there are 100 units of insulin per milliliter of fluid in the vial. Regular insulin is available in U-500 strength form, which is reserved for people with marked insulin resistance who take doses of more than 200 units per day [3, 4]. Concentrated insulin allows administration of smaller volumes per dose and may reduce the total number of daily injections. Until recently, regular U-500 insulin was the only concentrated insulin. Life-threatening dosing errors occurred due to lack of a U-500 syringe or availability of a U-500 insulin pen. Syringe specifically for insulin U-500 is now available; it has a green cover and 5-unit increment scale. U-500 disposable prefilled pens are also in the market [5].

New strength formulations of concentrated insulin such as glargine U-300, degludec U-200, and lispro U-200 are only available in a disposable prefilled pen; therefore, these do not carry the same safety concerns related to dosing and administration errors that U-500 insulin used to have [5, 6]. Most concentrated insulin pens give warning about not to transfer insulin from the pen into a syringe as severe overdose can happen.

Dosing errors can occur if patients are not properly educated in the use of syringes/vials and the different insulin strengths.

The syringes for administering insulin are specifically designed for each different strength. A U-100 syringe should only be used with U-100 insulin vial. Patients from North America flying overseas must bring their own insulin and syringes. In some countries the only insulin sold is in U-40 strength, syringes marked for U-40 should be used, and syringes for U-40 insulin most of the time have a red cover and red scale, rather than the orange needle cover and black scale of U-100 syringes.

Most insulin for animals is U-40 insulin and most pet owners use the specific insulin syringe U-40 to eliminate the need for dosage conversion required for a U-100 insulin syringe, which may reduce the risk of inaccurate dosing and waste [7].

(1) One unit of U-100 insulin is 0.01ml in volume.

(2) One unit of U-500 insulin is 0.002 ml in volume.

(2.1) Drawing 5-unit markings of insulin U-100 vial into a U-500 syringe is 5 times less concentration than the intended dose and can result in poorly controlled diabetes [3, 4].

(3) One unit of U-40 insulin is 0.025 ml.

(3.1) Drawing 5-unit markings of insulin U-100 vial into U-40 syringe is 2.5 times greater concentration than the intended dose, resulting in hypoglycemia which is what happened with our patient.

In countries like Turkey and India, availability of both U-40 and U-100 insulin vials and syringes increases the probability of dosing error resulting in hypoglycemia or poorly controlled diabetes unless patients are informed and acquainted with both types of vials and syringes at the time of initiating insulin therapy [8, 9]. In the United Kingdom where 80% of the diabetic population are seen at special diabetes clinics, patients were switched under the direct supervision of the physician. It was the doctor's responsibility to train the diabetic patient and to issue a prescription for U-100 materials. The pharmacist collected all the U-40 materials before filling the new prescription. Conversion to U-100 insulin was postponed if the patient failed to bring old insulin and syringes to the pharmacy [8].

4. Conclusion

Insulin plays a very important role in the management of diabetes; however, there are many variables that can be difficult to handle for patients who are initiating its use. Diabetes education is the cornerstone of diabetes management, because diabetes requires day-to-day knowledge of nutrition, exercise, monitoring, and medication. Education and training of insulin use prior initiation of therapy can prevent multiple complications; thus, a better understanding of the different strengths of insulins and use of prefilled disposable pens will prevent rare cases like our patient who had multiple episodes of hypoglycemia and erratic diabetes management due to use of veterinarian U-40 syringes to administer U-100 insulin.

References

[1] E. Selvin, C. M. Parrinello, N. Daya, and R. M. Bergenstal, "Trends in insulin use and diabetes control in the U.S.: 1988-1994 and 1999-2012," *Diabetes Care*, vol. 39, no. 3, pp. e33–e35, 2016.

[2] A. M. Drewes, "Diagnosis and treatment of diabetes mellitus in chronic pancreatitis," *World Journal of Gastroenterology*, vol. 19, no. 42, pp. 7276–7281, 2013.

[3] A. Clark, "U-500 insulin: not for ordinary use," *US Pharmacist, The Pharmacist's Resource for Clinical Excellence*, vol. 35, no. 5, pp. 14–17, 2010.

[4] S. Reutrakul, K. Wroblewski, and R. L. Brown, "Clinical use of U-500 regular insulin: Review and meta-analysis," *Journal of Diabetes Science and Technology*, vol. 6, no. 2, pp. 412–420, 2012.

[5] J. L. Rosselli, S. N. Archer, N. K. Lindley, and L. M. Butler, "U300 insulin glargine: a novel basal insulin for type 1 and type 2 diabetes," *Journal of Pharmacy Technology*, vol. 31, no. 5, pp. 234–242, 2015.

[6] A. J. Chabanuk, "U-200 humalog insulin now available in United States," *Home Healthcare Now*, vol. 34, no. 2, p. 102, 2016.

[7] A. Thompson, P. Lathan, and L. Fleeman, "Update on insulin treatment for dogs and cats: insulin dosing pens and more," *Veterinary Medicine: Research and Reports*, vol. 6, pp. 129–142, 2015.

[8] C. Selcuk and H. Aksahin, "U-40 syringe for U-100 insulin: a new cause of hypoglycemia in Turkey," *Turkish Journal of Endocrinology and Metabolism*, vol. 2, pp. 75-76, 2000.

[9] S. Chowdhury and P. Chakraborty, "Errors of insulin therapy: Real-life experiences from developing world," *Journal of Family Medicine and Primary Care*, vol. 6, no. 4, pp. 724–729, 2017.

38

Myocardial Infarction after Long-Term Treatment with a Tyrosine Kinase Inhibitor (TKI) with Anti-VEGF Receptor Activity

L. Paschke,[1] T. Lincke,[2] K. Mühlberg,[3] Tom H. Lindner,[4] and R. Paschke[5]

[1]*Division of Endocrinology, Department of Endocrinology and Nephrology, University Clinic Leipzig, Germany*
[2]*Division of Nuclear Medicine, Department of Radiology, University Clinic Leipzig, Germany*
[3]*Department of Angiology, University Clinic Leipzig, Germany*
[4]*Division of Nephrology, Department of Endocrinology and Nephrology, University Clinic Leipzig, Germany*
[5]*Department of Medicine, Division of Endocrinology, Departments of Oncology, Pathology, and Biochemistry and Molecular Biology & Arnie Charbonneau Cancer Institute Cumming School of Medicine, University of Calgary, Canada*

Correspondence should be addressed to R. Paschke; ralf.paschke@ucalgary.ca

Academic Editor: John Broom

TKIs including anti-VEGF receptor activity have been approved for the treatment of patients with radioiodine resistant thyroid carcinomas. For lenvatinib arterial thromboembolic events are listed as adverse events of special interest with lenvatinib. In the phase III study, arterial thromboembolic events were reported in 3% of lenvatinib-treated patients and 1% in the placebo group. Most of the patients had predisposing factors. Only one myocardial infarct was reported in the lenvatinib phase III study. We report a 73-year-old female patient with metastatic thyroid papillary carcinoma who was treated with total thyroidectomy. The operation was followed by four radioiodine therapies over a period of 6 years. At 6 years she developed lung metastasis without radioiodine uptake, one solitary liver metastasis and one solitary right renal metastasis. One year after the first diagnosis of radioiodine resistant lung metastasis the lung metastasis showed progression according to RECIST criteria. This treatment was resulting in prolonged partial response with disappearance of a hepatic and renal metastasis. A myocardial infarction occurred after 39 months of lenvatinib treatment resulting in implantation of 3 stents and a two chamber pacemaker. The treatment was discontinued. Except for well controlled hypertension there were neither predisposing diseases like diabetes nor symptoms of cardiac ischemia on exertion. However, the family history for cardiovascular diseases was positive for cardiac infarction reported for one brother. Another brother was treated for hypertension and the patient's mother suffered from a cerebral infarction at the age of 60. While only one myocardial infarct was reported in the lenvatinib phase III study with 392 patients this case suggests that long-term treatment with lenvatinib may be associated with an increased risk for myocardial infarct also in patients with no predisposing diseases except well controlled hypertension and positive family history for cardiovascular diseases.

1. Introduction

In 2015 lenvatinib, an inhibitor of vascular endothelial growth factor receptors 1, 2, and 3, fibroblast growth factor receptors 1 through 4, platelet-derived growth factor receptor α, RET, and KIT signaling networks [1, 2], has been approved by the FDA and EMA for the treatment of radioiodine refractory differentiated thyroid cancer.

A randomized, double-blinded phase III study involved patients with progressive thyroid cancer that was refractory to ^{131}iodine and randomly assigned 261 patients to receive lenvatinib (daily dose of 24 mg/d in 28-day cycles) and 131 patients to receive placebo. Compared with placebo, lenvatinib was associated with significant improvements in progression-free survival and the response rate among patients with ^{131}iodine-refractory thyroid cancer [3]. During the 13.8 months of median duration of treatment, treatment-related adverse events (all grades) occurred in 97.3% in the lenvatinib group; of these 75.9% were treatment-related adverse events of grade 3 or higher [3]. In the SELECT trial

3.0% of lenvatinib-treated patients presented arterial thromboembolic events. Most of the patients had cardiovascular risk factors. Only one myocardial infarct was reported.

Here, we report a patient with papillary thyroid cancer who suffered from a myocardial infarction during long-term treatment with lenvatinib. This case cautions that long-term treatment with lenvatinib can be associated with myocardial infarction also in patients who were asymptomatic and had no predisposing diseases except well controlled hypertension and a positive family history for cardiovascular diseases.

2. Patient

We report a 73-year-old female patient with metastatic thyroid papillary carcinoma who was treated with total thyroidectomy. The operation was followed by four radioiodine therapies over a period of 6 years. At 6 years she developed lung metastasis without radioiodine uptake, one solitary liver metastasis and one solitary right renal metastasis. One year after the first diagnosis of radioiodine resistant lung metastasis the lung metastasis showed progression according to RECIST criteria. The patient was therefore enrolled in the phase III study comparing lenvatinib to placebo. After the study ended the patient was unblinded. Lenvatinib treatment resulted in prolonged partial response with disappearance of the hepatic and renal metastasis. During further treatment with lenvatinib with dose reduction from initially 24 to 10 mg at 17 months of lenvatinib treatment a myocardial infarction occurred after 39 months of lenvatinib treatment resulting in implantation of 3 stents and a two chamber pacemaker. Treatment with lenvatinib was discontinued at the time of diagnosis of the myocardial infarction. Except for well controlled hypertension there were neither predisposing diseases like diabetes nor symptoms of cardiac ischemia on exertion. Quarterly repeated echocardiography at rest showed normal results during the first two years of lenvatinib treatment during the phase III study. However, the family history for cardiovascular diseases was positive for cardiac infarction reported for one brother. Another brother was treated for hypertension and the patients' mother suffered from a cerebral infarction at the age of 60.

3. Discussion

Tyrosine kinase inhibitors with anti-VEGF receptor activity are known for their potential to cause thromboembolic adverse events.

Sorafenib, an inhibitor of VEGFR-1, VEGFR-2, and VEGFR-3, RET (including RET/PTC translocations), RAF (including BRAFV600E point mutation), and platelet-derived growth factor receptor beta (PDGFRβ) [4], was approved for the treatment of radioiodine refractory DTC in 2014 by the EMA and FDA. Before it was also approved for the treatment of unresectable hepatocellular carcinoma and advanced renal-cell carcinoma.

A randomized, double-blind, placebo-controlled phase III study involving patients with advanced clear-cell renal-cell carcinoma reported cardiac ischemia or infarction in 12 patients in the sorafenib group (3%) and 2 patients in the placebo group (<1%) (P=0.01). Of these events, 11 (including 2 deaths in the sorafenib group and 1 death in the placebo group) were considered to be serious adverse events associated with treatment [5]. A phase 3, double-blinded, placebo-controlled study assigned 602 patients with advanced hepatocellular carcinoma who had not received previous systemic treatment to receive either sorafenib (at a dose of 400 mg twice daily) or placebo. Cardiac Ischemia or infarction appeared in 3% of the patients receiving sorafenib compared to 1% in the placebo group [6]. The median durations of sorafenib treatments in these studies were 10.6 months [4], 5.8 months [5], and 5.3 months [6].

Furthermore, soon after the introduction of bevacizumab-treatment for metastatic breast cancer the clinical incidence of arteriovascular events, i.e., cerebrovascular ischemia was reported in 2% of the patients and 1.6% of the patients suffering from heart failure and even more alarming 15% having severe hypertension [7]. In addition, meta-analysis showed that the addition of bevacicumab to chemotherapy increased the risk of arterial thrombotic events when compared to the chemotherapy alone [8]. Moreover a pooled analysis of five randomized trials encompassing 1745 patients randomly assigned to chemotherapy alone or chemotherapy plus bevacicumab for the treatment of metastatic colorectal cancer, breast cancer, and non-small-cell lung cancer showed that the increase of arterial thromboembolic events (ATEs) was further increased in elderly patients or patients with a history of ATEs. Patients with both risk factors developed ATEs in 17.9% [9].

A meta-analysis including 9711 patients from 19 randomized controlled trials with bevacicumab [10] revealed an overall incidence of ATEs of 1,5% whereof cardiac ischemia (67,4%), CNS ischemia (7,9%), and cerebrovascular accident (6,7%) were most common. The mortality of these ATEs was 8,2% [10].

Because of the thromboembolic potential of TKIs Conti et al. proposed in 2013 a cardiovascular assessment of patients undergoing a TKI treatment before treatment start and to include patients at high/highest risk according to established risk scores like the Global Registry of Acute Coronary Events (GRACE) score in a cardiovascular monitoring program [11].

Recently, a multicenter phase 2 study of sunitinib another antiangiogenic tyrosine kinase inhibitor in patients with locally advanced or metastatic differentiated, anaplastic or medullary thyroid carcinomas, revealed that during a median follow-up time of 9 months/25 months 14.1% of the patients suffered from cardiac events [12]. Out of 5 deadly adverse events 4 were cardiac events. Due to an expected increased risk of severe adverse cardiac events the follow-up of the study included systematic survey, a left ventricular ejection fraction (LVEF) ultrasound, and N-terminal probrain natriuretic peptide or N-terminal brain natriuretic peptide (probrain natriuretic peptide [BNP]/BNP) dosage. None of these specific parameters showed the potential to select patients more stringently [12].

Furthermore a meta-analysis on 4679 patients under treatment with sorafenib or sunitinib or pazopanib demonstrated an increased risk of fatal adverse events (RR 2.23) regardless of tumor type and drug used, when compared with control groups. Myocardial infarction represented the cause in 15% of all deaths attributable to VEGFR inhibitor [13].

Our case report suggests that lenvatinib should also be added to the list of TKIs with ATE potential. So far, most of the thromboembolic events appeared after short-term treatment median duration of 10.8 months with tyrosine kinase inhibitors and mostly in patients with predisposing factors. However, our patient suffered from her first myocardial infarction after long-term treatment with lenvatinib for 39 months, in absence of predisposing diseases except well controlled hypertension and a positive family history for cardiovascular diseases. These findings suggest that long-term treatment with lenvatinib may be associated with an increased risk for myocardial infarction. Therefore, as previously proposed by Conti et al. for other TKIs also patients with lenvatinib treatment should be assessed for cardiovascular risk and coronary ischemia before and during the treatment. However, as indicated by our patient not only patients with high/very high cardiovascular risk factors should be under closer clinical cardiovascular surveillance as our patient's GRACE score before study entry indicated only a low individual risk of death by myocardial infarction. The assessment of cardiovascular risk and coronary ischemia should include a family history for cardiovascular diseases, cardiac stress testing, and an initial and regular cardiac survey to identify those at increased risk for cardiac events. It should be performed before starting lenvatinib treatment and at annual intervals during lenvatinib therapy. In addition, further data on adverse events during long-term TKI treatment with anti-VEGF receptor activity should be systematically collected.

Disclosure

The Abstract was presented as a poster in 39th Annual Meeting of the European Thyroid Association.

References

[1] J. Matsui, Y. Yamamoto, Y. Funahashi et al., "E7080, a novel inhibitor that targets multiple kinases, has potent antitumor activities against stem cell factor producing human small cell lung cancer H146, based on angiogenesis inhibition," *International Journal of Cancer*, vol. 122, no. 3, pp. 664–671, 2008.

[2] J. Matsui, Y. Funahashi, T. Uenaka, T. Watanabe, A. Tsuruoka, and M. Asada, "Multi-kinase inhibitor E7080 suppresses lymph node and lung metastases of human mammary breast tumor MDA-MB-231 via inhibition of vascular endothelial growth factor-receptor (VEGF-R) 2 and VEGF-R3 kinase," *Clinical Cancer Research*, vol. 14, no. 17, pp. 5459–5465, 2008.

[3] M. Schlumberger, M. Tahara, L. J. Wirth et al., "Lenvatinib versus placebo in radioiodine-refractory thyroid cancer," *The New England Journal of Medicine*, vol. 372, no. 7, pp. 621–630, 2015.

[4] M. S. Brose, C. M. Nutting, B. Jarzab et al., "Sorafenib in radioactive iodine-refractory, locally advanced or metastatic differentiated thyroid cancer: a randomised, double-blind, phase 3 trial," *The Lancet*, vol. 384, no. 9940, pp. 319–328, 2014.

[5] B. Escudier, T. Eisen, W. M. Stadler et al., "Sorafenib in advanced clear-cell renal-cell carcinoma," *The New England Journal of Medicine*, vol. 356, no. 2, pp. 125–134, 2007.

[6] J. M. Llovet, S. Ricci, V. Mazzaferro et al., "Sorafenib in advanced hepatocellular carcinoma," *The New England Journal of Medicine*, vol. 359, no. 4, pp. 378–390, 2008.

[7] K. Miller, M. Wang, J. Gralow et al., "Paclitaxel plus bevacizumab versus paclitaxel alone for metastatic breast cancer," *The New England Journal of Medicine*, vol. 357, no. 26, pp. 2666–2676, 2007.

[8] V. Ranpura, S. Hapani Chuang J, and S. Wu, "Risk of cardiac ischemia and arterial thromboembol- ic events with the angiogenesis inhibitor bevacicumab in cancer patients: a meta-analysis," *Lancet Oncology*, vol. 10, pp. 559–568, 2009.

[9] F. A. Scappaticci, J. R. Skillings, S. N. Holden, H.-P. Gerber, K. Miller et al., "Arterial thromboembolic events in patients with metastatic carcinoma treated with chemotherapy and bevacicumab," *Journal of the National Cancer Institute*, vol. 99, pp. 1232–1239, 2007.

[10] W.-X. Qi, Z. Shen, L.-N. Tang, and Y. Yao, "Risk of arterial thromboembolic events with vascular endothelial growth factor receptor tyrosine kinase inhibitors: An up-to-date meta-analysis," *Critical Review in Oncology/Hematology*, vol. 92, no. 2, pp. 71–82, 2014.

[11] E. Conti, A. Romiti, M. B. Musumeci et al., "Arterial thrombotic events and acute coronary syndromes with cancer drugs: Are growth factors the missed link?: What both cardiologist and oncologist should know about novel angiogenesis inhibitors," *International Journal of Cardiology*, vol. 167, no. 6, pp. 2421–2429, 2013.

[12] A. Ravaud, C. de la Fouchardière, P. Caron et al., "A multicenter phase II study of sunitinib in patients with locally advanced or metastatic differentiated, anaplastic or medullary thyroid carcinomas: mature data from the THYSU study," *European Journal of Cancer*, vol. 76, pp. 110–117, 2017.

[13] F. A. Schutz, Y. Je, C. J. Richards, and T. K. Choueiri, "Meta-analysis of randomized controlled trials for the incidence and risk of treatment-related mortality in patients with cancer treated with vascular endothelial growth factor tyrosine kinase inhibitors," *Journal of Clinical Oncology*, vol. 30, no. 8, pp. 871–877, 2012.

39

Schwannoma Misdiagnosed as Adrenal Adenoma: A Case Report and Review of the Literature

Mussa H. AlMalki[1,2] **Metib Alotaibi,**[1] **Mohammad Maswood Ahmad**[1] **Muhammad Amin ur Rahman,**[3] **and Turki Alharthi**[4]

[1]*Obesity, Endocrine and Metabolism Center, King Fahad Medical City, Riyadh, Saudi Arabia*
[2]*King Fahad Medical City, College of Medicine, King Saud Bin Abdul Aziz University for Health Science, Riyadh, Saudi Arabia*
[3]*Department of Pathology and Laboratory Medicine Administration, King Fahad Medical City, Riyadh, Saudi Arabia*
[4]*Department of Endocrinology, Military Hospital, Jeddah, Saudi Arabia*

Correspondence should be addressed to Mussa H. AlMalki; m2malki@yahoo.com

Academic Editor: John Broom

Schwannoma is a benign neurogenic tumor originating from the neural sheath of Schwann cells. It is an extremely rare cause of adrenal adenoma which is very difficult to diagnose preoperatively. We report the case of a right adrenal schwannoma discovered incidentally in a 62-year-old woman during evaluation of right flank pain. The biochemical and hormonal evaluations were unremarkable. Radiological examination revealed a 4.8 cm lesion keeping with right adrenal adenoma. Surgical intervention was done due to the large size of the tumor, and laparoscopic right adrenalectomy was performed. The postoperative course was uneventful. Histological examination established the diagnosis of schwannoma, which was further confirmed by immunohistochemical staining. In conclusion, adrenal schwannoma is extremely rare and can be misdiagnosed as nonsecreting adrenal adenoma. Complete surgical excision is the treatment of choice which is associated with favorable outcome and also helps in clarifying its histopathological nature.

1. Introduction

Schwannoma is a rare, benign, and slowly progressive neurogenic tumor originating from the Schwann sheath of the nerves. It occurs predominantly in the head and neck regions [1]. Visceral schwannoma in the adrenal region is extremely rare, accounting for only 0.7% of the adrenal tumors [2]. These tumors are very difficult to diagnose preoperatively, usually present as incidental findings and are often misdiagnosed as adrenal adenoma [3]. Surgery is the treatment of choice, whenever feasible. Consequently, a definitive diagnosis can only be made upon histological and immunohistochemical studies of the resected lesion [4]. Herein, we report a case of large adrenal schwannoma mimicking adrenal adenoma with a brief review of the literature.

2. Case Presentation

A 62-year-old Saudi woman underwent medical assessment for right flank pain. She was referred to the endocrine clinic for further evaluation. Her medical history revealed hypothyroidism on levothyroxine replacement and bilateral knee osteoarthritis, while family history was unremarkable. Clinically, she was asymptomatic with a heart rate of 71 beats/minute and blood pressure of 128/75 mmHg. Examination of her abdomen revealed no palpable mass. Blood counts and biochemical panel were within normal limits. No hormonal overproduction was detected as 24 h urinary catecholamines, plasma renin activity, plasma aldosterone concentration, and cortisol values were within normal ranges.

A computed tomography (CT) scan (Figure 1) demonstrated a well-circumscribed, uniform, hypodense fat-containing lesion 4.8 cm in diameter with a Hounsfield unit of twelve on unenhanced CT. Also, its density measured 10 HU in the porto-venous phase and 15 HU on the delayed 15 minutes phase. The absolute and relative washout value at 15 minutes of more than 55% and 35% respectively, keeping with right adrenal adenoma. Due to the large size of the tumor, surgical intervention was decided and right

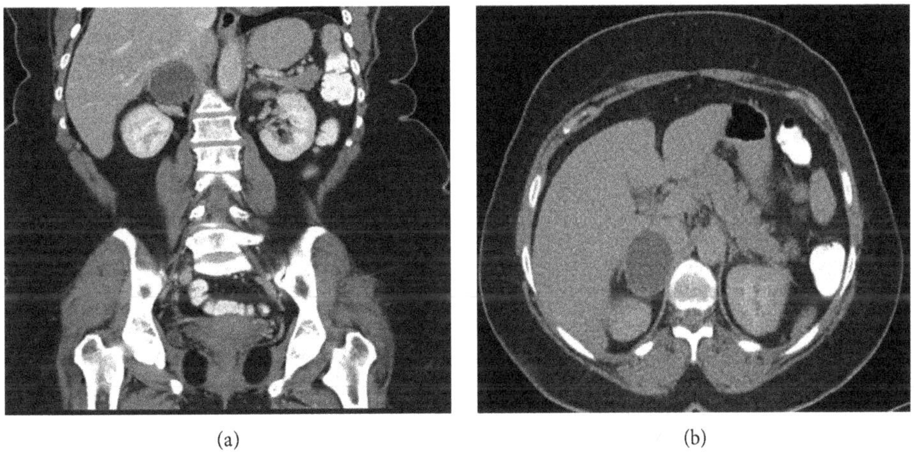

FIGURE 1: Preop CT adrenal: (a) coronal section and (b) axial section showed a 4.8 × 4.1 cm well-defined rounded right adrenal hypodense lesion. It has precontrast density of 12 HU. Its density measured 10 HU in the porto-venous phase and 15 HU on the delayed 15 minutes phase. No wall calcification. The left adrenal gland is within normal.

laparoscopic adrenalectomy was performed. The postoperative period was uneventful. On gross pathological examination, the tumor was 4.5 cm in size, encapsulated, and was present adjacent to the normal-appearing adrenal gland. A central cystic space was seen within the tumor mass.

Histologically (Figures 2–5), the tumor comprised spindle cell proliferation arranged in small fascicles of tumor cells with elongated to wavy nuclei and scanty eosinophilic cytoplasm with indistinct cell membranes, present in a fibrillary stroma. Most of the tumor appeared very cellular with only focal alternating hypocellular (Antoni B) areas (Figure 5). The stroma also showed a variable amount of thick collagen bundles. In some areas, the tumor cell nuclei were seen palisading around a fibrillary material (Verocay bodies). Foamy and hemosiderin-laden macrophages were also seen. The tumor cells were positive with S100 on immunohistochemistry. The morphology and immunohistochemistry were consistent with a diagnosis of a schwannoma, the cellular variant which is often seen in paravertebral locations, and it shows more cellularity than the classical variant. There were no features, such as increased mitoses, pleomorphism, or necrosis, to suggest malignancy.

The patient remained asymptomatic during the five-month follow-up period, and there was no evidence of any radiological recurrence or distant metastasis (Figure 6).

3. Discussions

Schwannoma is encapsulated, usually a benign, slow-growing tumor that arises from the Schwann cells surrounding the peripheral nerves [1]. It is usually located within the head and neck region or the peripheral extremities with lesser frequency in the retroperitoneum [5].

These tumors are rare and account only for 1–5% of retroperitoneal masses [6]. Schwannoma in the adrenal region is extremely rare, accounting for only 0.7% of the adrenal tumors with about 80 cases have been reported to date [2].

Malignant schwannoma is infrequent and typically found in the extremities and often in association with neurofibromatosis types 1 and 2 [7].

Due to their asymptomatic clinical course and non-secreting nature, preoperatively they are often misdiagnosed as nonfunctioning adrenal adenoma.

They can occur at any age but predominantly between the second and fifth decade of life. However, retroperitoneal schwannomas are most commonly seen between 40 and 60 years of age, with a slight female predominance [7, 8]. In one series of 33 cases, a median age at the diagnosis was 49 years (14–89 years) with a slight female predominance (F : M = 1.2 : 1) [9]. Similarly, Zhou et al. also found female predilection (F : M: 1.4 : 1) with a median age of 47 years [2]. Differential diagnosis of adrenal schwannomas includes adrenal adenoma, pheochromocytoma, myelolipomas, neuroblastoma, ganglioneuroma, cortical carcinomas, cysts, and metastases [9]. Although most of the patients with adrenal schwannoma have no clinical or biochemical evidence of hormonal overproduction, a complete hormonal evaluation is still required as for other adrenal masses, including serum electrolytes, low-dose dexamethasone suppression testing, serum aldosterone renin ratio, and a 24-hour urine collection for catecholamines and metanephrines.

In one case series of 33 patients, the majority was identified incidentally, and only 13 patients had abdominal pain, flank pain, or discomfort before a specific diagnosis. One case showed elevated urinary catecholamines [9]. Recently, in case series of 31 patients by Zhou et al. the majority (84%) was identified incidentally, and only five patients had symptoms. Of these, three patients were clinically suspicious for the diagnosis of cortisol-producing adenoma; one patient with symptoms prompting the possible diagnosis of aldosterone-producing adenoma; and one patient hospitalized for acute intermittent abdominal pain without evidence of adrenal-relevant hormonal abnormalities [2].

Imaging characteristics on CT scan may aid in diagnosis. Schwannomas usually appear as a well-circumscribed,

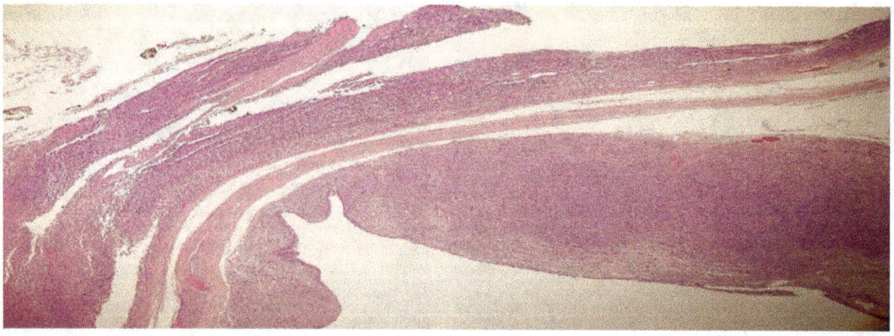

FIGURE 2: Low-power view of the adrenal gland (top) and schwannoma with capsule (middle) and cystic change (bottom). H&E ×40.

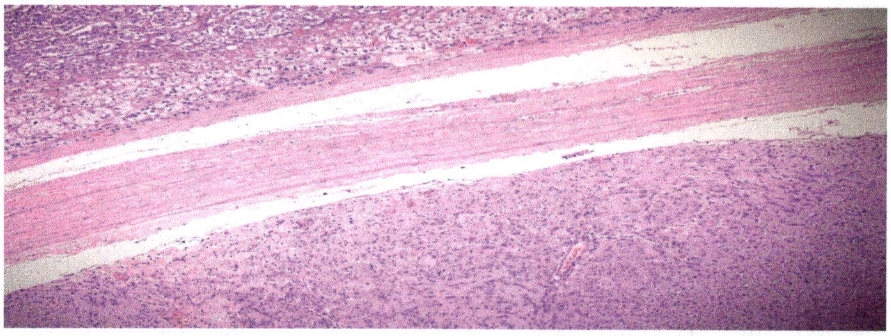

FIGURE 3: Adrenal (top), tumor capsule (middle), and schwannoma (bottom). H&E ×100.

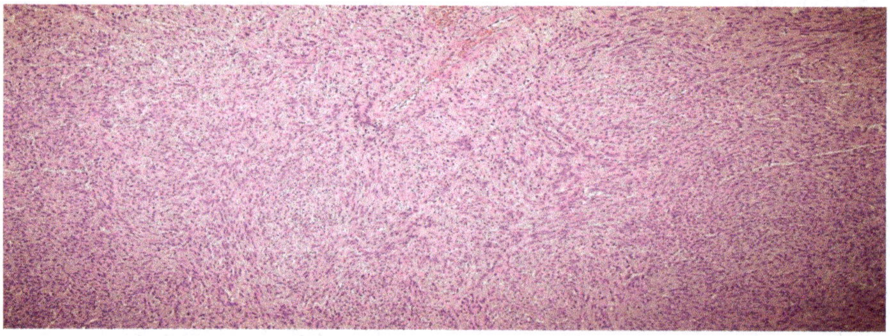

FIGURE 4: Schwannoma cell morphology, H&E ×200.

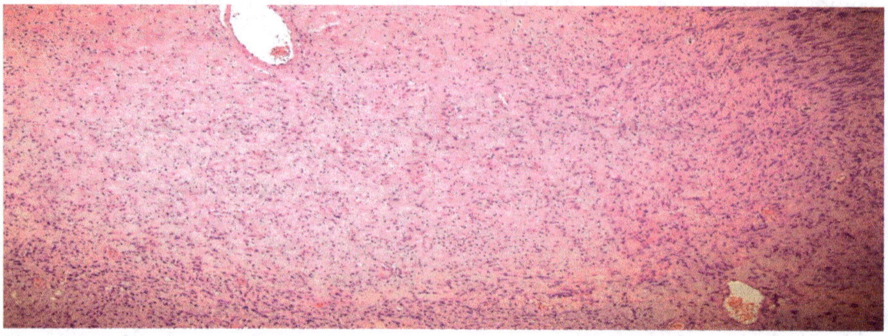

FIGURE 5: Schwannoma hypocellular areas (Antoni (B)) areas.

homogenous, and round or oval lesion, with slight enhancement on the CT scan with cystic degeneration or calcification [10]. In one study, it was found that the combination of necrosis with a minimal degree of tumor enhancement in the arterial phase of the CT scan increased the probability of ruling out schwannoma [11]. Furthermore, the schwannomas on MRI appear as a well-circumscribed mass with cystic degenerative changes with low

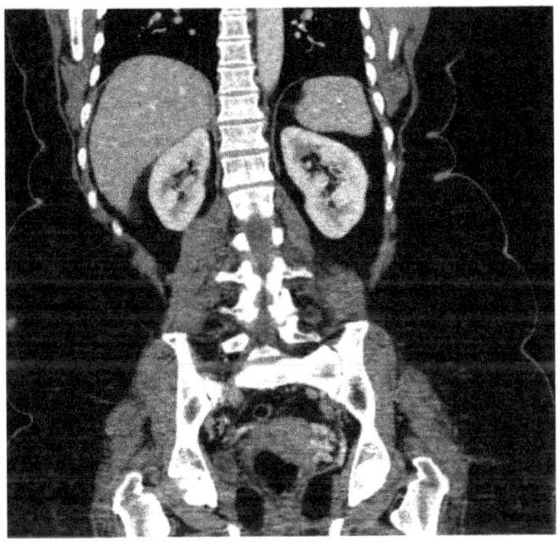

(a)

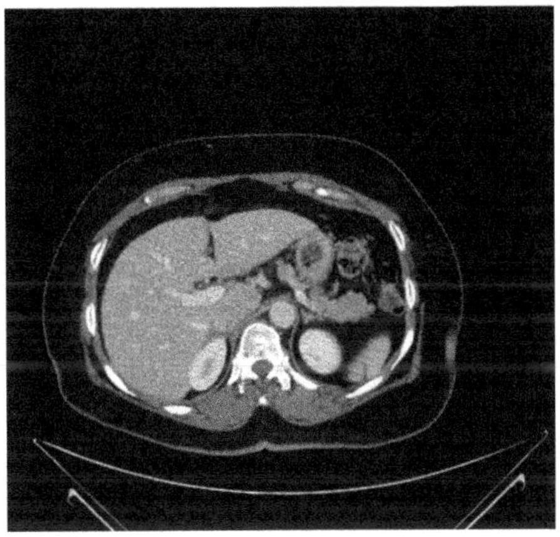

(b)

FIGURE 6: Postop CT adrenal: (a) coronal section and (b) axial section showed postresection of the right adrenal mass with no signs of residual or recurrent disease. The left adrenal gland is unremarkable.

signal intensity on T1-weighted images and heterogeneous high signal intensity on T2-weighted images. However, these imaging characteristics are not specific [12].

It should be noted that the preoperative diagnosis is not definitive due to limited hormonal disturbances and overlapping radiological features [13]. Therefore, it will remain unclear until after surgical intervention and histopathologic examination of the resected lesion. In our case, the clinical features and the location of the mass were strongly suggestive of an adrenal adenoma, and laboratory workup did not contribute any further other than ruling out hormonal overproduction. The final diagnosis could be uncovered only after histopathological evaluation of the resected lesion.

On gross examination, adrenal schwannomas appear as a well-circumscribed, firm, round, and tan-yellow to grayish-white mass. Although the majority of them are solid with homogenous consistency, some may have cystic areas and appear larger or may have areas of calcification or hemorrhage [14]. Histologically, schwannomas are diagnosed based on the detection of spindle cells with characteristic elongated to wavy nuclei, showing alternating cellular (Antoni A) and hypocellular (Antoni B) regions [15]. Immunohistochemically, these lesions stain positively for S100 antibodies with negative CD34, inhibin, and cytokeratin [16]. The cellular variant shows more hypercellular areas with rare to no hypocellular areas. Often there is no difficulty in histological diagnosis of schwannoma based on the characteristic morphology and S100 immunohistochemical staining.

Standard management of adrenal schwannomas is surgical resection as they are not sensitive to radiotherapy and chemotherapy [4]. The appropriate approach in adrenal schwannomas, either laparoscopic or open, remains debatable. However, Hobart et al. concluded that both techniques achieve similar results, but it remains controversial in larger schwannomas [9, 17]. Complete laparoscopic resection was achieved in our patients. The surgical histopathology consisted of spindle cell proliferation with morphological features as described above, consistent with a diagnosis of a schwannoma, cellular variant.

Prognosis is usually favorable after surgical resection. However, local recurrences have been observed in 33–50% of the cases [18]. Zhou et al. reported good survival without any evidence of recurrence or metastasis at follow-up from 7–115 months [2]. In our cases, the patient remained asymptomatic with no evidence of radiological recurrence or distant metastasis at five months after the surgery.

4. Conclusion

Adrenal schwannomas are rare tumors that are difficult to diagnose preoperatively. Definitive diagnosis can be made only by the histological and immunohistochemical examination of the resected lesion. Hence, complete surgical excision is the treatment of choice and is associated with a favorable outcome.

References

[1] W. Shabana, W. Raslan, S. Hassan, and T. Al-Tartir, "Schwannoma masquerading as adrenocortical tumor: a case report and review of literature," *Urology Case Reports*, vol. 26, Article ID 100926, 2019.

[2] J. Zhou, D. Zhang, W. Li et al., "Primary adrenal schwannoma: a series of 31 cases emphasizing their clinicopathologic features and favorable prognosis," *Endocrine*, vol. 65, no. 3, pp. 662–674, 2019.

[3] S. Damodaran, G. Mahimairaj, and K. Velaichamy, "A case series of two cases of juxta-adrenal schwannoma presenting as adrenal mass lesion and review of the literature," *Urology Annals*, vol. 7, no. 2, pp. 254–258, 2015.

[4] M. Abdessater, M. El Mokdad, J. Gas, W. Sleiman, P. Coloby, and S. Bart, "Juxta-adrenal schwannoma presenting as a giant adrenal tumor: a case report and a literature review," *International Journal of Surgery Case Reports*, vol. 53, pp. 132–136, 2018.

[5] S. K. Sharma, F. Koleski, A. Husain, D. Albala, and T. Turk, "Retroperitoneal schwannoma mimicking an adrenal lesion," *World Journal of Urology*, vol. 20, no. 4, pp. 232-233, 2002.

[6] A. D. Gubbay, G. Moschilla, B. N. Gray, and I. Thompson, "Retroperitoneal schwannoma: a case series and review," *ANZ Journal of Surgery*, vol. 65, no. 3, pp. 197–200, 1995.

[7] B. K. P. Goh, Y.-M. Tan, Y.-F. A. Chung, P. K. H. Chow, L. L. P. J. Ooi, and W.-K. Wong, "Retroperitoneal schwannoma," *The American Journal of Surgery*, vol. 192, no. 1, pp. 14–18, 2006.

[8] J. Cury, R. F. Coelho, and M. Srougi, "Retroperitoneal schwannoma: case series and literature review," *Clinics*, vol. 62, no. 3, pp. 359–362, 2007.

[9] Y. Mohiuddin and M. G. F. Gilliland, "Adrenal schwannoma: a rare type of adrenal incidentaloma," *Archives of Pathology & Laboratory Medicine*, vol. 137, no. 7, pp. 1009–1014, 2013.

[10] K. Suzuki, A. Nakanishi, Y. Kurosaki, J. Nogaki, and E. Takaba, "Adrenal schwannoma: CT and MRI findings," *Radiation Medicine*, vol. 25, no. 6, pp. 299–302, 2007.

[11] Y. Shen, Y. Zhong, H. Wang et al., "MR imaging features of benign retroperitoneal paragangliomas and schwannomas," *BMC Neurology*, vol. 18, no. 1, 2018.

[12] G. Dell'Aversano Orabona, D. Ricci, I. Emili, F. Serpi, V. Ferrara, and A. Vanzulli, "Adrenal schwannoma: a case report," *BJR Case Reports*, vol. 48, Article ID 20190044, 2019.

[13] S.-Q. Li, Y.-S. Zhang, J. Shi, and H.-Z. Li, "Clinical features and retroperitoneal laparoscopic resection of adrenal schwannoma in 19 patients," *Endocrine Practice*, vol. 21, no. 4, pp. 323–329, 2015.

[14] S. Kumar, V. S. Karthikeyan, C. S. Manohar, K. Sreelakshmi, and M. Shivalingaiah, "Adrenal schwannoma: a rare incidentaloma," *Journal of Clinical and Diagnostic Research*, vol. 10, no. 8, pp. PD01–PD02, 2016.

[15] J. D. Jakowski, P. E. Wakely Jr., and R. E. Jimenez, "An uncommon type of adrenal incidentaloma: a case report of a schwannoma of the adrenal medulla with cytological, histological, and ultrastructural correlation," *Annals of Diagnostic Pathology*, vol. 12, no. 5, pp. 356–361, 2008.

[16] M. Adas, F. Ozulker, G. Adas, B. Koc, T. Ozulker, and I. M. Sahin, "A rare adrenal incidentaloma: adrenal schwannoma," *Case Reports in Gastroenterology*, vol. 7, no. 3, pp. 420–427, 2013.

[17] K. K. Richter, R. Premkumar, H.-S. Yoon, and P. Mercer, "Laparoscopic adrenalectomy for a rare 14 cm adrenal schwannoma," *Surgical Laparoscopy, Endoscopy & Percutaneous Techniques*, vol. 21, no. 6, pp. e339–e343, 2011.

[18] A. Jeshtadi, N. Govada, S. B. Somalwar, and S. Nagulapally, "Schwannoma of the adrenal gland," *Journal of Medical and Allied Sciences*, vol. 4, pp. 77–80, 2014.

Maturity-Onset Diabetes of Young Type 5: Diabetes with Extrapancreatic Features

Adnan Haider,[1,2] Oksana Symczyk,[1,2] Ayesha Hassan,[3] Muhammad Atif Khan,[4] Inderpreet Madahar,[5] and Dylan Holland[1,2]

[1]*600 Suncrest Towne Center, Morgantown, WV 26505, USA*
[2]*Department of Endocrinology Department of Medicine, West Virginia University, Morgantown, WV, USA*
[3]*Department of Internal Medicine, West Virginia University, Morgantown, WV, USA*
[4]*Ohio State University, 281 W Lane Avenue, Columbus, OH 43210, USA*
[5]*West Virginia School of Medicine, Morgantown, WV 26506, USA*

Correspondence should be addressed to Adnan Haider; adnan.haider@hsc.wvu.edu

Academic Editor: Wayne V. Moore

Objective. This case involves a new-onset diabetes patient diagnosed during pregnancy with the congenital dysplastic right kidney. *Case Report.* Clinical presentation, biochemical features, imaging in a patient with diabetes diagnosed during pregnancy, and congenital dysplastic right kidney. *Discussion.* We present a case of a 22-year-old female with the congenital dysplastic right kidney diagnosed with gestational diabetes mellitus after failing a 1-hour oral glucose tolerance test, requiring insulin during pregnancy. Because of the family history of diabetes and morphologic renal abnormalities at young ages on the maternal side of the family, our patient was evaluated for maturity-onset diabetes of adult and was found to have HNF-1β mutation. *Conclusion.* This case highlights the importance of considering the diagnosis of maturity-onset diabetes of young and particularly MODY-5 in individuals with extrapancreatic features. MODY-5 should also be considered in a patient undergoing renal transplant at young ages with a family history of morphologic renal abnormalities.

1. Background

MODY-5 is caused by an autosomal dominant mutation in the HNF1b gene. Our objective is to report a case of a young female with a history of the dysplastic right kidney, diagnosed with gestational diabetes. Morphologic kidney abnormalities, electrolyte abnormalities (low magnesium and high urate), strong family history of diabetes, and renal abnormalities at young ages should alert the clinician of this diagnosis.

2. Case Report

A previously healthy 22-year-old female was diagnosed with gestational diabetes after failing her 1-hour glucose tolerance test at 28 weeks gestation with a blood glucose level of 241. Elevated glucose levels were noted on random basic metabolic panels done prior to pregnancy, but the patient did not meet criteria to diagnose diabetes mellitus. Patient had no other symptoms at the time of the abnormal oral glucose tolerance test. The pertinent medical history prior to pregnancy included ultrasounds showing a small multicystic dysplastic right kidney. Patient's left kidney showed compensatory hypertrophy and a small midpole cyst (Figure 1). Kidney function is followed by nephrology and has been unremarkable. The family history is positive for polycystic kidney disease in her mother and maternal grandmother.

Due to her diagnosis of gestational diabetes, prior elevated glucose readings, and pertinent medical history, a polycystic disease panel was performed to test for mature onset diabetes of the young (MODY). This panel came back positive for a pathologic mutation to HNF-1β with deletion of exons 1–9 with genomic coordinates chr17: 36047329_36105161 (GRCh37). The patient was

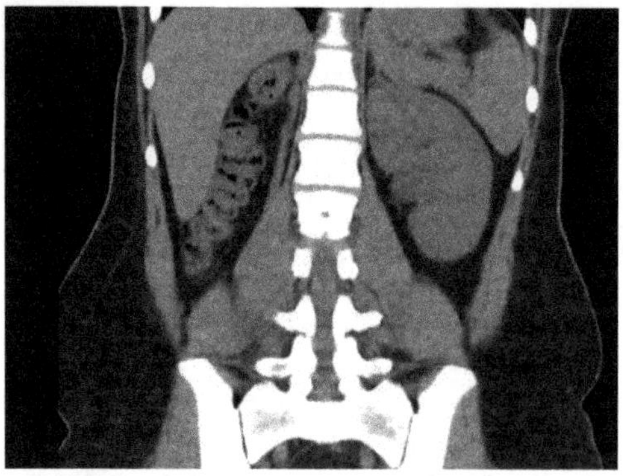

Figure 1: Absent right kidney with compensatory hypertrophy noted in the left kidney.

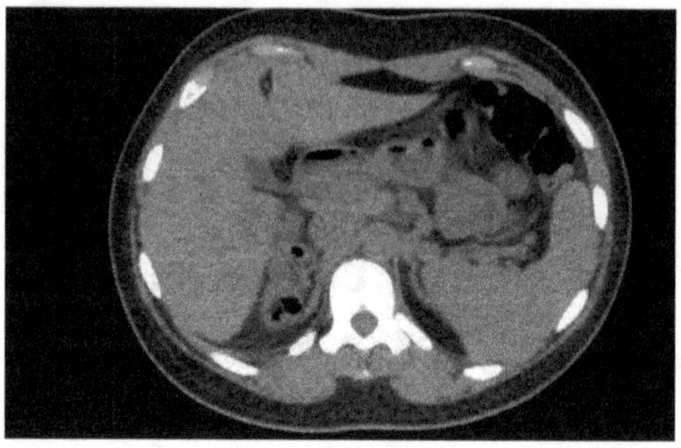

Figure 2: The uncinate process, head and body appear normal in size, but pancreatic tail is not visualized on noncontrast CT scan.

subsequently diagnosed with MODY-5. Patient was originally managing glycemic control with diet and exercise but eventually was placed on basal insulin and titrated to meet the glycemic targets during pregnancy. Patient has required no insulin since giving birth to her baby.

Patient did experience other extrapancreatic symptoms that included low magnesium (1.3 mg/dl), high uric acid (11.1 mg/dl), and pancreatic hypoplasia noted on previous CT done two years prior to her diagnosis. CT scan was done to rule out renal stones and did show pancreatic tail hypoplasia (Figure 2). Patient's most recent blood work done 6 weeks following delivery is given in Table 1. She delivered a healthy baby girl via spontaneous vaginal delivery at 39 weeks of gestation weighing 3170 g with APGAR score of 8 and 9 at 1 and 5 minutes, respectively. Her daughter has normal kidneys.

Table 1: Pertinent labs done on the patient, showing low magnesium and high uric acid levels.

Lab	Value	Normal range
Fasting glucose	113 mg/dl	<100 mg/dl
C-peptide	2.8 ng/ml	0.9–7.1 ng/ml
Magnesium	1.3 mg/dl	1.8–2.6 mg/dl
Calcium	9.9 mg/dl	8.5–10.0 mg/dl
Albumin	4.5 mg/dl	3.2–4.6 mg/dl
Uric acid	11.1 mg/dl	2.9–6.3 mg/dl
PTH	70.1 pg/ml	8.5–77 pg/ml
Creatinine	1.08 mg/dl	0.60–1.05 mg/dl
GFR	73 ml/min/BSA	<60 ml/min/BSA

3. Discussion

Monogenic forms of diabetes result from a single gene defect with an autosomal dominant pattern of inheritance. A high index of suspicion based on the strong family history of diabetes at young ages in at least three generations is suggestive of this diagnosis which can affect successful patient management, ensure healthy pregnancy in female patients, and offering genetic counselling to the families.

To date, fourteen different genes have been implicated in the etiology of MODY. GCK mutation is the most common culprit mutation accounting for 30–50% of all MODY [1]. Hepatic nuclear factor 1B gene identified in patients with MODY-5 comprises less than 5% of MODY subtypes [1].

Although the exact prevalence is not known, current estimates suggest that 1–5% of all diabetes cases in the United States and other developed countries are a monogenic form of diabetes [2, 3]. Often the diagnosis is overlooked and misdiagnosed as diabetes type 1 or type 2, and therefore, the true prevalence of MODY may be higher. Given the absence of a typical phenotype and the cost of genetic analysis, it is indeed a challenge to distinguish MODY from many people with young-onset type 2 and type 1 diabetes. Patients with MODY are often misdiagnosed as type 2 diabetes, mainly if hyperglycemia was first detected in adulthood. Several reasons such as the increasing prevalence of diabetes among youths, positive family history of diabetes, lack of characteristic clinical features, and therapeutic response to insulin secretagogues add to this confusion. Similarly, if they are present in their early teens, the default diagnosis is usually type 1 diabetes, and they are put on insulin, sometimes with multiple daily injections a day. Most MODY types do not involve extrapancreatic organs; in contrast, MODY-5 frequently comprises extrapancreatic organs [4].

The first case of MODY-5 was reported in 1997 in a Japanese family [5]. The HNF-1β is encoded by the human transcription factor 2 gene and is expressed in a wide variety of tissues, including the kidney, pancreas, genitourinary epithelium, liver, and lung during embryogenesis [6].

HNF1B-associated MODY is a multisystem disease and includes genital tract malformation, abnormal liver function test, hypomagnesemia, and hyperuricemia associated early gout; neurological features such as autism spectrum disorders and cognitive impairment are also seen in MODY-5. Renal cysts are the most frequently detected feature of HNF-1β-associated kidney disease, and MODY-5 is also known as renal cysts and diabetes (RCAD) syndrome.

Patients with a strong family history of diabetes at young ages and renal morphologic abnormalities diagnosed at or soon after birth should be considered for the HNF1B screen.

Diabetes prevalence was 80% and that of renal malformations was 91% in HNF-1β mutation. Diabetes can present with weight loss, polyuria, and polydipsia in about half of the patients; ketoacidosis was the initial presentation in 5% of the patients. A1c profile in MODY-5 patients showed A1c ranging from <7% in one-third of the patients to >13% in another 35% of the patients at the initial diagnosis [7].

Pancreatic hypoplasia with resulting beta-cell hypoplasia results in decreased insulin secretion and release, altered glucose-sensing, and increased hepatic insulin resistance which also play a major role in the development of diabetes. Severity of pancreatic hypoplasia determines the severity of hyperglycemia and possibility of ketoacidosis at initial presentation. Imaging of the pancreas is therefore helpful in MODY-5 patients. Nongenetic factors that affect insulin sensitivity (infection, puberty, pregnancy, and rarely obesity) can trigger diabetes onset and affect the severity of hyperglycemia in MODY but do not play a significant role in the development of MODY [8].

Renal functional decline is reported; a median yearly decrease in the estimated glomerular filtration rate (eGFR) of 2.45 ml/min/1.73 m2 was observed in a study of 27 adults with an HNF-1β mutation and a wide variety of renal phenotypes [9]. MODY-5 patient who develops ESRD should be considered for renal transplantation; however, these patients are at increased risk of developing post-transplant diabetes mellitus [10]. Like type 1 diabetes patients requiring renal replacement therapy, HNF-1β patient should be considered for simultaneous pancreatic and renal transplant [10]. Functional renal anomalies notably hypomagnesemia and hyperuricemia are also seen in MODY-5 patients. HNF-1β transcription functions over the FXYD domain containing ion transport regulator 2 (fxyd2), a gene that encodes sodium-potassium ATPase in the distal convoluted tubule, which plays an important role in magnesium reabsorption. HNF-1β is also responsible for transcription of uromodulin gene which is involved in urate transport [11]. Unlike asymptomatic hypomagnesemia, elevated uric acid levels can present as symptomatic monoarticular gout. Primary hyperparathyroidism has been identified because HNF-1β inhibits the transcription of parathormone hormone [12].

4. Conclusion

MODY-5 should be considered a multisystem disorder and should be considered in the differential in young patients with renal malformations.

Another group of patients where screening for HNF-1β will be helpful and can change management are young patients requiring renal transplantation secondary to morphologic renal abnormalities such as renal cysts. Retrospectively screening such a population for HNF1B mutation might provide exciting information about the prevalence of this mutation.

Abbreviations

MODY: Maturity onset diabetes of young
HNF-1β: Hepatocyte nuclear factor one beta
OGTT: Oral glucose tolerance test
GCK: Glucokinase.

References

[1] Y. Horikawa, "Maturity-onset diabetes of the young as a model for elucidating the multifactorial origin of type 2 diabetes mellitus," *Journal of Diabetes Investigation*, vol. 9, no. 4, pp. 704–712, 2018.

[2] S. Amed and R. Oram, "Maturity-onset diabetes of the young (MODY): making the right diagnosis to optimize treatment," *Canadian Journal of Diabetes*, vol. 40, no. 5, pp. 449–454, 2016.

[3] S.-H. Kim, "Maturity-onset diabetes of the young: what do clinicians need to know?" *Diabetes and Metabolism Journal*, vol. 39, no. 6, p. 468, 2015.

[4] H. Nishigori, S. Yamada, T. Kohama et al., "Frameshift mutation, A263fsinsGG, in the hepatocyte nuclear factor-1beta gene associated with diabetes and renal dysfunction," *Diabetes*, vol. 47, no. 8, pp. 1354-1355, 1998.

[5] N. Iwasaki, M. Ogata, O. Tomonaga et al., "Liver and kidney function in Japanese patients with maturity-onset diabetes of the young," *Diabetes Care*, vol. 21, no. 12, pp. 2144–2148, 1998.

[6] S. Decramer, O. Parant, S. Beaufils et al., "Anomalies of theTCF2Gene are the main cause of fetal bilateral hyperechogenic kidneys," *Journal of the American Society of Nephrology*, vol. 18, no. 3, pp. 923–933, 2007.

[7] J. C. Mateus, C. Rivera, M. O'Meara, A. Valenzuela, and F. Lizcano, "Maturity-onset diabetes of the young type 5 a MULTISYSTEMIC disease: a CASE report of a novel mutation in the HNF1B gene and literature review," *Clinical Diabetes and Endocrinology*, vol. 6, 2020.

[8] I. S. Haldorsen, M. Vesterhus, H. Rder et al., "Lack of pancreatic body and tail inHNF1Bmutation carriers," *Diabetic Medicine*, vol. 25, no. 7, pp. 782–787, 2008.

[9] S. Faguer, S. Decramer, N. Chassaing et al., "Diagnosis, management, and prognosis of HNF1B nephropathy in adulthood," *Kidney International*, vol. 80, no. 7, pp. 768–776, 2011.

[10] J. Halbritter, C. Mayer, A. Bachmann et al., "Successful simultaneous pancreas kidney transplantation in maturity-onset diabetes of the young type 5," *Transplantation*, vol. 92, no. 8, pp. e45–e47, 2011.

[11] T. C. Hart, "Mutations of the UMOD gene are responsible for medullary cystic kidney disease 2 and familial juvenile hyperuricaemic nephropathy," *Journal of Medical Genetics*, vol. 39, no. 12, pp. 882–892, 2002.

[12] S. Ferrè, E. M. H. F. Bongers, R. Sonneveld et al., "Early development of hyperparathyroidism due to loss ofPTH-Transcriptional repression in patients with HNF1β mutations?" *Journal of Clinical Endocrinology and Metabolism*, vol. 98, no. 10, pp. 4089–4096, 2013.

41

Recurrent Hypoglycemia in a Case of Congenital Analbuminemia

Martin Litzel,[1] Gianluca Caridi,[2] Francesca Lugani,[2] Monica Campagnoli,[3] Lorenzo Minchiotti,[3] and Stefan Fischli[1]

[1]*Division of Endocrinology, Diabetes and Clinical Nutrition, Luzerner Kantonsspital, Luzern 6000, Switzerland*
[2]*Laboratory of Molecular Nephrology, Istituto Giannina Gaslini, IRCCS, Genoa 16147, Italy*
[3]*Department of Molecular Medicine, University of Pavia, Pavia 27100, Italy*

Correspondence should be addressed to Stefan Fischli; stefan.fischli@luks.ch

Academic Editor: Lucy Mastrandrea

In congenital analbuminemia (CAA), mutations in the albumin gene result in a severe deficiency or absence of plasma albumin. Only about 90 cases have been reported to date, but the specific features of glucose and lipid metabolism in congenital analbuminemia have only been studied in a rat model of analbuminemia. We report the case of a female patient hospitalized for a streptococcal skin infection who showed recurrent hypoglycemia. A diagnosis of CAA was confirmed by mutation analysis and by the detection of a single base variation in the *ALB* gene. Hypoglycemia was first documented after a fasting period during acute illness. Recurrent hypoglycemia persisted despite good general condition and normal nutrition during antimicrobial therapy with moxifloxacin. Several contributing factors causing this hypoglycemia can be discussed. Individuals with CAA are prone to adverse drug effects caused by changes in drug-protein binding properties. It is unclear if specific changes of glucose and lipid metabolism in CAA constitute a risk factor for hypoglycemia.

1. Background

Congenital analbuminemia (CAA; OMIM # 616000) is a rare, autosomal recessive inherited disorder that is usually characterized by mutations in the albumin gene (*ALB*; NCBI Genomic Sequence: NC_00004.12), which lead to undetectable or low levels of the circulating protein [1]. Despite the condition being easily detected by routine serum protein electrophoresis, it is very rare, with only ~90 cases having so far been identified worldwide [1]. Thus, the estimated prevalence is <1 in 1 million [1]. CAA is relatively well tolerated in adulthood but can lead to serious consequences in the pre- and perinatal periods, during which it can cause preterm birth or neonatal or early childhood death [1]. Typical clinical findings in CAA include lower extremity edema and lipodystrophy, which are more obvious in women, and orthostatic hypotension. CAA should be suspected in the presence of a low or undetectable plasma albumin concentration in the absence of renal or gastrointestinal albumin loss or hepatic disease. Electrophoresis of plasma proteins characteristically shows a small albumin fraction and larger alpha-1, alpha-2, beta, and gamma fractions. Nonalbumin plasma proteins, such as immunoglobulins, coagulation factors, hormone-binding proteins, and lipoproteins, are present in higher concentrations as a compensatory mechanism. Hypercholesterolemia, with a high concentration of low-density lipoprotein (LDL) cholesterol, is a typical finding, but it is as yet unclear whether the dyslipidemia in CAA is associated with higher cardiovascular morbidity and mortality. Hypercholesterolemia can be reversed by administration of albumin indicating an interplay between albumin and lipid metabolism [2]. Total serum calcium is usually low, while ionized calcium is in the normal range, and symptomatic hypocalcemia has not been described in CAA [1].

The effects of analbuminemia on glucose and lipid metabolism have previously been studied in a rat model. Analbuminemic rats (NAR) were intolerant of carbohydrate deprivation and showed earlier mortality than normal rats (NR) during fasting [3]. One recognized mechanism is an impairment in lipid metabolism, associated with free fatty acid (FFA) deficiency. Normally, fasting induces gluconeogenesis, glycogenolysis, ketogenesis, and FFA oxidation. However, FFAs in plasma are largely bound to albumin, and an albumin deficiency causes lower intravascular lipolysis as well as reductions in FFA availability and transportation to target tissues. However, albumin administration to NAR reduces this FFA deficiency [4]. In addition, glucose metabolism in NAR is affected. In comparison to NR, glycogenolysis, as well as gluconeogenesis in albumin-deficient NAR is upregulated. Liver glycogen after a fasting period of 6 or 14 hours was significantly lower in NAR compared to NR. The injection of a gluconeogenic substrate caused a faster rise of glucose concentrations in NAR compared to NR. Glucose tolerance tests showed a more rapid return of glucose concentration to normal levels in the analbuminemic rats. These findings could be attributed to an enhanced islet responsiveness with increased insulin secretion of NAR compared to NR [5].

Individuals with CAA are vulnerable to the adverse effects of drugs that have high protein-binding affinities and that are acidic due to alterations in the pharmacokinetics and bioavailability of these drugs [1]. Hypoglycemia is a recognized side effect of fluoroquinolones, such as moxifloxacin, and is due to a blockade of pancreatic islet ion channels, which causes an increase in insulin secretion [6, 7]. A large proportion of moxifloxacin is bound to plasma proteins and specifically to albumin [8].

2. Case Report

2.1. Clinical Findings. A 40-year-old woman with a previous clinical diagnosis of CAA [9] was hospitalized for severe lower leg cellulitis. The cellulitis was diagnosed by her general physician five days before and treated with oral amoxicillin/clavulanic acid. She reported redness and pain in both lower legs of 6 days' duration. Because of general sickness, nausea, and loss of appetite, food intake was reduced to a minimum since six days. Clinical examination revealed obesity (height: 158 cm; weight: 100 kg; body mass index: 40 kg/m^2), normal vital signs (temperature: 36.5°C; blood pressure: 111/67 mmHg; heart rate: 91 bpm), and bilateral lipodystrophy of the lower extremities, with edema, tenderness, redness, and warmth.

A clinical diagnosis of CAA was proposed when the patient was 23 years old and hospitalized for treatment of a popliteal deep vein thrombosis and lower leg cellulitis [9]. Capillary serum protein electrophoresis confirmed the near-complete absence of the albumin peak and a compensatory increase in the other protein fractions (data not shown). Her family history was suggestive of analbuminemia in her younger brother and mild hypoalbuminemia in her older brother, suggesting a heterozygous state [9]. Her personal history included recurrent deep vein thrombosis, severe bilateral lower limb lipedema, and dyslipidemia. Liposuction had been performed several times on both legs and had been complicated by postoperative cellulitis. Her current medication consisted of oral amoxicillin/clavulanic acid, rivaroxaban, diclofenac, and a statin/ezetimibe combination. With hospital admission, oral amoxicillin/clavulanic acid was replaced by intravenous application, and clindamycin was added two days later. Because of poor response of the cellulitis to the previous therapy, piperacillin/tazobactam was initiated and amoxicillin/clavulanic acid and clindamycin was stopped after 15 days. At the initial in-hospital examination, capillary glucose measurement identified severe hypoglycemia (1.7 mmol/l). Despite oral administration of dextrose, recurrent low-glucose concentrations were identified while the patient was hospitalized (Figure 1). However, her cellulitis and general condition improved gradually, and she was discharged after 3 weeks. The antimicrobial treatment was then switched to oral moxifloxacin.

The patient then attended the endocrine outpatient clinic for evaluation of the recurrent hypoglycemia. Glucose monitoring using a flash-glucose monitoring system (FreeStyle libre®, Abbott Diabetes Care, Alameda, California) over 14 days confirmed frequent hypoglycemia, with a minimum of 2.8 mmol/l (Figure 2). The patient never showed signs of neuroglycopenia. Renal or hepatic insufficiency and hypocortisolism were excluded (Table 1a), and she was not using any hypoglycemic drugs. One month after the discontinuation of moxifloxacin, continuous flash-glucose monitoring was repeated, which showed an increase in her glucose concentrations, but there were still several values close to or below the lower limit of the normal range (Figure 2). In addition, a 10 h fasting test was performed, but her plasma glucose, free fatty acids, and hydroxybutyrate concentrations were normal (Table 1b). However, the levels of free fatty acids were clearly lower than in a comparable reference group of fasting obese subjects without insulin resistance [10]. In a follow-up conversation 8 months later, the patient reported general well being. There were no possible symptoms of hypoglycemia.

2.2. Mutation Analysis of the ALB Gene. Because low serum albumin can have causes other than CAA, the clinical diagnosis of this disorder requires confirmation by mutation analysis of the *ALB* gene [1]. Genomic DNA from the proband and from two unrelated healthy volunteers, used as controls, was extracted from whole blood, as described by Watkins et al. [11]. The other family members refused consent for the genetic study. The 14 coding exons of *ALB* and their intron–exon junctions [12] were PCR-amplified from genomic DNA using specific primer pairs [11]. All the 14 coding exons of the *ALB*, encompassing the intron–exon junctions, were amplified, and the products were screened for variations by single-strand conformational polymorphism (SSCP) and heteroduplex analysis (HA). The only differences identified by heteroduplex and SSCP analysis were detected in the 381 bp PCR product obtained with primers A07A and A08A, encompassing exon 4, and the intron 3–exon 4 and exon 4–intron 4 junctions (Figure 3(a), lanes 1 and 1′). The electrophoretic behavior was identical to that previously reported for a boy of nonconsanguineous Swiss parents [13]. The variant region was submitted for DNA sequence analysis, which identified a C-to-T change at position c.412 (c.412C > T) in the homozygous proband (Figure 3(b)). This alters the codon CGA encoding Arg 114 to a stop codon, TGA, resulting in premature termination

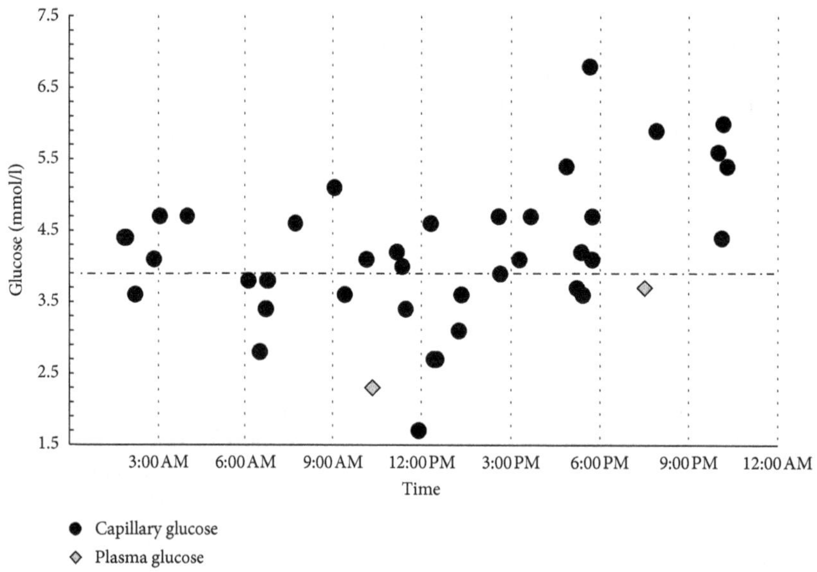

FIGURE 1: Capillary and plasma glucose values that were recorded during 7 days of hospitalization. All values are projected to a 24-hours view. These values were recorded on the first presentation at hospital admission. The dashed line marks the cutoff value for hypoglycemia with 3.9 mmol/l.

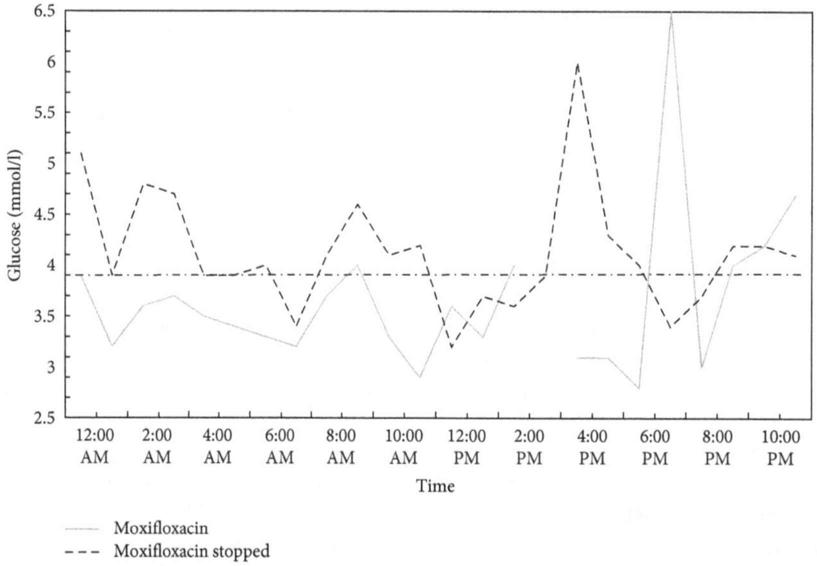

FIGURE 2: Hourly glucose concentration minima obtained using the sensor flash-glucose monitoring system during treatment with moxifloxacin and 4 weeks after it was stopped. The lines show the lowest glucose levels that were recorded for each hour. Each monitoring period covered 14 days. The dashed line marks the cutoff value for hypoglycemia with 3.9 mmol/l.

and is, therefore, responsible for the analbuminemic trait. The putative protein product (p.Arg138Ter) should consist of only 113 residues, but it could not be isolated from the patient's serum. The same molecular defect has been previously reported to cause analbuminemia in two unrelated individuals: the above-mentioned Swiss boy [13] and an American woman [14].

3. Discussion

The analbuminemic patient reported here presented with a streptococcal skin infection, which was first treated with amoxicillin/clavulanic acid, later in combination with clindamycin, still later with piperacillin/tazobactam, and finally with oral moxifloxacin. At admission, capillary glucose measurement revealed marked hypoglycemia, with a level of 1.7 mmol/l. Several hypoglycemic glucose levels were documented in the following days of hospitalization (Figure 1), but neuroglycopenic symptoms never occurred. When the antimicrobial therapy was switched to moxifloxacin, recurrent hypoglycemia persisted with a minimum of 2.8 mmol/l (Figure 2). Hypoglycemia has never been reported in patients with CAA in the literature so far. Several mechanisms causing recurrent hypoglycemia in this patient

Table 1: Biochemical parameters.

Parameter	Result	Reference range
(a) Baseline		
Albumin	10	35–52 g/l
Total plasma protein	59	66–87 g/l
Alkaline phosphatase	145	35–105 U/l
Serum cortisol (1600 h)	238	74–286 nmol/l
Thyroid-stimulating hormone	3.58	0.27–4.20 mU/l
Free triiodothyronine	3.8	3.1–6.8 pmol/l
Free thyroxine	12.5	12–22 pmol/l
Gamma glutamyltransferase	52	6–42 U/l
Alanine aminotransferase	31	<35 U/l
Glycated hemoglobin (HbA1c)	4.4	<6.5%
Creatinine	63	45–84 μmol/l
Ionized calcium	1.18	1.15–1.29 mmol/l
Phosphorus	0.91	0.87–1.45 mmol/l
25-OH vitamin D3	9	75–220 nmol/l
Immunoglobulin A	9.63	0.7–4.0 g/l
(b) After 10 hours of fasting		
Total cholesterol	9.66	<5.2 mmol/l
High-density lipoprotein cholesterol	1.84	>1.0 mmol/l
Low-density lipoprotein cholesterol	8.05	<2.59 mmol/l
Triglycerides	1.31	<2.0 mmol/l
Free fatty acids	0.24	0.10–0.45 mmol/l
Acetoacetic acid	24	<150 μmol/l
3-hydroxybutric acid	27	<120 μmol/l
Glucose	4.1	3.9–5.5 mmol/l
Insulin	3.6	3.0–25.0°mU/l
C-peptide	408	270–1,270°pmol/l
HOMA[1]	0.7	<2.5

[1]Homeostasis model assessment (Matthews et al. 1985).

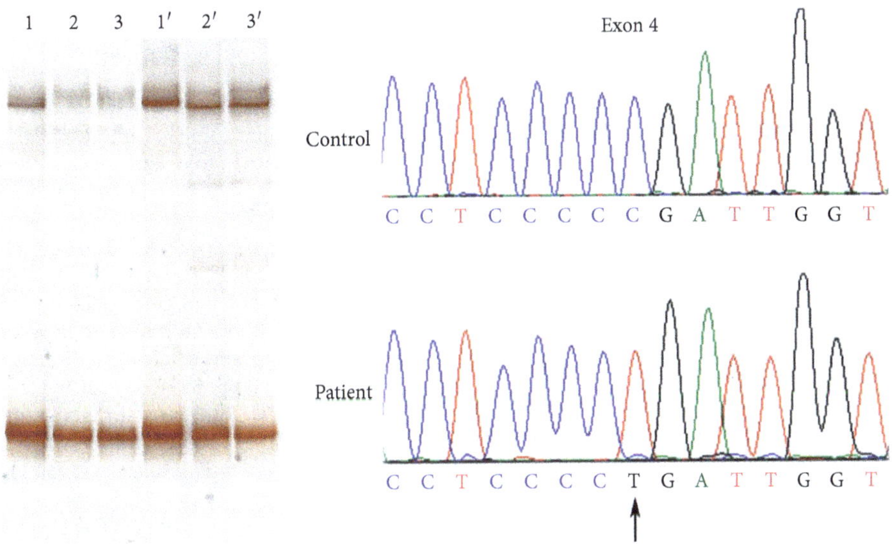

(a) (b)

Figure 3: HA, SSCP, and DNA sequence analysis of exon 4 of the *ALB* gene of the patient reported herein. (a) Heteroduplex analysis (HA) and single-strand conformational polymorphism (SSCP) analysis. The DNA sequences encompassing exon 4 and the exon–intron junctions from the patient and two controls were amplified using primers A07A and A08A, and the fragments were electrophoresed on a non-denaturing polyacrylamide gel: lane 1, proband; lanes 2 and 3, and controls. The same samples were denatured and cooled before loading: lane 1′, proband, lanes 2′ and 3′, and controls. (b) DNA sequence of the mutated region of exon 4 in the patient. The arrow indicates the homozygous C-to - transition at position c.412 (c.412C > T).

can be discussed. First, the inflammatory state, with a high metabolic rate and prolonged fasting, likely depleted her glycogen stores. In this situation free fatty acid oxidation plays an important role for energy homeostasis. Disorders of free fatty acid metabolism are associated with occurrence of hypoglycemia [15]. Studies from analbuminemic rats have shown improved insulin sensitivity, increased insulin secretion, faster depletion of liver glycogen stores during fasting, free fatty acid deficiency with reduced rates of hepatic lipogenesis, triglyceride secretion, and limited lipoprotein lipase activity [4, 5]. It is unclear if these abnormalities can contribute to the occurrence of hypoglycemia under certain conditions in humans, but an association of hypoglycemia and low albumin levels has been reported for inpatient medical patients recently [16, 17]. Later in the course of this case, antimicrobial treatment with moxifloxacin may have induced hypoglycemia by increasing endogenous insulin secretion. There was no therapy with any other hypoglycemic drug. Further there was no history of gastric surgery like roux-en-Y gastric bypass that is associated with endogenous hyperinsulinism. The period between hospital admission and last sensor glucose measurement was about 4 months. The clearly lowest glucose levels were documented at the time of hospital admission. At least at this time point, a simple connection of hypoglycemia to inflammation and critical illness cannot be excluded. Unfortunately the levels of free fatty acids or ketone bodies were not measured when our patient first presented to the hospital after prolonged food deprivation. As neuroglycopenic symptoms never occurred and the patient reported well being after recovery from the cellulitis, she was not willing to undergo further evaluations for hypoglycemia such as a 72-hour fasting test.

Giving the rarity of CAA and possible other causes of low albumin levels, sequencing of the *ALB* gene should always be performed to confirm a suspected diagnosis. Mutation analysis confirmed the diagnosis of our patient, which was based on clinical and laboratory findings obtained 19 years ago. The cytosine mutated in our case is in a CpG sequence, which was supposed to be a hypermutable site in the *ALB* gene [1]. This molecular defect, c.412 C > T, was previously identified in two unrelated analbuminemic subjects [13, 14]. A different variation at that position, c.412C > G, is known to cause albumin Yanomama (p.Arg138Gly), an alloalbumin present in polymorphic (>1%) frequency in an Amazonian Indian tribe [18]. Our finding of a fourth mutation at that cytosine residue confirms the hypothesis of a high tendency of this region to variation.

We report the first case of recurrent hypoglycemia in a female patient with known CAA. It remains to further investigations if metabolic abnormalities associated with analbuminemia can contribute to occurrence of hypoglycemia. Furthermore, this case demonstrates possible consequences of altered pharmacokinetics in the presence of low albumin levels, which in our case likely caused drug-induced hypoglycemia.

All data generated or analyzed during this case report study are included in this published article. The genetic studies described in this case report were performed in accordance with the ethical principles of the Declaration of Helsinki.

Authors' Contributions

ML and SF were responsible for the outpatient care of the patient. They contributed to the major work on the manuscript. GC, FL, MC, and LM performed the mutation analysis of the albumin gene. LM contributed also to the drafting of the text. All the authors read and approved the final version of this article.

Acknowledgments

GC and FL acknowledge the support of the "Compagnia di San Paolo" (ROL9849). The work performed in Pavia was supported by a grant from the Italian Ministry of Education, University and Research (MIUR) to the Department of Molecular Medicine of the University of Pavia under the initiative Dipartimenti di Eccellenza (2018–2022).

References

[1] L. Minchiotti, G. Caridi, M. Campagnoli et al., "Diagnosis, phenotype, and molecular genetics of congenital analbuminemia," *Frontiers in Genetics*, vol. 10, 2019.

[2] T. A. Waldmann, R. S. Gordon, and W. Rosse, "Studies on the metabolism of the serum proteins and lipids in a patient with analbuminemia," *The American Journal of Medicine*, vol. 37, no. 6, pp. 960–968, 1964.

[3] T. Kawaguchi, M. Shimode, H. Matsushita, and S. Nagase, "Frequent administration of uric acid extends survival of fasting analbuminemic rats under cold environment," *The Japanese Journal of Physiology*, vol. 36, no. 2, pp. 295–303, 1986.

[4] T. R. Figueira, A. E. Vercesi, and H. C. Oliveira, "Lack of plasma albumin impairs intravascular lipolysis and explains the associated free fatty acids deficiency and hypertriglyceridemia," *Lipids in Health and Disease*, vol. 9, no. 1, p. 146, 2010.

[5] T. R. Figueira, R. A. Ribeiro, L. M. Ignacio-Souza, A. E. Vercesi, E. M. Carneiro, and H. C. F. Oliveira, "Enhanced insulin secretion and glucose tolerance in rats exhibiting low plasma free fatty acid levels and hypertriglyceridaemia due to congenital albumin deficiency," *Experimental Physiology*, vol. 97, no. 4, pp. 525–533, 2012.

[6] N. Maeda, T. Tamagawa, I. Niki et al., "Increase in insulin release from rat pancreatic islets by quinolone antibiotics," *British Journal of Pharmacology*, vol. 117, no. 2, pp. 372–376, 1996.

[7] H.-Y. Qiu, S.-S. Yuan, F.-Y. Yang et al., "HERG protein plays a role in moxifloxacin-induced hypoglycemia," *Journal of Diabetes Research*, vol. 2016, Article ID 6741745, 6 pages, 2016.

[8] H. Stass, A. Dalhoff, D. Kubitza, and U. Schühly, "Pharmacokinetics, safety, and tolerability of ascending single doses of moxifloxacin, a new 8-methoxy quinolone, administered to healthy subjects," *Antimicrobial Agents and Chemotherapy*, vol. 42, no. 8, pp. 2060–2065, 1998.

[9] B. Gössi, D. Kleinert, and U. Gössi, "A further case of analbuminemia," *Schweizerische Medizinische Wochenschrift*, vol. 130, no. 16, pp. 583–589, 2000.

[10] P. Arner and M. Rydén, "Fatty acids, obesity and insulin resistance," *Obesity Facts*, vol. 8, no. 2, pp. 147–155, 2015.
[11] S. Watkins, J. Madison, M. Galliano, L. Minchiotti, and F. W. Putnam, "A nucleotide insertion and frameshift cause analbuminemia in an Italian family," *Proceedings of the National Academy of Sciences*, vol. 91, no. 6, pp. 2275–2279, 1994.
[12] P. P. Minghetti, D. E. Ruffner, W. J. Kuang et al., "Molecular structure of the human albumin gene is revealed by nucleotide sequence within q11-22 of chromosome 4," *The Journal of Biological Chemistry*, vol. 261, pp. 6747–6757, 1986.
[13] M. Campagnoli, A. Sala, S. Labò et al., "Analbuminemia in a Swiss family is caused by a C $\longrightarrow$ T transition at nucleotide 4446 of the albumin gene," *Clinical Biochemistry*, vol. 38, no. 9, pp. 819–823, 2005.
[14] S. Watkins, J. Madison, M. Galliano, L. Minchiotti, and F. W. Putnam, "Analbuminemia: three cases resulting from different point mutations in the albumin gene," *Proceedings of the National Academy of Sciences*, vol. 91, no. 20, pp. 9417–9421, 1994.
[15] J. L. Merritt II, M. Norris, and S. Kanungo, "Fatty acid oxidation disorders," *Annals of Translational Medicine*, vol. 6, no. 24, p. 473, 2018.
[16] I. Khanimov, J. Wainstein, M. Boaz et al., "Reduction of serum albumin in non-critically ill patients during hospitalization is associated with incident hypoglycaemia," *Diabetes & Metabolism*, vol. 46, no. 1, pp. 27–32, 2019.
[17] E. Leibovitz, J. Wainstein, and M. Boaz, "Association of albumin and cholesterol levels with incidence of hypoglycaemia in people admitted to general internal medicine units," *Diabetic Medicine*, vol. 35, no. 12, pp. 1735–1741, 2018.
[18] N. Takahashi, Y. Takahashi, T. Isobe et al., "Amino acid substitutions in inherited albumin variants from Amerindian and Japanese populations," *Proceedings of the National Academy of Sciences*, vol. 84, no. 22, pp. 8001–8005, 1987.

42

Antibody-Mediated Extreme Insulin Resistance: The Importance of Pre-Treatment Screening

Tina Mosaferi[1] **Sahar Sherf**[2] **Laura Y. Sue**[2] **and Ines Donangelo**[2]

[1]*Department of Medicine, David Geffen School of Medicine, University of California Los Angeles, Los Angeles, CA, USA*
[2]*Division of Endocrinology, David Geffen School of Medicine, University of California Los Angeles, Los Angeles, CA, USA*

Correspondence should be addressed to Ines Donangelo; idonangelo@mednet.ucla.edu

Academic Editor: Wayne V. Moore

We report the case of a 56 year-old Hispanic male with a 10-year history of type 2 diabetes who presented with abrupt onset of hyperglycemia resistant to escalating doses of intravenous insulin infusion (>2500 units daily). He was diagnosed with antibody-mediated insulin resistance given the presence of hyperglycemia despite receiving >200 units insulin/day, a lack of identifiable precipitants for diabetic ketoacidosis or hyperosmolar hyperglycemic state, and elevated insulin antibodies. He underwent pre-immunomodulatory therapy screening for infections, rheumatologic disorders, and malignancy, which uncovered a new diagnosis of latent tuberculosis. While concurrently being treated for latent tuberculosis, he successfully responded to immunomodulatory therapy with rituximab, dexamethasone, and cyclophosphamide. Insulin was discontinued completely, and he maintained appropriate glycemic control on oral diabetic agents (metformin and pioglitazone). This case supports the use of immunomodulatory therapy for the treatment of antibody-mediated insulin resistance and highlights the importance of pre-immunomodulatory therapy screening to uncover occult infection or identify underlying neoplastic/rheumatologic disease prior to immunosuppression.

1. Introduction

Antibody-mediated extreme insulin resistance is characterized by hyperglycemia despite the use of >200 units of insulin/day and is often divided into two subtypes, insulin receptor antibody-mediated (Type B insulin resistance) and insulin antibody-mediated insulin resistance. Although the exact prevalence remains unknown, concern for high mortality has been reported [1]. The National Institutes of Health (NIH) published an immunomodulatory protocol for the treatment of Type B insulin resistance in 2010 [2], yet little has been documented to guide pretreatment screening. This article aims to present a case of antibody-mediated insulin resistance that highlights the challenge of subtype diagnosis and emphasizes the importance of pretreatment screening.

2. Case Report

A 56 year-old Hispanic male with hypertension and a 10-year history of diabetes was hospitalized for abrupt worsening of glycemic control and diabetic ketoacidosis (DKA). His diabetes was initially managed on metformin and sitagliptin, with insulin added six years after diagnosis. His glycemic control had been stable with home self-monitored blood glucoses (SMBG) averaging around 160 mg/dL, however there was an abrupt rise in SMBG to around 400 mg/dL starting six months prior to presentation. After hospitalization at another institution two months prior for DKA, he was discharged on detemir insulin 20 units every morning, detemir insulin 40 units every evening, and aspart insulin 15 units before each meal.

He presented to our emergency department with 18-kg weight loss, initial blood glucose 427 mg/dL, and a hemoglobin A1c 12.4% (112 mmol/mol) with bicarbonate 15 mmol/L (20–30 mmol/L), anion gap 18, moderate serum ketones, and 2+ urine ketones. On physical exam he weighed 57.9 kg, with a BMI of 24.93 kg/m^2. He was normotensive with regular heart rate. No acanthosis nigricans, dorsoclavicular fat pad, abdominal striae, or skin lesions were present. He was started on intravenous regular insulin infusion. Despite prompt normalization of the metabolic acidosis, he continued to have markedly high insulin needs to keep serum glucose levels between 150–250 mg/dL. The peak insulin infusion rate was 2,526 units/24 hours (Figure 1). There was no meaningful reduction

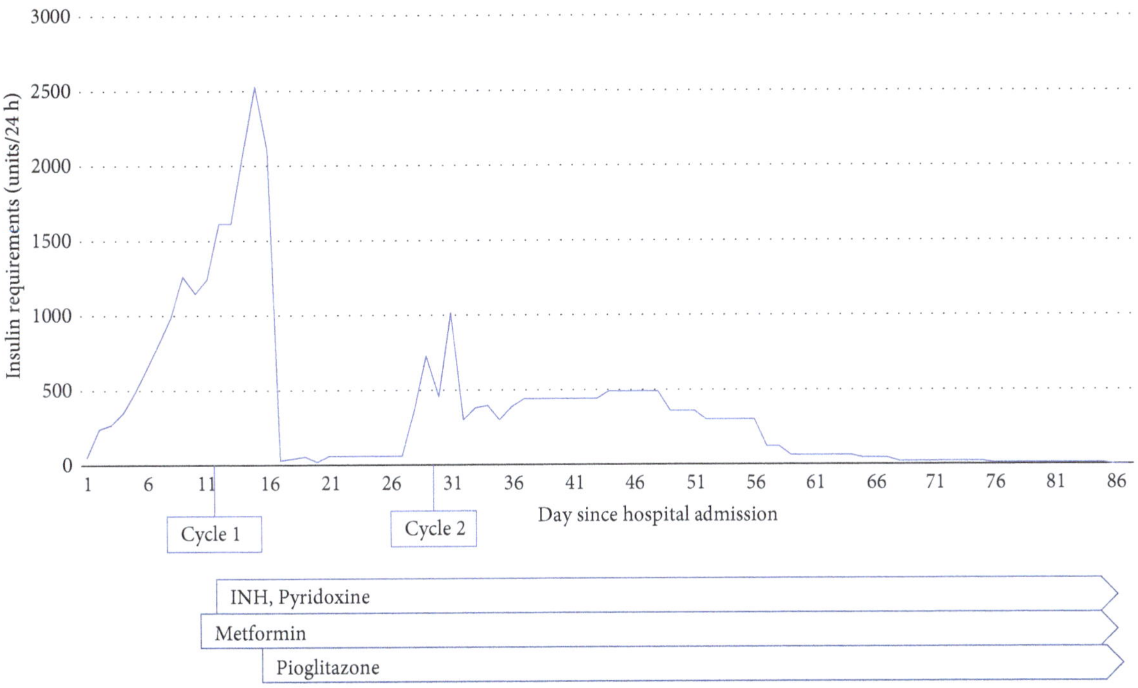

FIGURE 1: Clinical course defined by daily insulin requirements and initiation of oral antihyperglycemic therapy, diagnosis of latent tuberculosis, and initiation of immunomodulatory therapy. Cycle 1 of immunomodulatory therapy was initiated concomitantly with latent tuberculosis treatment.

in daily insulin requirements that occurred with the addition of metformin 500 mg oral twice daily or concentrated U-500 regular insulin (up to 300 units before each meal). Adiponectin level was normal at 18 mcg/mL (4–20 mcg/mL) with intact C-peptide of 3.0 ng/mL (1.1–4.3 ng/mL) and concomitant serum glucose level of 226 mg/dL. He was diagnosed with antibody-mediated insulin resistance with evidence of elevated insulin antibody levels (12.4 U/mL, normal range 0.0–0.4 U/mL). No commercial assay was available to measure the insulin receptor antibody level. Despite being unable to confirm the presence of insulin receptor antibodies, the decision was made to initiate the NIH treatment protocol for Type B insulin resistance [2, 3], which includes rituximab, dexamethasone, and cyclophosphamide. Evaluation for malignancy, rheumatologic disease, and infection was performed prior to initiating immunosuppression. Computed tomography (CT) of the chest, abdomen, and pelvis was negative for malignancy. Serum and urine protein electrophoresis was negative for monoclonal gammopathy, and flow cytometry was negative for lymphoproliferation. Prostate specific antigen was normal at 0.44 ng/mL (0–3.5 ng/mL). Autoimmune workup revealed mildly elevated antinuclear antibody titer (1:80, normal <1:40) and double stranded DNA antibody level (220 IU/mL, normal ≤200 IU/mL) but was otherwise unremarkable (negative for glutamic acid decarboxylase-65, thyroid peroxidase, SSA, SSB, smith, smooth muscle, centromere B, cyclic citrulline, RNP, scleroderma, and Jo 1 antibodies). Infectious workup revealed positive *Mycobacterium tuberculosis* Quantiferon-GOLD TB-Nil > 10 IU/mL (positive ≥0.35 IU/mL), but subsequent acid-fast culture and stain and respiratory *Mycobacterium tuberculosis* PCR were negative. CT of the chest did not show evidence of active tuberculosis. Remaining infectious disease studies were negative (Hepatitis B core Ig, Hepatitis B surface antigen, Hepatitis C antibody, Hepatitis A IgM, HIV-1/2 Ag/Ab, strongyloides IgG, coccidioides IgG/IgM, and urine histoplasma antigen). After initiation of treatment for latent tuberculosis with isoniazid and pyridoxine, he underwent cycle 1 of the NIH immunomodulatory protocol with marked reduction in daily insulin requirements (Figure 1). Pioglitazone 45 mg daily was then initiated. One month following two treatment cycles, insulin therapy was discontinued and blood glucose levels were controlled on metformin and pioglitazone alone (Figure 1).

3. Discussion

The abrupt, marked insulin resistance in this case drew suspicion for an autoimmune etiology and antibody-mediated insulin resistance was ultimately diagnosed. We were unable to further distinguish between Type B insulin resistance and insulin antibody-mediated insulin resistance. Prior case reports have discussed that in Type B insulin resistance presentation with DKA is rare, and that it is often associated with elevated adiponectin levels, female sex, black ethnicity, presence of acanthosis nigricans, and concomitant rheumatologic diagnoses [1–3] (Table 1). Our patient presented with DKA, lacked acanthosis nigricans and had normal adiponectin levels, therefore not the typical presentation of Type B insulin resistance. However, there is no definite set of clinical characteristics that assist in differentiating between the two subtypes [4].

Table 1: Case reports of antibody-mediated insulin resistance

	Age, sex (years, M/F)	Race/ethnicity	Acanthosis nigricans	Triglyceride (mg/dL)	HbA1c (%) [mmol/mol]	C-peptide (ng/mL)	Adiponectin (mcg/mL)	Insulin antibody titer	Insulin receptor antibody	Maximum documented insulin requirement	Associated rheumatologic/ malignancy diagnosis
Our case	56, M	Hispanic	N	85	12.4 [112]	3	18	Elevated		2526 U/day	
Malek et al, Case B-30 [2]*	20, F	Black	Y	42	11.9 [107]		54.4		Y	18000 U/day	Mixed connective tissue disorder
Malek et al, Case B-33 [2]	50, F	Black		68	9 [75]		21.3		Y	1300 U/day	Systemic lupus erythematosus
Malek et al, Case B-34 [2]	62, M	Black		36	9.2 [77]		12.5		Y	1250 U/day	Systemic lupus erythematosus
Malek et al, Case B-35 [2]**	17, F	Black	Y	41	6.8 [51]		8.3		Y	0 U/day	
Malek et al, Case B-36 [2]	64, M	Canadian		102	11.7 [104]		15.2		Y	1800 U/day	Systemic lupus erythematosus
Malek et al, Case B-37 [2]	58, F	Black		92	10.2 [88]		24.8		Y	7000 U/day	
Malek et al, Case B-38 [2]	21, F	Black		41	13.5 [124]		43.4		Y	750 U/day	
Kim et al, Case 1 [4]***	63, M	Black	N	52	9.6 [81]	4.2	23	Borderline elevated	Y	21000 U/day	
Kim et al, Case 2 [4]	61, F	Jamaican	Y	39	15.5 [146]	3.03	29		Y	11650 U/day	
Kim et al, Case 3 [4]	60, M	Black	N	103	10.8 [95]	1.75	16	Elevated	N	1500 U/day	
Liminet et al. [5]	83, M		N		11–12 [97–108]	3.0		Elevated	N	100 U/hr	Lymphocytic lymphoma
Mizuhashi et al. [6]	62, M				10.4 [90]			Elevated			Pulmonary adenocarcinoma
Takaya et al. [7]	66, M				11.9 [107]	5.24		Elevated	N	>150 U/day	
Greenfield et al. [8]	68, F	White	N	442	12.4 [112]	0.98	1.7	Elevated	N	>300 U/day	
Lahtela et al. [9]	27, M				12.6 [114]	0		Elevated		360 U/day	
Rhie et al, Case 1 [10]	71, M	White						Elevated	N	440 U/day	Waldenstrom macroglobulinemia
Rhie et al, Case 2 [10]	69, M							Elevated	N	2050 U/day	Multiple myeloma
Segal et al. [11]	12, M	White			12.5 [113]	0		Elevated		6000 U/day	
Willard et al. [12]	39, F	Nigerian	Y	72	12 [108]	8.56	9		Y	>1000 U/day	Systemic lupus erythematosus

Y = yes; N = no; *Malek et al. [2] mentions 7 additional cases that are not included in this table given paucity of reported data. **Case B-35 uniquely with normoglycemia, but nevertheless with acanthosis nigricans, hyperinsulinemia, and positive insulin receptor antibody. ***Insulin antibody titer listed as "borderline elevated" given reported titer of 0.4 U/ml and listed normal reference range 0.4 U/ml.

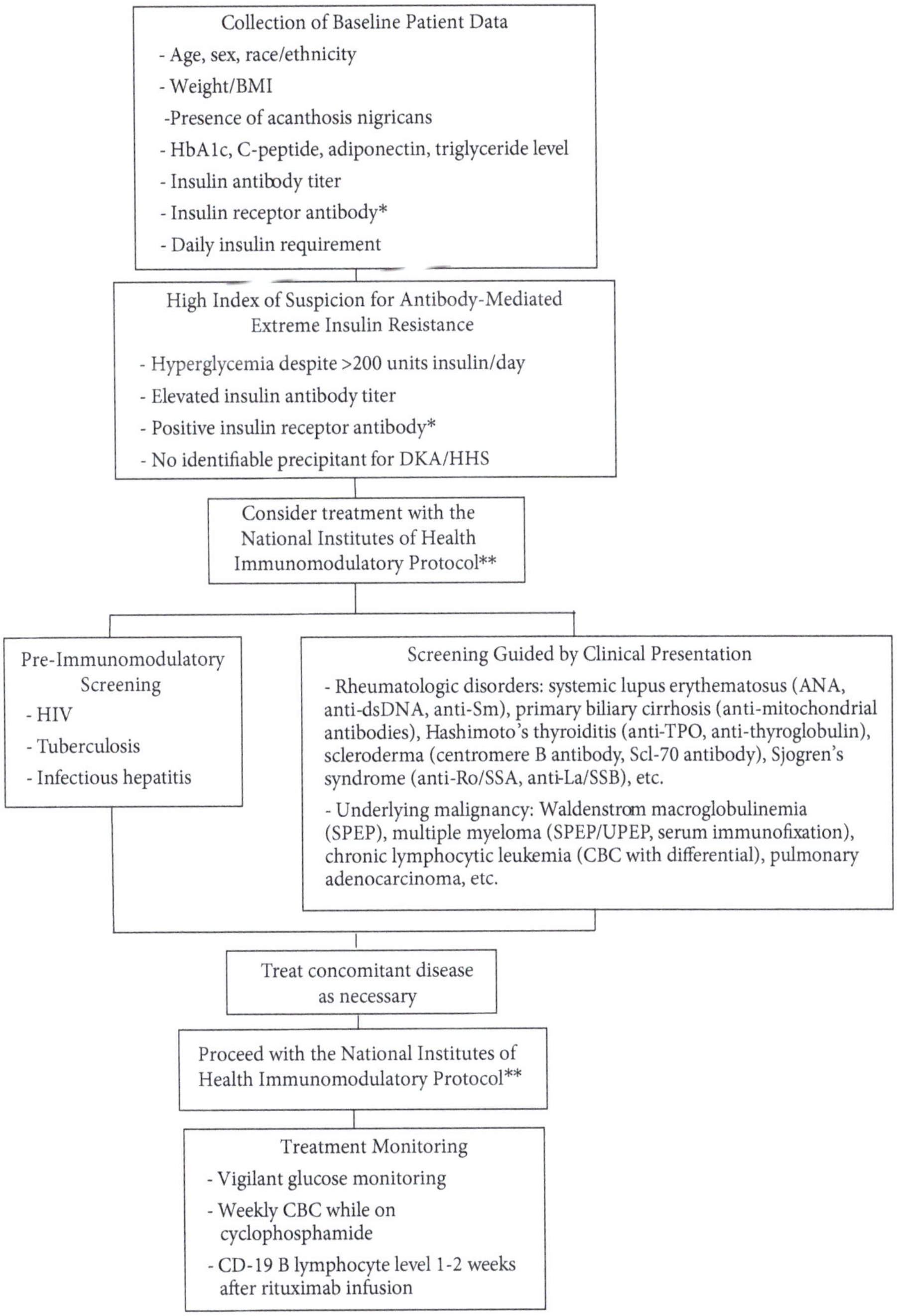

FIGURE 2: Pre-Immunomodulatory Therapy Screening Protocol. BMI = body mass index; HbA1c = glycated hemoglobin; DKA = diabetic ketoacidosis; HHS = hyperosmolar hyperglycemic state; HIV = Human Immunodeficiency Virus; ANA = antinuclear antibodies; anti-dsDNA = anti-double stranded DNA; anti-Sm = anti Smith antibody; anti-TPO = anti-thyroid peroxidase antibody; Scl-70 antibody = anti-topoisomerase 1 antibody; SPEP = serum protein electrophoresis; UPEP = urine protein electrophoresis; CBC = complete blood count. *There is no commercially available insulin receptor antibody assay in the United States of America at this time. **National Institutes of Health Immunomodulatory Protocol originally detailed by Malek et al. [2]. Immunotherapy cycles consist of rituximab infusion, 2 mg/mL in 0.9% sodium chloride, 750 mg/m^2 body surface area (Day 1); dexamethasone 40 mg once daily by mouth (Day 1–4); and cyclophosphamide 100 mg once daily by mouth (Day 1 through remission).

From a serologic perspective, our patient had elevated insulin antibody levels but we were unable to evaluate for the presence of an insulin receptor antibody. To our knowledge, at this time a commercial assay for insulin receptor antibody remains unavailable in the United States of America. Presence of both insulin receptor antibody and a borderline elevated insulin antibody titer has been reported in one case (Table 1). Elevated plasma adiponectin levels may indicate insulin receptor dysfunction, therefore supporting a diagnosis of Type B insulin resistance; however, lack of an accepted reference standard limits the comparison of adiponectin levels attained by different laboratory assays [13].

Differentiating between Type B insulin resistance and insulin antibody-mediated insulin resistance should not deter the initiation of therapeutic planning. Kim et al. [4] were the first to report the successful use of the NIH immunomodulatory protocol developed for Type B insulin resistance in a patient with insulin antibody-mediated insulin resistance, suggesting efficacy in both autoimmune pathologies. Similarly, the excellent clinical outcome in our case supports that distinguishing the precise subtype of antibody-mediated extreme insulin resistance should not delay immunomodulatory therapy implementation. Our patient responded favorably to two cycles of the NIH immunomodulatory protocol and now has good glycemic control on metformin and pioglitazone alone.

This case adds to the literature by emphasizing the importance of pre-immunomodulatory treatment screening. Our investigation resulted in a diagnosis of latent tuberculosis, prompting initiation of isoniazid and pyridoxine in conjunction with immunomodulatory therapy. In an effort to encourage standardized data collection and enhance safe immunomodulatory administration, we drew from our own treatment experience as well as prior case reports (Table 1) to create a pre-immunomodulatory therapy screening protocol (Figure 2). Considering that cases of antibody-mediated insulin resistance have shown both associations and causal relationships with rheumatologic disorders and malignancies (Table 1), investigation into such pathologies should be guided by clinical suspicion based on a patient's presenting history, physical exam, and basic laboratory findings. We also suggest that all patients should be assessed for HIV, tuberculosis, and infectious hepatitis considering the detrimental implications of a missed diagnosis in the setting of iatrogenic immunosuppression.

In conclusion, our case reiterates the challenge of distinguishing between Type B insulin resistance and insulin antibody-mediated insulin resistance while supporting the use of the NIH immunomodulatory protocol in cases of suspected antibody-mediated insulin resistance [2–4]. Although striving to distinguish the precise subtype of antibody-mediated extreme insulin resistance should not delay therapy, pretreatment screening is indicated to diagnose possible underlying rheumatologic disorders and malignancy as well as to detect occult infectious processes that could otherwise result in deleterious health consequences. Our proposed pre-immunomodulatory therapy screening protocol has not been validated, yet we hope it will serve as a guide for future clinical encounters.

Disclosure

This work was presented at the 101st Annual Meeting of the Endocrine Society in March 2019.

References

[1] E. Arioglu, A. Andewelt, C. Diabo, M. Bell, S. I. Taylor, and P. Gorden, "Clinical course of the syndrome of autoantibodies to the insulin receptor (Type B insulin resistance): a 28-year perspective," *Medicine*, vol. 81, no. 2, pp. 87–100, 2002.

[2] R. Malek, A. Y. Chong, B. C. Lupsa et al., "Treatment of Type B insulin resistance: a novel approach to reduce insulin receptor autoantibodies," *The Journal of Clinical Endocrinology & Metabolism*, vol. 95, no. 8, pp. 3641–3647, 2010.

[3] J. Klubo-Gwiezdzinska, M. Lange, E. Cochran et al., "Combined immunosuppressive therapy induces remission in patients with severe type B insulin resistance: a prospective cohort study," *Diabetes Care*, vol. 41, no. 11, pp. 2353–2360, 2018.

[4] H. N. Kim, B. Fesseha, L. Anzaldi, A. Tsao, P. Galiatsatos, and A. Sidhaye, "Antibody-mediated extreme insulin resistance: a report of three cases," *The American Journal of Medicine*, vol. 131, no. 1, pp. 102–106, 2018.

[5] C. Liminet, J. Vouillarmet, K. Chikh, and E. Disse, "Antibody-mediated insulin resistance: when insulin and insulin receptor act as autoantigens in humans," *Canadian Journal of Diabetes*, vol. 40, no. 5, pp. 462–465, 2016.

[6] S. Mizuhashi, K. Nakamura, Y. Mori, M. Noda, and K. Nakanishi, "Insulin allergy and immunologic insulin resistance caused by interleukin-6 in a patient with lung cancer," *Diabetes Care*, vol. 29, no. 7, pp. 1711–1712, 2006.

[7] M. Takaya, M. Nagao, S. Takemitsu et al., "Severe insulin-resistant diabetes due to insulin antibodies associated with eosinophilia," *Internal Medicine*, vol. 54, no. 18, pp. 2367–2371, 2015.

[8] J. R. Greenfield, A. Tuthill, M. A. Soos et al., "Severe insulin resistance due to anti-insulin antibodies: response to plasma exchange and immunosuppressive therapy," *Diabetic Medicine*, vol. 26, no. 1, pp. 79–82, 2009.

[9] J. T. Lahtela, M. Knip, R. Paul, J. Antonen, and J. Salmi, "Severe antibody-mediated human insulin resistance: successful treatment with the insulin analog lispro: a case report," *Diabetes Care*, vol. 20, no. 1, pp. 71–73, 1997.

[10] F. H. Rhie, O. P. Ganda, M. M. Bern, J. Soeldner, B. Gerson, and F. Azizi, "Insulin resistance and monoclonal gammopathy," *Metabolism*, vol. 30, no. 1, pp. 41–45, 1981.

[11] T. Segal, E. A. Webb, R. Viner, C. Pusey, G. Wild, and J. Allgrove, "Severe insulin resistance secondary to insulin antibodies: successful treatment with the immunosuppressant MMF," *Pediatric Diabetes*, vol. 9, no. 1, pp. 250–254, 2008.

[12] D. Willard, J. Upadhyay, C. Kim, and D. Steenkamp, "Diabetic ketoacidosis without diabetes," *The Journal of Clinical Endocrinology & Metabolism*, vol. 101, no. 11, pp. 3870–3873, 2016.

[13] R. K. Semple, E. K. Cochran, M. A. Soos et al., "Plasma adiponectin as a marker of insulin receptor dysfunction: clinical utility in severe insulin resistance," *Diabetes Care*, vol. 31, no. 5, pp. 977–979, 2008.

43

Severe Dental Disease as a Presenting Sign of Relapsed 6q24-Related Transient Neonatal Diabetes Mellitus

Anna Delamerced,[1] **Lauren J. Massingham**,[2] **and Jose Bernardo Quintos**[2]

[1]*The Warren Alpert Medical School of Brown University, Providence, RI, USA*
[2]*The Warren Alpert Medical School of Brown University, Rhode Island Hospital, Hasbro Children's Hospital, 593 Eddy Street, Providence, Rhode Island 02903, USA*

Correspondence should be addressed to Jose Bernardo Quintos; jbquintos@brown.edu

Academic Editor: Lucy Mastrandrea

Transient neonatal diabetes mellitus (TNDM) is a rare form of diabetes that presents in infancy and is characterized by intrauterine growth restriction and hyperglycemia without ketones on urinalysis. Patients are treated with insulin until remission, usually within the first year. Relapse to a permanent state may occur later in life, with a mean age of 14 years. The most common cause of TNDM is a chromosome 6q24 mutation that affects pancreatic β-cell function. Reports of relapse have been limited. We describe a case of an adolescent female with TNDM due to 6q24 hypomethylation who relapsed at 15 years of age with severe dental disease as the presenting sign.

1. Introduction

Transient neonatal diabetes mellitus (TNDM) associated with 6q24 chromosomal aberrations is a rare type of diabetes that presents in the neonatal period within the first six weeks of life [1]. Suggestive findings include severe intrauterine growth restriction (IUGR), hyperglycemia, dehydration, and lack of ketoacidosis [1]. When insulin is no longer needed, remissions occur during infancy by 18 months of age, with the mean age of remission at 4.5 months of age [2]. Patients can relapse in late childhood, adolescence, or adulthood [3, 4]. 6q24-related TNDM occurs in approximately 1 in 400,000 live births [5].

There are more than 20 known genetic causes. The most common cause of TNDM, in approximately 70% of affected patients, is a mutation in chromosome 6q24 that affects pancreatic β-cell function. Diagnosis is established with genetic testing [1].

The mean age of relapse is 14 years, although relapse has been reported to occur as early as at 4 years of age [2]. Relapsed TNDM is characterized by decreased insulin secretion, lack of autoantibodies, and no obesity. Approximately 50% of patients with 6q24-related TNDM may relapse, with no standard treatment for relapse [6, 7]. There are few case reports documenting relapse presentation in 6q24-related TNDM.

We describe a case showing severe dental disease as the primary presenting sign of relapsed 6q24-related TNDM. Initial clinical presentation, presentation at relapse, workup, and management are discussed.

2. Case Presentation

The patient is a 19-year-old female with a history of 6q24-related TNDM and Hashimoto's thyroiditis who was diagnosed with neonatal diabetes mellitus at birth.

She was born to a 25-year-old G3P2 mother, with a weight of 1927 grams, at 36 weeks of gestation via vaginal delivery after induction due to IUGR at an outside hospital. The pregnancy was significant for intrauterine growth restriction noted at 5 months of gestation. The pediatrician was at the delivery, and no resuscitation was needed. Apgar scores were 8 at 1 minute and 9 at 5 minutes. Macroglossia was noted. Umbilical hernia and hypotonia were not found.

The infant was noted to have hypoglycemia on day of life one and was given intravenous glucose and went on to develop hyperglycemia. Glucose levels were the 400 mg/dl, and an insulin drip was started. The infant was transferred to the NICU from the outside hospital due to hyperglycemia and concerns for necrotizing enterocolitis (NEC). Due to concerns for NEC, oral feeds were discontinued and she was placed on TPN, providing a steady glucose load. No surgical intervention was necessary for the NEC. Glucose was difficult to control even while on TPN with blood sugar levels ranging from the 100s to >200 mg/dl. At about 1 month of age, glucose levels started dropping and insulin was weaned. During this time, due to an IV infiltrate, IV insulin was briefly discontinued and blood glucose was 268 mg/dl. Insulin infusion was restarted and was discontinued at about 1 month of age. Blood sugar levels ranged between 80 and 150 mg/dl. The infant was discharged shortly afterward, feeding ad lib and checking blood sugar before meals. She required intermittent subcutaneous insulin at home, which was finally discontinued at approximately 4 months of age. Since then, the patient did not require insulin or have diabetes symptoms. All developmental milestones were on time. At 15 years of age, she chipped her tooth and went to the dentist for evaluation. The dentist noted extensive tooth decay. Jaw X-rays showed bone loss of nearly 80% in the left mandible. Due to her history of TNDM, she was sent to her primary care provider for further workup and diabetes screening where blood glucose was 369 mg/dl and urinalysis showed positive ketones. She was sent to the emergency department, and laboratory examination showed blood glucose of 361 mg/dl, Na+ of 131 mEq/L, *K*+ of 3.4 mmol/L, bicarbonate of 19 mmol/L, 2+ urine ketones, anion gap of 16, and pH of 7.4. HbA1c was 15.4% during her admission. The diabetes autoimmune panel was negative (ICA-512, GAD-65, and Insulin Antibodies).

She endorsed long-standing polydipsia, polyphagia, and polyuria. She denied weight loss, nausea, vomiting, abdominal pain, confusion, blurry vision, fatigue, fever, and difficulty breathing. Family history was negative for autoimmune diseases except for hypothyroidism in the paternal grandmother and maternal great-grandmother. Physical exam showed a weight of 58.4 kg (70th percentile), height of 163 cm (55th percentile), and BMI of 21.98 kg/m^2 (70th percentile). She was a well-appearing adolescent without thyromegaly and acanthosis nigricans and had Tanner Stage 5 breast. She was started on basal bolus insulin regimen consisting of 23 units of Glargine at bedtime and fast-acting insulin Lispro 1 unit per 10 grams of carbohydrates with meals.

She received the appropriate diabetes education. Laboratory examination also noted a TSH of 66 IU/ml (reference range: 0.35–5.5 uIU/ml); free T4 was 0.94 ng/dl (reference range: 0.8–1.8 ng/dl), and positive antibodies to thyroid peroxidase was 8580 IU/ml. She was treated with 75 mcg Levothyroxine that was titrated to a dose of 100 mcg. The 6q24 methylation-specific multiplex ligation-dependent probe amplification (MPLA) genetic test for transient neonatal diabetes identified hypomethylation within the 6q24 region. Deletion/duplication analysis ruled out paternal duplication of 6q24. Therefore, the hypomethylation could be the result of either paternal uniparental disomy of chromosome 6 (UPD6) or hypomethylation of the maternal allele. Via testing, UPD6 has been confirmed, meaning both copies of the 6q24 chromosome region in our patient were paternally inherited. This results in an epigenetic phenomena where both copies are still active. Typically, the paternal copy is active and the maternal copy is methylated and turned off. Epigenetic changes are typically de novo, as they depend on the parent of origin and are reset with each pregnancy, rather than DNA sequencing changes. Thus, risk of recurrence for parents, siblings, and offspring is unlikely. After diagnosis and her initial HbA1c of 15.4%, her HbA1c has ranged since then from 6.3% to 6.8%.

3. Discussion

We present a 19-year-old female with a history of TNDM who presented with neonatal diabetes mellitus in the newborn period, went into remission at 4 months of age, and presented with severe dental disease when she relapsed at 15 years of age. To the best of our knowledge, there have been no case reports of severe dental disease as the initial presenting sign of 6q24-related TNDM relapse.

Clinical features, management, and prognosis are influenced by the gene involved. The majority of TNDM cases is caused by a mutation in chromosome 6q24 that affects pancreatic β-cell function. 6q24-related TNDM can be caused by three mechanisms: paternal uniparental disomy of chromosome 6, duplication of the paternal 6q24 allele, or loss of maternal methylation [8].

Initial presentations of TNDM have been documented and usually involve hyperglycemia and excessive dehydration, within the first week of life, which gradually resolves between 3 and 18 months. In particular, 6q24-related TNDM is characterized by low birth weight and intrauterine growth restriction. One study found that 30% of 6q24-related TNDM patients were born at the time of less than 37 weeks of gestation [2]. The low birth weight is likely due to the failure of insulin secretion, which is important for intrauterine growth [1]. Additional characteristics that may present in patients include an umbilical hernia, macroglossia, or hypotonia. Less frequently reported features include renal and cardiac abnormalities [2].

Data on 6q24-related TNMD relapse are scarce. Presenting symptoms of relapse have not been documented extensively. Relapse may be due to increased physiologic stress or increased insulin demand, including childhood illness, the onset of puberty, or pregnancy. The median age of TNDM relapse is 14 years, but the age and presenting signs of relapse vary widely and can occur as early as at 4 years of age or as late as 27 years of age [3, 9]. Only a few cases of 6q24-related TNDM have been reported and were diagnosed incidentally or by routine laboratory investigation. These cases of relapsed diabetes were incidentally discovered after a routine glucose test (Table 1).

Our patient presented with a unique finding of severe dental disease as the main clinical presentation for relapsed 6q24-related TNDM. No previous cases have reported severe dental disease, gum disease, dental caries, or bone loss of the

Table 1: Review of the literature of 6q24-related TNDM at relapse.

Reference	Age of relapse	HbA1c or fasting glucose level at relapse	Genetic variant	Treatment
Schimmel [10]	15 years	198 mg/dl	Uniparental paternal isodisomy of chromosome 6	Sulfonylurea
Yorifuji et al. [7]	12 years	7–7.5%	Paternal duplication at 6q24	Initially alpha-glucosidase inhibitor, then DPP4-inhibitor
Fu et al. [11]	14 years	8.2%, 204 mg/dl	Hypomethylation of the maternal allele	Insulin glargine and lifestyle modifications, transitioning to sulfonylurea

jaw as primary features for TNDM relapse. An elevated TSH and positive anti-thyroid peroxidase antibodies, consistent with acquired hypothyroidism, could have contributed to bone loss of the jaw, as thyroid hormones play a role in bone mineral density.

After relapse, some patients have transitioned to oral hypoglycemic agents. While sulfonylureas have been used to treat relapsed TNDM, no specific guidelines exist for management of relapse. Possible treatments include targeting the GLP-1 pathway because these patients still have the ability to produce and respond to insulin through *G* protein-coupled pathways [6]. We plan to transition our patient to an oral hypoglycemic agent and to wean off and discontinue insulin.

In summary, little is known of the clinical presentation for 6q24-related TNDM relapse. We present a patient who was diagnosed with neonatal diabetes mellitus as an infant, went into remission at 4 months of age, and relapsed at 15 years of age with dental caries as the primary characteristic. Accumulation of further cases is needed to increase knowledge of management of 6q24-related diabetes relapse with insulin or hypoglycemic agents.

References

[1] I. K. Temple and D. J. Mackay, "Diabetes mellitus, 6q24-related transient neonatal. 2005," in *GeneReviews®*, M. P. Adam, H. H. Ardinger, R. A. Pagon et al., Eds., p. 2020, University of Washington, Seattle, WA, USA, 1993.

[2] L. E. Docherty, S. Kabwama, A. Lehmann et al., "Clinical presentation of 6q24 transient neonatal diabetes mellitus (6q24 TNDM) and genotype-phenotype correlation in an international cohort of patients," *Diabetologia*, vol. 56, no. 4, pp. 758–762, 2013.

[3] I. K. Temple, R. J. Gardner, D. J. Mackay, J. C. Barber, D. O. Robinson, and J. P. Shield, "Transient neonatal diabetes: widening the understanding of the etiopathogenesis of diabetes," *Diabetes*, vol. 49, no. 8, pp. 1359–1366, 2000.

[4] M. B. Lemelman, L. Letourneau, and S. A. W. Greeley, "Neonatal diabetes mellitus," *Clinics in Perinatology*, vol. 45, no. 1, pp. 41–59, 2018.

[5] R. H. Gore, M. E. Nikita, P. G. Newton, R. G. Carter, J. Reyes-Bautista, and C. L. Greene, "Duplication 6q24: more than just diabetes," *Journal of the Endocrine Society*, vol. 4, no. 5, 2020.

[6] D. J. G. Mackay and I. K. Temple, "Transient neonatal diabetes mellitus type 1," *American Journal of Medical Genetics Part C: Seminars in Medical Genetics*, vol. 154, no. 3, p. 335, 2010.

[7] T. Yorifuji, Y. Hashimoto, R. Kawakita et al., "Relapsing 6q24-related transient neonatal diabetes mellitus successfully treated with a dipeptidyl peptidase-4 inhibitor: a case report," *Pediatric Diabetes*, vol. 15, no. 8, p. 606, 2014.

[8] I. K. Temple and J. P. H. Shield, "6q24 transient neonatal diabetes," *Reviews in Endocrine and Metabolic Disorders*, vol. 11, no. 3, p. 199, 2010.

[9] D. Carmody, F. A. Beca, C. D. Bell et al., "Role of noninsulin therapies alone or in combination in chromosome 6q24-related transient neonatal diabetes: sulfonylurea improves but does not always normalize insulin secretion: table 1," *Diabetes Care*, vol. 38, no. 6, pp. e86–e87, 2015.

[10] U. Schimmel, "Long-standing sulfonylurea therapy after pubertal relapse of neonatal diabetes in a case of uniparental paternal isodisomy of chromosome 6," *Diabetes Care*, vol. 32, no. 1, p. e9, 2009.

[11] J.-L. Fu, T. Wang, and X.-H. Xiao, "Relapsed 6q24-related transient neonatal diabetes mellitus successfully treated with sulfonylurea," *Chinese Medical Journal*, vol. 132, no. 7, p. 846, 2019.

44

A Case of Diabetic Ketoacidosis in a Patient on an SGLT2 Inhibitor and a Ketogenic Diet: A Critical Trio not to be Missed

Samantha Steinmetz-Wood, Matthew Gilbert, and Katherine Menson

Department of Medicine, Larner College of Medicine at the University of Vermont, 111 Colchester Ave, Burlington, VT, USA

Correspondence should be addressed to Samantha Steinmetz-Wood; samantha.steinmetz-wood@uvmhealth.org, Matthew Gilbert; matthew.gilbert@uvmhealth.org, and Katherine Menson; katherine.menson@uvmhealth.org

Academic Editor: Lucy Mastrandrea

Results from major clinical trials have shown significant cardiorenal-protective benefits of SGLT2 inhibitors in patients with type 2 diabetes (T2DM), leading to increased popularity. A rare but serious side effect of SGLT2 inhibitors is euglycemic diabetic ketoacidosis (EDKA), which presents more covertly but has been described. Identification and report of modifiable risk factors would be an important step in helping clinicians appropriately counsel patients. In this case report, we present DKA in a patient on an SGLT2 inhibitor and ketogenic diet (KD). A 47-year-old male with a history of poorly controlled T2DM on metformin and empagliflozin presented to the emergency department (ED) with several days of pharyngitis, dyspnea, emesis, abdominal pain, and anorexia. Of note, one month prior to this event, he presented to the ED with malaise and was found to have an anion gap of 21, a bicarbonate level of 13 mmol/L, a pH level of 7.22, 3+ ketonuria, and a glucose level of 7 mmol/L (127 mg/dl). Additional workup was negative, and findings were attributed to his KD. His use of empagliflozin was not identified on his medication list. At second presentation, the patient was tachypneic and tachycardic and had mild abdominal tenderness. Labs revealed anion gap 28, bicarbonate 5 mmol/l, pH 6.94, 3+ ketonuria, glucose 14.9 mmol/L (269 mg/dl), and beta-hydroxybutyrate 8.9 mmol/L. The patient was diagnosed with DKA and was treated accordingly. With closure of anion gap, the patient was transitioned to insulin and metformin, and his empagliflozin was discontinued indefinitely. Before prescribing this medication class, physicians should inquire about low-carbohydrate diets given the higher risk for DKA, though knowledge of this risk is still not widespread.

1. Introduction

Recent results from major clinical trials such as CANVAS, CREDENCE, EMPA-REG OUTCOME, and DAPA-HF have shown significant cardiovascular and renal protective benefits of SGLT2 inhibitors [1–4]. These findings have led to increased use of this class of medication in patients with type 2 diabetes (T2DM). Although reported as rare, a serious side effect of SGLT2 inhibitors is diabetic ketoacidosis (DKA), which can present more covertly with euglycemic DKA and has been described numerous times. There are some thoughts about patients that might be at greater risk for developing this condition such as longer duration of diabetes, insulin deficiency, or even possible variants of the SGLT molecule [5, 6]. Identification of additional modifiable risk factors such as special diets would be an important step in helping clinicians choose which patients should avoid using this medication. In this case report, we present a case of profound DKA in a patient on an SGLT2 inhibitor on a ketogenic diet.

2. Case Presentation

A 47-year-old male, with a 10-year history of T2DM, presented to the emergency department (ED) with several days of sore throat, dyspnea, nonbloody emesis, abdominal pain, and poor oral intake. He denied any fever, chills, cough, chest pain, or diarrhea. He had a urinary tract infection (UTI) 2 weeks prior, which had resolved with a course of antibiotics. Over several months, he had made significant changes in his diet which resulted in a 60 lb weight loss. The patient reported that he was following an Atkins or ketogenic diet. In addition to diet control, he had been on metformin and empagliflozin started approximately 5 months ago. His last hemoglobin A1c was 76 mmol/dl (9.1%). Of note, one month prior to this presentation, he presented to the emergency department with weakness, intermittent chest discomfort, and shortness of breath with an anion gap of 21, a bicarbonate level of 13 mmol/L, a pH level of 7.22, and 3+ urinary ketones with a glucose level of 7 mmol/L (127 mg/dl). Cardiac workup was negative, lactate was normal, and liver enzymes and D-dimer were within normal limits. The patient was given 1 L fluid bolus with some improvement. Findings were attributed to a keto diet. The patient was discharged with recommendations to increase carbohydrate intake for 2 weeks and repeat electrolytes. His use of empagliflozin was not identified on his medication list in the emergency department nor was it mentioned in the ED notes. His repeat labs one week later did result in closure of his anion gap to 10. When this second presentation to the emergency department 24 days later, he was afebrile, tachypneic with a respiratory rate of 30, and tachycardic with a heart rate of 130 beats per minute, blood pressure was 160/89 mmHg, and SpO2 was 100% on room air. Other than respiratory discomfort, the exam only showed mild abdominal discomfort to palpation. Labs were significant for an anion gap of 28, a pH level of 6.94, with a bicarbonate level of 5 mmol/L, 3+ urinary ketones, a beta-hydroxybutyrate level of 8.9 mmol/L, and a glucose level of 14.9 mmol/L (269 mg/dl), as well as acute kidney injury with a creatinine level of 107 umol/L (1.21 mg/dl). His glutamic acid decarboxylase antibody assay ordered during this admission eventually returned negative. His C-peptide was 0.77 nmol/L (2.3 ng/ml). Cardiac workup was negative. CT scan did reveal possible aspiration pneumonitis. The patient was diagnosed with diabetic ketoacidosis, received several litres of fluid, started on insulin drip, and admitted to the medical ICU. With closure of anion gap, on the following day, the patient was transitioned to insulin basal bolus regimen, and metformin was eventually restarted. His empagliflozin was stopped indefinitely. Hospital course was also complicated by development of a new UTI, and the patient was treated with ceftriaxone/cephalexin. Finally, he was deemed medically stable for discharge with plans to follow up with endocrinology and his primary care provider.

3. Discussion

Our case illustrates a case of profound DKA of a patient on an SGLT2 inhibitor and following a ketogenic diet. Interestingly, our patient also developed a UTI twice in the same month, which is another reported side effect of this medication. Randomized control trials studying SGLT2 inhibitors have indicated DKA to be a rare side effect, with an estimated incidence rate of DKA varying from 0.13 to 0.76 events per 1000 patient years [6].

On review of the literature, this is not the first case of DKA in a patient on an SGLT2 inhibitor following a ketogenic or low-carbohydrate diet [7–10]. Another case reports a similar story of a 44-year-old man who had been on sitagliptin, metformin, and an Atkins diet, and 3-4 days after starting canagliflozin, he developed euglycemic DKA which was first missed by the ED and later recognized by his primary internist [10]. As in our case, our patient had already presented with euglycemic DKA to the ED, which was diagnosed as dehydration and starvation ketosis. Luckily, at that time, he recovered by one week with change in diet. Later, he presented with profound dehydration and severe anion gap metabolic acidosis with a bicarbonate level of <5 mEq/L, requiring inpatient critical care. Recognition of the association of this medication with euglycemic DKA and asking about medications is most important.

Studies have measured patients on SGLT2 inhibitors to have low-grade asymptomatic ketonemia [11, 12], and in a Japanese multicenter, randomized, 3-arm parallel comparative study, patients with T2DM assigned to low-carbohydrate diet on luseogliflozin had significantly higher serum ketone bodies than their study counterparts on higher carbohydrate diets [12]. Although ketonemia may be perceived as a negative effect of SGLT2 inhibitors, this seems to be their main mechanism of benefit. SGLT2 inhibitors are thought to act through calorie-restriction mimicry and by a proketogenic effect [13]. This also decreases the insulin to glucagon ratio, thereby improving insulin sensitivity. Ketone bodies are additionally a more efficient source of fuel for cardiac muscle [13].

A Canadian clinical literature review reviewed 46 cases of SGLT2-associated DKA and found that the most common precipitants of DKA were inappropriate insulin reduction or cessation, surgery, excessive alcohol intake, excessive physical exercise, and dietary restriction such as low-carbohydrate or reduced intake [14]. As SGLT2 inhibitors themselves mimic a low-carbohydrate diet and promote ketosis, it follows that the pairing of SGLT2 inhibitors and a ketogenic diet, in addition to stressors, may more easily precipitate a ketoacidotic state.

4. Conclusion

Before prescribing this medication class which is now starting to be more widely prescribed, physicians should ask whether patients are following low-carbohydrate diets as this likely puts them at higher risk for DKA. Knowledge of this risk is still not widespread.

References

[1] B. Neal, V. Perkovic, and D. R. Matthews, "Canagliflozin and cardiovascular and renal events in type 2 diabetes," *New England Journal of Medicine*, vol. 377, no. 21, p. 2099, 2017.

[2] V. Perkovic, M. J. Jardine, B. Neal et al., "Canagliflozin and renal outcomes in type 2 diabetes and nephropathy," *New England Journal of Medicine*, vol. 380, no. 24, pp. 2295–2306, 2019.

[3] B. Zinman, C. Wanner, J. M. Lachin et al., "Empagliflozin, cardiovascular outcomes, and mortality in type 2 diabetes," *New England Journal of Medicine*, vol. 373, no. 22, pp. 2117–2128, 2015.

[4] J. J. V. McMurray, S. D. Solomon, S. E. Inzucchi et al., "Dapagliflozin in patients with heart failure and reduced

ejection fraction," *New England Journal of Medicine*, vol. 381, 2019.

[5] F. M. Finucane, "SGLT2 inhibitor-induced euglycaemic diabetic ketoacidosis may be due to abrupt, severe and transient impaired glucose sensing in susceptible individuals with a hitherto unrecognised beta cell SGLT variant," *Medical Hypotheses*, vol. 114, pp. 11-12, 2018.

[6] N. Erondu, M. Desai, K. Ways, and G. Meininger, "Diabetic ketoacidosis and related events in the canagliflozin type 2 diabetes clinical program," *Diabetes Care*, vol. 38, no. 9, pp. 1680–1686, 2015.

[7] T. Smyth, "Acute illness while on a SGLT2 inhibitor and keto diet," *Medicine Matters*, 2018.

[8] N. H. Tougaard, "Very low carbohydrate diet and SGLT-2-inhibitor: double jeopardy in relation to ketoacidosis," *BMJ Case Report*, vol. 12, no. 4, 2019.

[9] T. Hayami, Y. Kato, H. Kamiya et al., "Case of ketoacidosis by a sodium-glucose cotransporter 2 inhibitor in a diabetic patient with a low-carbohydrate diet," *Journal of Diabetes Investigation*, vol. 6, no. 5, pp. 587–590, 2015.

[10] M. Sood, "Euglycemic diabetic ketoacidosis with SGLT2 inhibitor use in a patient on the Atkins diet: a unique presentation of a known side effect," *American Association of Clinical Endocrinologists Journals*, vol. 4, no. 2, 2018.

[11] S. H. Min, T. J. Oh, S.-I. Baek et al., "Degree of ketonaemia and its association with insulin resistance after dapagliflozin treatment in type 2 diabetes," *Diabetes & Metabolism*, vol. 44, no. 1, pp. 73–76, 2018.

[12] D. Yabe, M. Iwasaki, H. Kuwata et al., "Sodium-glucose cotransporter-2 inhibitor use and dietary carbohydrate intake in Japanese individuals with type 2 diabetes: a randomized, open-label, 3-arm parallel comparative, exploratory study," *Diabetes, Obesity and Metabolism*, vol. 19, no. 5, pp. 739–743, 2017.

[13] S. Kalra, A. Jain, J. Ved, and A. Unnikrishnan, "Sodium-glucose cotransporter 2 inhibition and health benefits: the Robin Hood effect," *Indian Journal of Endocrinology and Metabolism*, vol. 20, no. 5, pp. 725–729, 2016.

[14] R. M. Goldenberg, L. D. Berard, A. Y. Y. Cheng et al., "SGLT2 inhibitor-associated diabetic ketoacidosis: clinical review and recommendations for prevention and diagnosis," *Clinical Therapeutics*, vol. 38, no. 12, pp. 2654–2664, 2016.

Critical Low Catastrophe: A Case Report of Treatment-Refractory Hypoglycemia following Overdose of Long-Acting Insulin

Rashi Sandooja,[1] **John M. Moorman**,[2] **Monisha Priyadarshini Kumar**,[1] **and Karla Detoya**[3]

[1]*Department of Internal Medicine, Cleveland Clinic Akron General, Akron, OH, USA*
[2]*Department of Pharmacy Practice, Northeast Ohio Medical University, Rootstown, OH, USA*
[3]*Department of Endocrinology, Cleveland Clinic Akron General, Akron, OH, USA*

Correspondence should be addressed to Rashi Sandooja; sandoor@ccf.org

Academic Editor: Osamu Isozaki

Overdose of long-acting insulin can cause unpredictable hypoglycemia for prolonged periods of time. The initial treatment of hypoglycemia includes oral carbohydrate intake as able and/or parenteral dextrose infusion. Refractory hypoglycemia following these interventions presents a clinical challenge in the absence of clear guidelines for management. Octreotide has sometimes been used, but its use is generally limited to sulfonylurea overdose. In this case report, we present a case of refractory hypoglycemia following an overdose of 900 units of long-acting insulin glargine that failed to respond to usual modes of therapy mentioned above. Stress-dose corticosteroids were then initiated, followed by subsequent improvement in IV dextrose and glucagon requirements and blood glucose levels. Hence, corticosteroids may serve as an adjunctive therapy in managing hypoglycemia and can be considered earlier in the course of treatment in patients with refractory hypoglycemia to prevent volume overload, especially when large volumes of dextrose infusions are required.

1. Introduction

Insulin is a mainstay of treatment in patients with type 1 diabetes mellitus (T1DM), and a significant proportion of patients with type 2 diabetes mellitus (T2DM) are insulin-dependent [1–3]. At the same time, insulin therapy is associated with multiple adverse effects, with hypoglycemia being one of the most common. For example, in the U.K. Prospective Diabetes Study, the prevalence of hypoglycemia in patients with T2DM who were taking insulin was 11.2%, as compared to 3.3% in those taking sulfonylureas and 2.4% in those taking metformin [4]. However, these prevalences represent usual medication use and do not account for the potential for insulin overdose, either intentional or unintentional. Management of insulin overdose poses a clinical challenge and may require modified treatment strategies, given the lack of consensus and guidelines. The objective of this report is to describe a case of intentional insulin overdose associated with refractory hypoglycemia and to discuss the integrative approach to managing this case.

2. Case Report

A 27-year-old female with a history of bipolar 1 disorder, borderline personality disorder, posttraumatic stress disorder (PTSD), previous history of multiple suicide attempts, T2DM, and obesity (weight 160 kg; body mass index 56 kg/m^2) status-postsleeve gastrectomy in 2016 presented to the emergency department (ED) following a suicide attempt. She was brought to the ED by self-notifying emergency services after having shortness of breath and dizziness following self-injection of 900 units of insulin glargine U-100 (Lantus®) subcutaneously into her abdomen three hours prior. This represented her third intentional insulin overdose in the preceding six months. She was previously insulin-requiring, on Lantus, but was weaned off insulin four years ago after sleeve gastrectomy and subsequent 68 kg weight loss over the preceding five years. The patient's most recent hemoglobin A1c (HbA1c) ten months prior to presentation, while off insulin or any other hypoglycemic agents, was 4.7%. Home medications at this time included duloxetine 120 mg daily, bupropion 300 mg daily, lithium 900 mg daily, prazosin 5 mg at bedtime, trazodone 150 mg at bedtime, and mirtazapine 30 mg at bedtime.

The patient reported suicidal ideation and worsened depression for three months prior to presentation and decided to inject three full insulin glargine U-100 pens (300 units each), which she had at home from her prior insulin prescription. The initial fingerstick blood glucose taken by paramedics prior to arrival to the ED was 131 mg/dL. At that time, she was closely monitored, but not medically treated, and was sent to the ED. Her fingerstick blood glucose level upon presentation to the ED was 113 mg/dL, at which time she was somnolent but arousable and answering questions appropriately. Her physical examination upon arrival was unremarkable and did not reveal any areas of fluctuance at the reported injection sites.

Figure 1 depicts the patient's course of therapy from the time of ED presentation. An intravenous (IV) 10% dextrose (D10) infusion was started at 300 mL/hour 30 minutes after ED arrival to prevent hypoglycemia. A regular diet was started and carbohydrate intake was encouraged. Fingerstick glucose levels were monitored every 15 minutes for the first seven hours and every 30 minutes thereafter. The patient's blood glucose readings first approached the hypoglycemic range of <70 mg/dL approximately three hours after presentation (fingerstick blood glucose = 74 mg/dL). She received two 50-gram ampules of dextrose 50% (D50) IV, along with three 1 mg doses of intramuscular (IM) glucagon, over the next four hours in addition to the D10 IV infusion. The patient was then transferred to the medical intensive care unit (MICU) for close observation.

Due to persistent hypoglycemia and inability to wean the D10 IV infusion, a standing order for glucagon 1 mg IM for blood glucose <70 mg/dL was added. During the first 48 hours of her admission, she required eleven 1 mg IM glucagon doses in addition to the D10 IV infusion but continued to experience hypoglycemia with the lowest recorded blood glucose reading of 64 mg/dl. She was transitioned from a standard diet to a bariatric diet due to suspected reactive hypoglycemia associated with her postbariatric surgery status, which consisted of 56 grams of carbohydrate and 18 grams of protein per day. An IV glucagon infusion was started at 1 mg/hr on hospital day two (approximately 44 hours after presentation) in a continued effort to minimize IV fluid volume. In addition, a trial dose of hydrocortisone 100 mg IV bolus was given at the time the IV glucagon infusion was started. The IV glucagon infusion was titrated to 2 mg/hr as the D10 IV infusion was weaned off, which was done on hospital day three (approximately 73 hours after presentation). However, the patient's glucose levels began trending towards the hypoglycemic range, requiring further titration of the IV glucagon infusion to 4 mg/hr. Hydrocortisone 100 mg IV every 8 hours was then started to reduce the IV and IM glucagon requirements. The IV glucagon infusion was weaned off on hospital day four after three additional doses of hydrocortisone on days 3 and 4. The patient became hyperglycemic following the last dose of hydrocortisone (blood glucose = 309 mg/dL), which prompted discontinuation of the stress-dose steroids. Following discontinuation of medical therapy for hypoglycemia, her blood glucose ranged from 130 to 150 mg/dL, and the patient was transferred out of the MICU to a medical floor for observation without recurrence of hypoglycemia.

3. Discussion

Patients who experience an insulin overdose can present with prolonged, refractory hypoglycemia, especially with the administration of long-acting insulin [5]. Although the duration of action of insulin glargine is reported to be 24 to 30 hours [6], these parameters were observed with doses of 0.3 to 0.5 units/kg, whereas the patient in the present case self-administered a dose of 5.6 units/kg [7]. In cases of overdose, the duration of action may be affected by a number of factors, including the route and site of administration, injection volume, solution concentration (e.g., U-100 vs. U-300), local blood supply, and presence of lipodystrophy or cutaneous amyloidosis at the injection site. For example, insulin injections of larger volumes are more slowly absorbed from the subcutaneous space than smaller volumes, which may result in delayed hypoglycemia following the injection [8]. Other factors, such as the presence of insulin autoantibodies and renal dysfunction, can prolong the duration of hypoglycemia as well. Therefore, it may be difficult to predict the duration of hypoglycemia in cases of insulin overdose. Based on case reports involving insulin overdose, hypoglycemia has been reported up to several days after injection [5, 9, 10].

In patients who present with hypoglycemia, current clinical practice guidelines suggest a tiered approach to treatment based on the initial blood glucose level and the patient's ability to self-treat [11, 12]. The initial treatment for hypoglycemia should primarily involve oral carbohydrate ingestion [11]. However, if the patient is unable to ingest carbohydrates or if hypoglycemia persists despite this, parenteral dextrose and/or glucagon may be administered [12]. This should be accompanied by frequent monitoring of serum glucose levels and electrolytes, especially serum potassium. Continuous infusions of dextrose (e.g., 5% or 10% solutions) may be necessary depending on the patient's response to initial therapy and the ability to eat food [12].

In cases where hypoglycemia persists despite standard treatment modalities, other treatment options can be explored. The somatostatin analog octreotide has been tried in previous cases of insulin overdose [13, 14]. However, its use was associated with inconsistent results and is usually reserved for hypoglycemia secondary to sulfonylurea use [15]. Another uncommon approach to cases of insulin overdose includes excision of the insulin depot at the injection site when clear fluctuance is present. This theoretically can help in preventing delayed absorption of insulin and associated prolonged hypoglycemia and has been utilized successfully

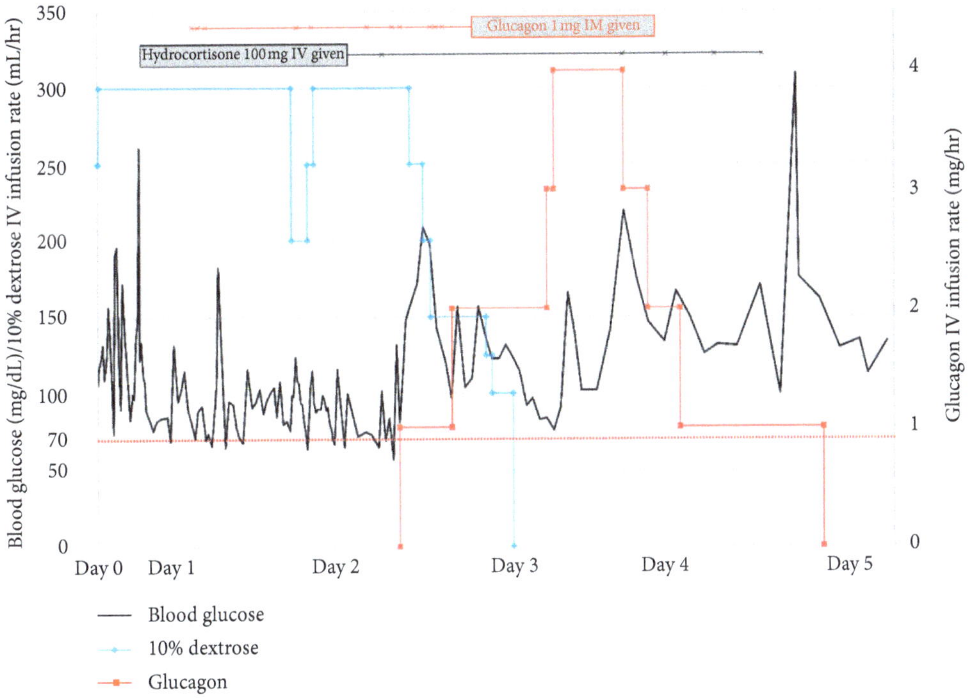

FIGURE 1: Blood glucose trends over time starting at ED presentation (black line, left axis), along with IV dextrose infusion rate (blue line, left axis), IV glucagon infusion rate (red line, right axis), hydrocortisone IV doses (black horizontal line across the top), and glucagon IM doses (red horizontal line across the top).

in previous cases [16, 17]. However, in cases such as the present one where an area of fluctuance is not visible on physical examination, this option is not possible.

Another treatment strategy that may be underutilized involves the use of glucocorticoids. These agents promote hepatic gluconeogenesis and decrease peripheral glucose uptake and are frequently associated with hyperglycemia as a result. Hence, glucocorticoids may serve as an adjunctive therapy option in managing refractory hypoglycemia in cases of insulin overdose. This approach has been utilized in a prior case of refractory hypoglycemia associated with insulin overdose where hydrocortisone was administered to prevent volume overload associated with the infusion of large volumes of dextrose-containing IV fluids [14]. Early initiation of steroids in cases with persistent hypoglycemia may reduce the duration of intensive care unit stay, avoid invasive procedures like central line placement for 25% or 50% dextrose infusions, and prevent volume overload from large volume dextrose infusions [18].

This patient presented with intentional insulin overdose after injecting 900 units (~5.6 units/kg) of insulin glargine U-100 (Lantus®). Her blood glucose levels first approached the hypoglycemic range of <70 mg/dL about six hours after she reported injecting the insulin. The initial management of her hypoglycemic episodes followed guideline recommendations, starting with oral carbohydrate ingestion and parenteral dextrose administration [11, 12]. One concern raised with this approach was regarding her history of sleeve gastrectomy and that the carbohydrate ingestion could lead to excess endogenous insulin release and subsequent worsening of hypoglycemia symptoms [19]. Therefore, the decision was made to place her on a high protein, low carbohydrate bariatric diet to help mitigate this potential issue. Adjunctive measures were required due to her persistent hypoglycemia, and she was therefore given IM glucagon injections in addition to oral and parenteral carbohydrates. An IV glucagon infusion was tried as well, which proved ineffective at completely resolving hypoglycemia.

In the setting of persistent hypoglycemia three days after the reported overdose and concern for volume overload, other treatment modalities were considered. Octreotide was not given due to the inconsistent results from previous cases along with its high cost and because sulfonylurea coingestion was not suspected [13, 14]. Excision of the insulin depot was not possible in our patient because she did not have a clear site of fluctuance at the injection site. Consistent with use of hydrocortisone in a previous case report [14], a trial of stress-dose hydrocortisone was started. Hydrocortisone was chosen due to its shorter duration of action compared to other glucocorticoids, thereby reducing the risk of subsequent hyperglycemia. Following the administration of four doses of hydrocortisone, she was able to be weaned off both the D10 and glucagon infusions and was able to maintain euglycemia.

There are some important limitations to the present case that should be considered as well. We were unable to obtain the insulin product to verify its identity, and there was no recent prescription history to reconcile since the patient was no longer on insulin. Therefore, it is possible that the insulin product administered was not as stated and/or the insulin product was expired. However, given the timeline of events and the intensive medical therapy that she required, it seems reasonable to assume that long-acting insulin with adequate potency was used. We did not rule out other secondary causes of hypoglycemia, such as postprandial hyperinsulinemic hypoglycemia associated with bariatric surgery. However, this is more commonly associated with Roux-en-Y gastric bypass than sleeve gastrectomy and was thought to be more likely associated with the insulin overdose in the present case given the temporal association with insulin administration [19]. Given the prior cases involving the use of glucocorticoids for insulin-induced hypoglycemia, we felt that the administration of hydrocortisone contributed towards the resolution of hypoglycemia and reduced the continued need for parenteral dextrose and glucagon in the present case. However, given the delay in the administration of hydrocortisone until three days after presentation, it is also possible that the hypoglycemia resolved due to the clearance of the exogenous insulin, as opposed to the effect of glucocorticoid administration. Finally, while the efficacy of IV glucagon infusion is more established in pediatrics with T1DM and in neonatal hypoglycemia, the efficacy of continuous infusions of IV glucagon for the treatment of insulin-induced hypoglycemia in adults is unclear given the absence of strong supporting evidence in this population [14, 20, 21]. Glucagon acts by promoting glycogenolysis and gluconeogenesis and thus has limited use once glycogen stores have been depleted. On the other hand, insulin itself promotes the conversion of glucose to glycogen for storage in the liver. Importantly, this was this patient's third suicide attempt with insulin, the first with 300 units of insulin lispro U-100 and the second with 300 units of insulin glargine U-100. These previous overdoses were managed successfully with IV glucagon infusions; therefore, it was reasonable to attempt the use of an IV glucagon infusion for persistent hypoglycemia during the present case. However, her prior suicide attempts involved much smaller doses of insulin, which may explain why the IV glucagon infusion alone failed to resolve hypoglycemia in the present case, thereby requiring hydrocortisone administration.

4. Conclusions

Insulin overdose often requires intensive care admission and frequent monitoring of blood glucose and electrolytes. Prolonged continuous D10 IV infusions can lead to volume overload, and parenteral administration of higher concentrations of dextrose (e.g. 25% or 50%) requires invasive procedures to obtain central venous access [18]. This case adds to the literature supporting the use of glucocorticoids in the management of refractory hypoglycemia associated with overdoses of long-acting insulin. Additionally, this case involved a patient who was not being treated for diabetes mellitus following sleeve gastrectomy and could be extrapolated to such patients. Early initiation of hydrocortisone should be considered in cases of refractory hypoglycemia secondary to overdose of long-acting insulin products to prevent unnecessary interventions, decrease IV fluid requirements, and reduce the risks associated with prolonged hypoglycemia.

References

[1] G. r. Jermendy, D. Erdesz, L. Nagy et al., "Outcomes of adding second hypoglycemic drug after metformin monotherapy failure among type 2 diabetes in Hungary," *Health and Quality of Life Outcomes*, vol. 6, no. 1, p. 88, 2008.

[2] C. D. Miller, L. S. Phillips, D. C. Ziemer, D. L. Gallina, C. B. Cook, and I. M. El-Kebbi, "Hypoglycemia in patients with type 2 diabetes mellitus," *Archives of Internal Medicine*, vol. 161, no. 13, pp. 1653–1659, 2001.

[3] T. Stargardt, L. Gonder-Frederick, K. J. Krobot, and C. M. Alexander, "Fear of hypoglycemia: defining a minimum clinically important difference in patients with type 2 diabetes," *Health Qual Life Outcomes*, vol. 7, p. 91, 2009.

[4] The United Kingdom Prospective Diabetes Study Group, "U.K. prospective diabetes study 16. Overview of 6 years' therapy of type II diabetes: a progressive disease," *Diabetes*, vol. 44, no. 11, pp. 1249–1258, 1995.

[5] R. Arem and W. Zoghbi, "Insulin overdose in eight patients," *Medicine*, vol. 64, no. 5, pp. 323–332, 1985.

[6] "Basaglar (insulin glargine) (prescribing information). Indianapolis, IN: Lilly, USA, LLC," 2019.

[7] L. Heinemann, R. Linkeschova, K. Rave, B. Hompesch, M. Sedlak, and T. Heise, "Time-action profile of the long-acting insulin analog insulin glargine (HOE901) in comparison with those of NPH insulin and placebo," *Diabetes Care*, vol. 23, no. 5, pp. 644–649, 2000.

[8] T. Søeborg, C. H. Rasmussen, E. Mosekilde, and M. Colding-Jørgensen, "Absorption kinetics of insulin after subcutaneous administration," *European Journal of Pharmaceutical Sciences*, vol. 36, no. 1, pp. 78–90, 2009.

[9] Y. Shibutani and C. Ogawa, "Suicidal insulin overdose in a type 1 diabetic patient: relation of serum insulin concentrations to the duration of hypoglycemia," *Journal of Diabetes and its Complications*, vol. 14, no. 1, pp. 60–62, 2000.

[10] T. S. Tofade and E. A. Liles, "Intentional overdose with insulin glargine and insulin aspart," *Pharmacotherapy*, vol. 24, no. 10, pp. 1412–1418, 2004.

[11] American Diabetes Association, "6. Glycemic targets: standards of medical care in diabetes—2020," *Diabetes Care*, vol. 43, no. Suppl 1, pp. S66–S76, 2020.

[12] G. E. Umpierrez, R. Hellman, M. T. Korytkowski et al., "Management of hyperglycemia in hospitalized patients in non-critical care setting: an Endocrine Society clinical practice guideline," *The Journal of Clinical Endocrinology & Metabolism*, vol. 97, no. 1, pp. 16–38, 2012.

[13] C. M. Groth and E. R. Banzon, "Octreotide for the treatment of hypoglycemia after insulin glargine overdose," *The Journal of Emergency Medicine*, vol. 45, no. 2, pp. 194–198, 2013.

[14] K. Tariq, S. Tariq, and A. M. Denney Queen, "Role of steroids in refractory hypoglycemia due to an overdose of 10,000 units of insulin glargine: a case report and literature review," *AACE Clinical Case Reports*, vol. 4, no. 1, pp. e70–e74, 2018.

[15] C. J. Fasano, G. O'Malley, P. Dominici, E. Aguilera, and D. R. Latta, "Comparison of octreotide and standard therapy versus standard therapy alone for the treatment of sulfonylurea-induced hypoglycemia," *Annals of Emergency Medicine*, vol. 51, no. 4, pp. 400–406, 2008.

[16] J. Droste, V. Hundia, A. Pettit, N. Narayan, and A. Nejim, "Excision of injection site substantially reduced serum insulin concentration in a potentially life-threatening insulin analogue overdose," *Practical Diabetes*, vol. 29, no. 6, pp. 243–245, 2012.

[17] D. Warriner, M. Debono, R. A. Gandhi, E. Chong, and F. Creagh, "Acute hepatic injury following treatment of a long-acting insulin analogue overdose necessitating urgent insulin depot excision," *Diabetic Medicine*, vol. 29, no. 2, pp. 232–235, 2012.

[18] F. Josh, "Treatment of massive insulin poisoning refractory to glucose," 2017, https://emcrit.org/pulmcrit/insulin-poisoning/.

[19] D. Eisenberg, D. E. Azagury, S. Ghiassi, B. T. Grover, and J. J. Kim, "ASMBS position statement on postprandial hyperinsulinemic hypoglycemia after bariatric surgery," *Surgery for Obesity and Related Diseases*, vol. 13, no. 3, pp. 371–378, 2017.

[20] M. White, M. R. Zacharin, G. A. Werther, and F. J. Cameron, "Intravenous glucagon in a deliberate insulin overdose in an adolescent with type 1 diabetes mellitus," *Pediatric Diabetes*, vol. 17, no. 1, pp. 66–69, 2016.

[21] R. E. Miralles, A. Lodha, M. Perlman, and A. M. Moore, "Experience with intravenous glucagon infusions as a treatment for resistant neonatal hypoglycemia," *Archives of Pediatrics & Adolescent Medicine*, vol. 156, no. 10, pp. 999–1004, 2002.

46

Insulin Autoimmune Syndrome in a 25-Year-Old, Previously Healthy Kuwaiti Man

Einas Alrashidi[1] and Thamer Alessa [2]

[1]*Department of Internal Medicine, Al-Farwaniya Hospital, Kuwait*
[2]*Division of Endocrinology, Diabetes and Metabolism, Jaber Al-Ahmad Hospital, Kuwait*

Correspondence should be addressed to Thamer Alessa; thamermd@gmail.com

Academic Editor: Michael P. Kane

Insulin autoimmune syndrome (IAS) is a disease characterized by hyperinsulinaemic hypoglycaemia associated with autoantibodies against endogenous insulin. We have described a case of a 25-year-old, previously healthy Kuwaiti man who was admitted to the Mubarak Al-Kabeer hospital with a history of recurrent hypoglycaemia. The patient revealed that he had taken several different injectable anabolic steroids and growth hormone with oral amino acids and other tablets (fat burners) for bodybuilding in the last two months. He denied knowingly using insulin or insulin analogues. The patient had elevated fasting insulin level (>301 uIU/mL) and elevated insulin autoantibodies (>100.0 IU/mL). After appropriate work-up, he was diagnosed with IAS. After treatment with prednisolone (1 mg/kg/day), the patient had complete recovery. In patients with repeated hypoglycaemia, IAS should be considered in the differential diagnosis. Glucocorticoid therapy can be effective for the treatment of hypoglycaemia in patients with IAS.

1. Case Report

A 25-year-old, previously healthy Kuwaiti man was brought by ambulance to the Mubarak Al-Kabeer Hospital in May 2014 after he became unconscious. A capillary glucose value of <2 mmol/L was measured by the emergency medical service. He was managed in the emergency department with intravenous 5% dextrose infusion and recovered with no sequelae, after which he was admitted to the medical ward for further investigation.

The patient mentioned a 2-months history of recurrent episodes of palpitation, dizziness, light-headedness, and sweating and had recurrent visits to the emergency room in April 2014 with documented values of hypoglycaemia (capillary glucose value reached as low as 3.5 mmol/L) which improved after receiving intravenous dextrose infusion. Those symptoms developed usually late after meals and after prolonged hours with no carbohydrate intake and improved after eating. The episodes never happened immediately postprandial. There were no signs of seizures. The symptoms also improved after transient use of oral dexamethasone in high doses daily for several days in mid-April 2014 which were prescribed by an endocrinologist empirically to treat possible adrenal insufficiency. After stopping the dexamethasone, the hypoglycaemic episodes recurred.

The patient was previously healthy but did report an uncertain amount of weight gain and also a history of erectile dysfunction for 1 month that was not investigated and had not been treated. He had no previous surgeries. There was no family history of insulinoma or any other significant disease. The patient revealed that he took several different injectable anabolic steroids and growth hormone together with oral amino acids, and other tablets (fat burners) for bodybuilding in the previous two months. He denied knowingly using insulin or insulin analogues. The patient is single with 4 pack-year smoking history and works in a private company.

2. Investigations

In the medical ward, he still required 5% dextrose infusion and then 10% to maintain normoglycaemia; however, several additional but less frequent hypoglycaemic episodes occurred. On admission, his weight was 66 kg, height was 170 cm, body mass index was as 22.83 kg/m^2, blood pressure was 125/75 mm Hg, and pulse rate was 65 beats per minute. The physical

Table 1: Results of 72-hour fasting test.

Symptoms of hypoglycaemia	Yes
Glucose (reference range 3.9–6.1 mmol/L)	2.4 mmol/L
Insulin (reference range 1.9–23 uIU/ml)	>301 uIU/mL
C-peptide (reference range 33–1458 pmol/L)	681 pmol/L
Proinsulin (reference range <11.0 pmol/L)	2.7 pmol/L
Beta-hydroxybutyrate (reference range 30–300 mmol/L)	27.8 mmol/L
Circulating oral hypoglycaemic agents	Not available
Antibodies to insulin IgG (reference range 0–10 IU/ml) by enzyme-linked immunosorbent assay (ELISA)	>100.0 IU/mL

Table 2: Other laboratory investigations.

Test	Result	Reference range
Haemoglobin A1c	5.1%	Nondiabetic (<5.7%)
Anti-GAD Ab	Negative	0–10 IU/mL
Anti-IA2 Ab	Negative	0–10 IU/mL
Anti-islet cells Ab	Negative	0–10 IU/mL
Insulin-like growth factor 1 (IGF-1)	33	29–85 nmol/L (adults 20–30 years)
Cortisol morning	467	185–624 nmol/L
Cortisol evening	255	150–276 nmol/L
Adrenocorticotropic hormone (ACTH)	42.3	10–46 pg/mL
LH	0.7	1.24–8.68 IU/L
FSH	1.6	1.27–19.26 IU/L
Prolactin	317	57–281 mIU/L
Total testosterone	4.2	6.1–27.1 nmol/L

examination showed a nonpalpable thyroid and no features of hyperpigmentation. Testicular exam revealed normal size testes and phallus with normal hair distribution.

Urine sulfonylurea screen was not available at our hospital. When intravenous dextrose infusion was held, the patient was kept fasting and under close observation in the ward with plasma glucose measured repeatedly using glucose meter (Abbott Diabetes care Ltd, range road, Witney, Oxon, UK), and after 24 hours of fasting in a planned 72 hours fasting test to assess the hypoglycaemic event, the patient had a hypoglycaemic attack with symptoms of dizziness, palpitation, and sweating. The capillary glucose value was 2.5 mmol/L. and several laboratory blood tests to assess the hypoglycaemic event was performed (Table 1).

During the hypoglycaemia, serum insulin was elevated (>301 uIU/ml), while C-peptide was within the reference range (681 pmol/L) and proinsulin was below normal (2.7 mmol/L) as well as beta-hydroxybutyrate (27.8 mmol/L). Anti-insulin antibody titer (IgG) was significantly elevated (>100.0 IU/mL).

Other laboratory investigation results (Table 2), including those of full blood count, liver function test, renal function test, and thyroid profile, were normal. Adrenocorticotropic hormone (ACTH) and nonstimulated morning cortisol levels were normal. ACTH stimulation test was not done as features of hyperinsulinism were evident on laboratory results during the hypoglycaemic event. Total testosterone and luteinising hormone (LH) levels, tested one week before admission by the out-patient clinic, were below the reference range (4.2 nmol/L [reference range 6.1–27.1 nmol/L] and 0.7 IU/L [reference range 1.24–8.68 IU/L], respectively). This could be explained by his previous use of recreational anabolic steroids. The prolactin level was only mildly elevated (317 mIU/L [reference range 57–281 mIU/L]), and follicular stimulating hormone (FSH) level was within reference range (1.6 IU/L [reference range 1.27–19.26 IU/L]). Magnetic resonance imaging (MRI) of the abdomen, including the pancreas, and the *sella turcica*, showed no abnormalities.

Given the high levels of anti-insulin antibodies, hyperinsulinaemia, late postprandial hypoglycaemia, and clinical presentation in coincidence with intake of anabolic steroids and other products like thiol and amino acids, and with exclusion of other differential diagnoses of hypoglycaemia, anti-insulin antibodies-induced hypoglycaemia syndrome, also called Insulin autoimmune syndrome (IAS), was the most likely explanation of patient's condition and continued hypoglycaemia.

3. Treatment

The patient was started on a high dose of glucocorticoid therapy with prednisolone 1 mg/kg/day while in the medical ward. The patient then travelled abroad less than a month later for further medical work-up and care in the United States (US) before his planned follow up visit in the endocrine clinic. A similar diagnosis of IAS was made based on the same work-up done at our hospital while no further hypoglycaemic events occurred, and the patient was kept on prednisolone (1 mg/kg/day) and was asked to continue the therapy for several weeks with tapering dose until discontinuing it.

4. Outcome and Follow Up

The patient returned to Kuwait after the two weeks visit to the US and then attended the endocrine clinic after 5 weeks of therapy with prednisolone. The patient never had any further hypoglycaemic attack during the course of therapy and was asked to start tapering down the dose at that point. After discontinuing the glucocorticoid therapy, the patient never developed any hypoglycaemia symptoms indicating remission of the condition. His last anti-insulin antibody titer test was done in July 2014 with negative results (Figure 1).

5. Discussion

IAS, or Hirata disease, is a rare cause of endogenous hyperinsulinaemic hypoglycaemia, characterized by autoantibodies to endogenous insulin in individuals without previous exposure to exogenous insulin [1]. The condition is known as Hirata's disease (HD), after Yukimasa Hirata, the author who first described the syndrome in 1970 [2]. It is now recognized as the third most common cause of hypoglycaemia in Asian patients [3] following insulinoma and nonpancreatic neoplasia as the first and second most common aetiologies, respectively [3]. The syndrome affects both sexes equally [4] and is more

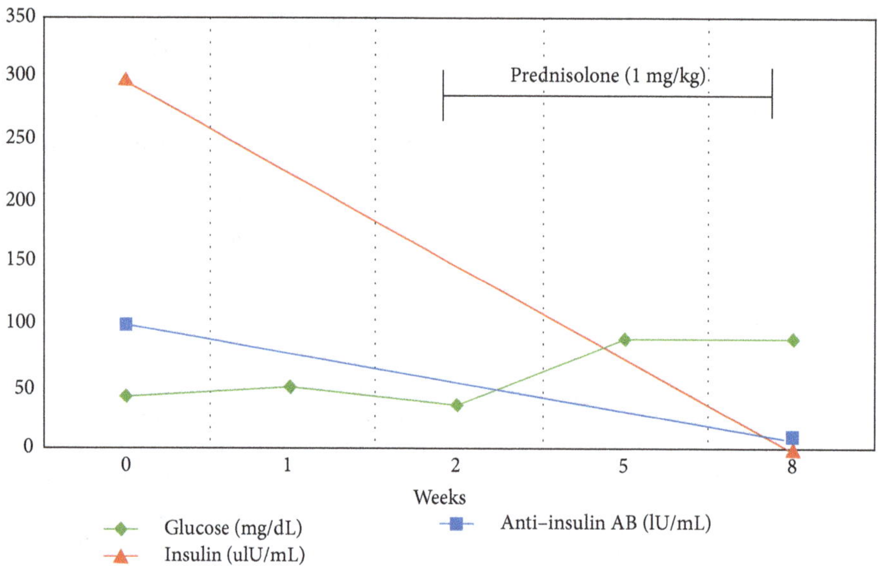

FIGURE 1: Resolution of hypoglycaemia and anti-insulin antibodies after starting prednisolone in our patient.

frequent in patients over 40 years of age. Interestingly, our patient was much younger, and this condition is rarely reported among children or at a young age.

The mechanism of hypoglycaemia in IAS is unknown but the most widely accepted hypothesis is a mismatch between blood glucose and free insulin concentration, secondary to the binding and release of secreted insulin by autoantibodies [5]. Usually, after a meal, glucose concentration rises which stimulates insulin secretion. In this disorder, autoantibodies bind to insulin molecules and inhibit their effect, leading to hyperglycaemia [4, 5]. As glucose concentration eventually falls, insulin secretion also subsides, and the total insulin level decreases. At this time, insulin molecules spontaneously dissociate from the autoantibodies giving rise to a high free insulin level inappropriate for the glucose concentration, thus provoking hypoglycaemia [5]. Due to this insulin-glucose mismatch, on several occasions insulinoma is suspected instead of IAS [6]. When insulin autoantibodies bind to insulin, the half-life increases from 5 minutes to hours [7], while the half-life of the C-peptide usually remains shorter and unaffected (30–35 minutes) giving rise to an elevated insulin level while having a nonelevated C-peptide and proinsulin and changing the insulin to C-peptide ratio to >1. It is also possible that the insulin autoantibody is capable of binding to endogenous proinsulin and C-peptide as well, delaying their half-lives, and possibly keeping the insulin to C-peptide ratio in the normal range of <1 [8, 9]. In our patient, the proinsulin was below reference range indicating an inhibitory effect on the proinsulin synthesis due to the hyperinsulinaemic period or a possible nonextended half-life of proinsulin which helped to clear it before the onset of hyperinsulinaemia. Furthermore, the C-peptide level was within the reference range, indicating a similar nonextended half-life with possible insulin to C-peptide ratio >1, but the insulin level could not be measured beyond 301 uIU/mL.

Also, high serum insulin levels can be accompanied by low proinsulin and C-peptide levels, misleading the diagnosis as injectable insulin administration [3]. Our patient denied using exogenous insulin while proinsulin was below the reference range and the C-peptide level was normal.

The anti-insulin antibody could not be detected beyond 100 IU/mL. In case of recurrence, further detailed evaluation can be conducted by sending the antibody for laboratory testing abroad.

IAS has an association with other autoimmune diseases such as Graves' disease, rheumatoid arthritis, and HLA DR4, which has been demonstrated in 96% of Japanese patients with IAS [1]. The most common drug associated with IAS is methimazole, while the use of other drugs such as carbimazole, glutathione, tiopronin, tolbutamide, gold thioglucose, interferon-α, captopril, diltiazem, hydralazine, procainamide, isoniazid, D-penicillamine, imipenem, and penicillin has been associated with this condition [4, 5, 10]. A few case reports of IAS associated with the use of alpha lipoic acid (ALA) were also reported [10, 11]. Also, insulin autoantibodies may be triggered by exposure to viruses like mumps, rubella, Coxsackie B influenza, hepatitis C, chickenpox, and measles by acting as super-antigens or they may manifest spontaneously [3].

Our patient had a history of anabolic steroids, growth hormone, and oral amino acids use which may have contributed to his condition. Further information on the supplements used by the patient was not known; such information would have helped us in evaluating this case since some health supplements have been reported to be triggers for IAS. Furthermore, our patient did not have any previous exposure to exogenous insulin. To our knowledge, this is the first documented case of IAS in a young healthy male without any associated condition or autoimmune disease in the Arabian Gulf region.

Although a spontaneous improvement of the symptoms was reported in the literature [4], most patients were treated differently by various investigators [4]. Management of IAS as reported by different case reports included using different immunosuppressive regimens, such as prednisolone [12], hydrocortisone [13], cyclophosphamide [14], azathioprine [15], rituximab [16], mycophenolate mofetil [17], and plasmapheresis [18, 19]. Our patient had a complete recovery after 8-weeks course of prednisolone, although many case reports documented a recovery period after 12-weeks of prednisolone [20, 21].

IAS could be a misleading condition and careful diagnosis is needed to rule out other causes of hyperinsulinaemic hypoglycaemia, especially in patients with previous history of bariatric surgery or signs of insulinoma. The patient history of supplements intake and use of recreational hormones is important in the evaluation of IAS as precipitating factors with the possibility of additional unknown triggers.

Consent

Written informed consent was obtained from the patient.

Authors' Contributions

Alrashidi E. wrote the article. Alessa T. contributed to the writing and discussion of the article and was the named physician involved in the care of the patient. All authors read and approved the final manuscript.

References

[1] Y. Uchigata and Y. Hirata, "Insulin autoimmune syndrome (IAS, Hirata disease)," *Annales de medecine interne*, vol. 150, no. 3, pp. 245–253, 1999.

[2] Y. Hirata, "Insulin autoimmunity in a case of spontaneous hypoglycemia," *Journal of the Japan Diabetes Society*, vol. 1970, no. 13, pp. 312–319, 1970.

[3] A. A. Ismail, "The insulin autoimmune syndrome (IAS) as a cause of hypoglycaemia: an update on the pathophysiology, biochemical investigations and diagnosis," *Clinical Chemistry and Laboratory Medicine*, vol. 54, no. 11, pp. 1715–1724, 2016.

[4] B. C. Lupsa, A. Y. Chong, E. K. Cochran, M. A. Soos, R. K. Semple, and P. Gorden, "Autoimmune forms of hypoglycemia," *Medicine*, vol. 88, no. 3, pp. 141–153, 2009.

[5] J. B. Redmon and F. Q. Nuttall, "Autoimmune hypoglycemia," *Endocrinology and Metabolism Clinics of North America*, vol. 28, no. 3, pp. 603–618, 1999.

[6] D. L. Willard, M. Stevenson, and D. Steenkamp, "Type B insulin resistance syndrome," *Current Opinion in Endocrinology, Diabetes, and Obesity*, vol. 23, no. 4, pp. 318–323, 2016.

[7] A. A. Ismail, "The double whammy of endogenous insulin antibodies in non-diabetic subjects," *Clinical Chemistry and Laboratory Medicine*, vol. 46, no. 2, 2008.

[8] M. R. Lebowitz and S. A. Blumenthal, "The molar ratio of insulin to C-peptide. an aid to the diagnosis of hypoglycemia due to surreptitious (or inadvertent) insulin administration," *Archives of Internal Medicine*, vol. 153, no. 5, pp. 650–655, 1993.

[9] S. L. Wong, A. Priestman, and D. T. Holmes, "Recurrent hypoglycemia from insulin autoimmune syndrome," *Journal of General Internal Medicine*, vol. 29, no. 1, pp. 250–254, 2014.

[10] M. Lidar, R. Rachmani, E. Half, and M. Ravid, "Insulin autoimmune syndrome after therapy with imipenem," *Diabetes Care*, vol. 22, no. 3, pp. 524–525, 1999.

[11] Y. Hirata, "Methimazole and insulin autoimmune syndrome with hypoglycemia," *Lancet (London, England)*, vol. 2, no. 8357, pp. 1037–1038, 198329.

[12] S. M. Bae, M. N. Bae, E. Y. Kim et al., "Recurrent insulin autoimmune syndrome caused by alpha-lipoic acid in type 2 diabetes," *Endocrinology and Metabolism (Seoul, Korea)*, vol. 28, no. 4, pp. 326–330, 2013.

[13] A. Matsuyoshi, S. Shimoda, K. Tsuruzoe et al., "A case of slowly progressive type 1 diabetes with unstable glycemic control caused by unusual insulin antibody and successfully treated with steroid therapy," *Diabetes Research and Clinical Practice*, vol. 72, no. 3, pp. 238–243, 2006.

[14] T. Ishizuka, S. Ogawa, T. Mori et al., "Characteristics of the antibodies of two patients who developed daytime hyperglycemia and morning hypoglycemia because of insulin antibodies," *Diabetes Research and Clinical Practice*, vol. 84, no. 2, pp. e21–e23, 2009.

[15] D. Micic, S. Brkic, A. Kendereski et al., "Immunological resistance to human biosynthetic insulin - effects of immunosuppression and plasmapheresis," *Diabetes Research and Clinical Practice*, vol. 19, no. 1, pp. 83–89, 1993.

[16] D. R. Saxon, M. T. McDermott, and A. W. Michels, "Novel management of insulin autoimmune syndrome with rituximab and continuous glucose monitoring," *The Journal of Clinical Endocrinology and Metabolism*, vol. 101, no. 5, pp. 1931–1934, 2016.

[17] T. Segal, E. Webb, R. Viner, C. Pusey, G. Wild, and J. Allgrove, "Severe insulin resistance secondary to insulin antibodies: successful treatment with the immunosuppressant MMF," *Pediatric Diabetes*, vol. 9, no. 3, pp. 250–254, 2008.

[18] N. Dozio, M. Scavini, A. Beretta et al., "Imaging of the buffering effect of insulin antibodies in the autoimmune hypoglycemic syndrome," *The Journal of Clinical Endocrinology and Metabolism*, vol. 83, no. 2, pp. 643–648, 1998.

[19] M. Philippon, S. Sejil, M. Mugnier et al., "Use of the continuous glucose monitoring system to treat insulin autoimmune syndrome: quantification of glucose excursions and evaluation of treatment efficacy," *Diabetic Medicine*, vol. 31, no. 7, pp. e20–e24, 2014.

[20] J.-C. Maiza, M. Caron-Debarle, C. Vigouroux, and S. Schneebeli, "Anti-insulin receptor antibodies related to hypoglycemia in a previously diabetic patient," *Diabetes Care*, vol. 36, no. 6, e77 pages, 2013.

[21] J. P. Chu, X. W. Zheng, J. Lu et al., "Insulin-induced autoimmune syndrome: a case report," *Experimental and Therapeutic Medicine*, vol. 12, no. 5, pp. 3359–3362, 2016.

47

A Case of Glycogenic Hepatopathy as a Complication of Poorly Controlled Type 1 Diabetes Mellitus

Samhitha Munugoti,[1] Vamsee Reddy,[1] Gaurav Patel,[1] Maneesh Gaddam,[2] and Triveni Abburi[1]

[1]*Department of Internal Medicine, Prime Health Care Consortium at St. Mary's and St. Clare Denville Hospital Program, Denville, NJ, USA*
[2]*Division of Pulmonary, Critical Care, and Sleep Medicine, Tufts Medical Center, Boston, MA, USA*

Correspondence should be addressed to Samhitha Munugoti; samhithamunugoti@gmail.com

Academic Editor: Osamu Isozaki

A 23-year-old African American male with a medical history significant for poorly controlled type 1 diabetes mellitus (T1DM) presented with abdominal pain and vomiting. His laboratory workup was consistent with diabetic ketoacidosis (DKA). An acute elevation of liver enzymes was noted as the DKA resolved, with the alanine transferase and aspartate transferase levels elevated to more than 50 times the normal limit within the next 24 hours. Because abnormal liver function tests are found frequently in patients with type 1 diabetes mellitus, it is important to have a broad differential diagnosis. Furthermore, a low threshold of suspicion is required to identify a relatively underdiagnosed etiology like glycogenic hepatopathy (GH). This case report describes how patterns and trends of liver function tests provide important clues to the diagnosis of GH; how imaging modalities like ultrasonography, computerized tomography (CT) scan, and magnetic resonance imaging (MRI) scan could be used to differentiate GH from nonalcoholic fatty liver disease (NAFLD); and how the diagnosis of GH can be made without the need for invasive liver biopsy. The knowledge about GH should prevent its delayed diagnosis and improve the outcomes by appropriately managing uncontrolled type 1 DM.

1. Introduction

Patients with type 1 diabetes are frequently associated with abnormal liver function tests. Therefore, further investigation is often required to evaluate for associated hepatic abnormalities such as abnormal glycogen deposition, nonalcoholic fatty liver disease (NAFLD), fibrosis, and cirrhosis [1]. The most frequent etiology of elevated aminotransferases in type 1 diabetes is NAFLD [2]. However, a rare, underdiagnosed but important cause of liver injury is glycogenic hepatopathy (GH), first documented as a component of Mauriac syndrome in 1930 [3]. Since then, many cases due to other etiologies have been reported. These include poorly controlled diabetes mellitus, dumping syndrome after gastrectomy, anorexia nervosa, use of high-dose corticosteroids, and high doses of insulin [4–7]. While GH has been traditionally diagnosed by liver biopsy, less invasive alternatives have been suggested [8]. Improvement of hyperglycemia and hepatomegaly is commonly noted with GH. Diagnosis can be made based on clinical and radiological data, and liver biopsy becomes essential when other hepatic disorders needed to be ruled out.

2. Case Presentation

A 23-year-old African American male with type I diabetes mellitus diagnosed at the age of 3 presented with abdominal pain and vomiting for two days. His home insulin regimen included 40 units/day of regular insulin in divided doses along with insulin lispro with meals, the dosage of which he was not aware. The patient did not recall when he took his last dose of insulin but reported frequent episodes of high glucose levels previously. His family members confirmed his noncompliance to the insulin regimen, primarily due to a lack of understanding of his medical condition and poor socioeconomic status.

On presentation, the patient was hemodynamically stable and afebrile along with normal heart and respiratory rates. He was of tall, thin build with a BMI of 19. He was alert and awake with an unremarkable cardiac and respiratory examination. Abdominal examination revealed no guarding, rigidity, or tenderness but was noted to have hepatomegaly.

On initial laboratory studies, his complete blood count was unremarkable. The basic metabolic profile revealed sodium of 132 mEq/L, potassium of 5.3 mEq/L, chloride of 89 mEq/L, carbon dioxide of 14 mEq/L, blood urea nitrogen of 19.4 mg/dL, creatinine of 1.3 mg/dL, and an anion gap of 29 mEq/L. His glucose levels were found to be 566 mg/dL. Arterial blood gas showed a pH of 7.3, pCO2 of 24 mm of Hg, pO2 of 107 mm of Hg, HCO3 of 11.7 mmol/L, and lactate of 2.4 mmol/L. He was noted to have positive acetones and ketones. This was consistent with diabetic ketoacidosis in the setting of poor compliance, with the Hba1c levels of 17%.

The patient was initially given 8 units of regular insulin and was started on an insulin drip at 0.1 U/Kg. Over the next 12 hours, the patient's DKA resolved and he was transitioned to subcutaneous insulin. Liver function tests at that time revealed aspartate aminotransferase (AST) of 816 U/L, alanine aminotransferase (ALT) of 569 U/L, and alkaline phosphatase (ALP) of 132 U/L. An extensive workup for elevated aminotransferases was pursued. Further history was obtained with no recent travel, acetaminophen ingestion, and any other substances including alcohol, herbal, or over-the-counter medications. There was no family history or past medical history for any liver disease. Drug screens for salicylates, acetaminophen, amphetamines, barbiturates, benzodiazepines, cocaine, ethanol, and cannabinoids were negative. Serology was negative for viral hepatitis A, B, and C. Antismooth muscle antibodies were negative ruling out autoimmune hepatitis. A normal ceruloplasmin level of 28 mg/dL with no Kayser–Fleischer rings on examination, no neurological or psychiatric manifestations, or family history of Wilson's disease made the diagnosis of Wilson's disease unlikely.

Over the next 24 hours, his liver enzymes continued to increase dramatically with AST of 10,499 U/L, ALT of 2,486 U/L, and ALP of 230 U/L. The synthetic liver function tests which included serum albumin, prothrombin time, and international normalized ratio were within normal limits. Extreme elevations of aminotransferases can be precipitated by ischemic hepatopathy. However, there were no episodes of hypotension, and lactic acid was mildly elevated to 2.4 mmol/L during his hospitalization. Ultrasonography of the abdomen was performed which was consistent with hepatomegaly but no steatosis or cirrhosis. Nonalcoholic fatty liver disease (NAFLD) and glycogenic hepatopathy (GH) were the two major considerations at this point. A CT scan of the abdomen/pelvis revealed hyperdense hepatomegaly and the density was greater than the spleen (Figure 1). The ratio of liver-to-spleen (L/S) Hounsfield units (HU) was 1.56. Although pointing towards GH and against NAFLD, an MRI scan was performed for hepatomegaly. On this imaging, there was no significant difference in liver intensity between the in-phase and opposed-phase sequences, confirming the diagnosis of GH (Figure 2). Although liver biopsy is considered the gold standard for diagnosing GH, there was enough clinical and radiological evidence to diagnose the patient with GH.

The patient's aminotransferases started trending down as the blood glucose levels were better controlled during the admission with 17 units of insulin glargine once daily and 6-8 units of insulin lispro premeal (Figure 3). A follow-up after 10 days confirmed improving aminotransferases with well-controlled blood sugar levels.

3. Discussion

Patients who present with frequent episodes of DKA and treated with high doses of insulin may often have GH. However, the incidence is unknown as GH is relatively underdiagnosed and therefore underestimated. The presentation is nonspecific and can range from abdominal pain, nausea, and vomiting to an asymptomatic elevation of aminotransferases [9]. Hepatomegaly is the most common finding noted on physical examination [9].

GH is caused by a reversible accumulation of excess glycogen in the liver. This excessive accumulation in the liver causes hepatomegaly and hepatocyte injury leading to elevated liver enzymes [10–12]. Glycogenesis and glycogenolysis are the two processes occurring in the liver to balance the glycogen, which is the reservoir of glucose. Elevated serum glucose levels in poorly controlled diabetes lead to the diffusion of glucose into the hepatocytes facilitated through the GLUT 2 transporter, which occurs independently of insulin [13]. The glucose is then trapped in the hepatocytes after irreversible phosphorylation by the enzyme glucokinase to glucose-6-phosphate. Upon initiating treatment with insulin, the glucose-6-phosphate is now polymerized to glycogen by the enzyme glycogen synthase, which continues for some time despite a drop in insulin levels [13, 14]. This continued accumulation of glycogen leads to hepatomegaly. This acute presentation of hepatomegaly occurs when prolonged or marked hyperglycemia is treated with exogenous insulin [15, 16]. Therefore, it is only obvious that the description of Mauriac syndrome in 1930 happened only shortly after the availability of insulin treatment [17].

Given the rarity of this condition, a high index of suspicion is required to diagnose GH. The diagnosis should be suspected when elevated liver enzymes are noted in a patient with uncontrolled T1DM, especially with exaggerated hemoglobin A1c levels [18]. The pattern of the elevated liver enzymes provides important clues to differentiate the various hepatic abnormalities. GH is associated with the following patterns of abnormal liver enzymes:

(1) Elevations in ALT and AST in out of proportion to ALP and bilirubin indicating predominant hepatocellular injury [13, 16, 18].

(2) AST is higher than ALT [19].

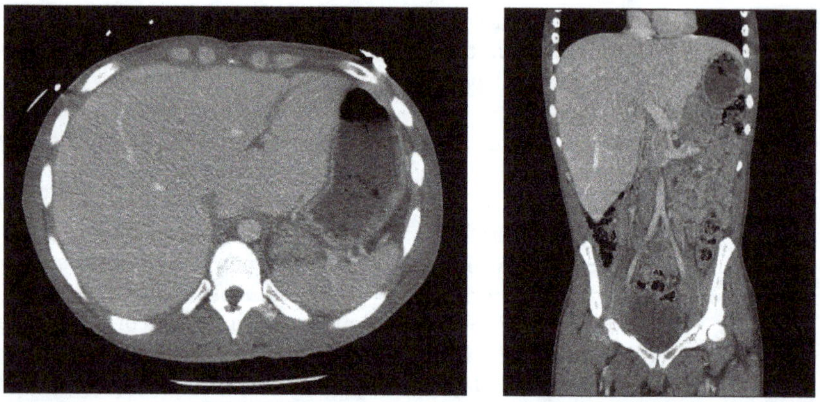

Figure 1: Axial and coronal sections of the abdominal CT scan showing hepatomegaly with a hyperdense liver.

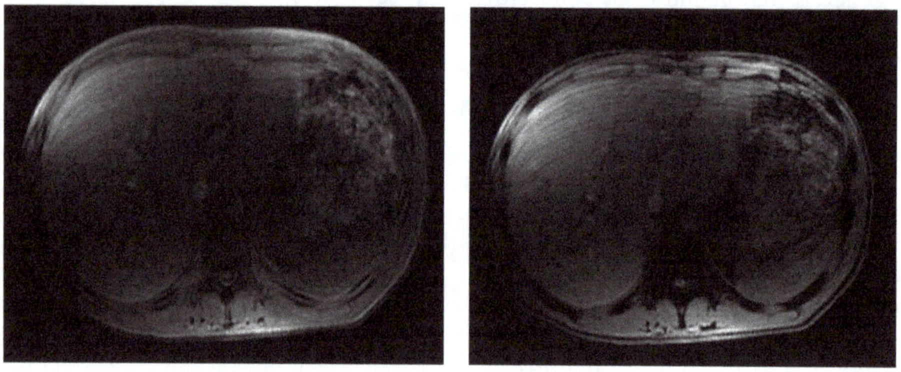

(a) (b)

Figure 2: T1-MRI images showing no difference in the signal intensities between the in-phase (a) and opposed-phase (b).

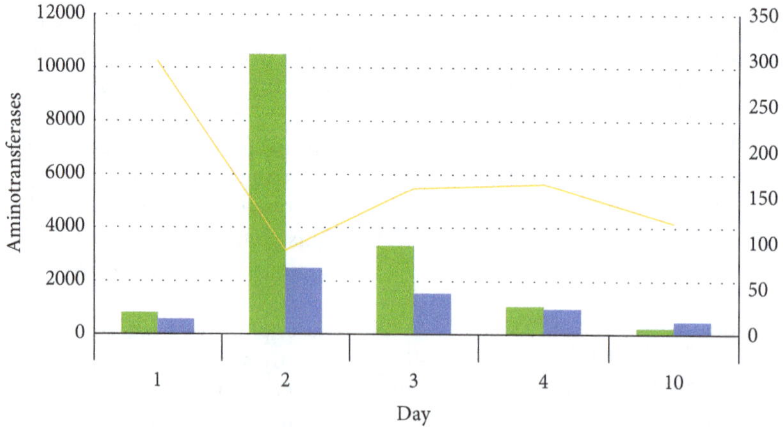

	1	2	3	4	10
AST (U/L)	816	10,499	3333	1069	239
ALT (U/L)	569	2486	1555	975	485
Blood glucose (mg/dL)	299	92	160	165	122

AST (U/L)
ALT (U/L)
Blood glucose (mg/dL)

Figure 3: Relationship between the trends of aminotransferases and blood glucose levels. AST: aspartate aminotransferase; ALT: alanine aminotransferase.

(3) Synthetic function of the liver is preserved, that is, normal albumin and INR levels [13, 20, 21].

GH is usually noted to have aminotransferases elevated about 13 times the upper normal limit [19]. Our patient had a pattern of liver enzymes similar to that described above. Although ALT (which is present in the highest concentration in the liver) is more specific for liver injury than AST (which is found in the liver, cardiac muscle, skeletal muscle, kidneys, brain, pancreas, lungs, leukocytes, and erythrocytes), there are few other liver conditions where the AST is higher than ALT. Common etiologies include alcoholic liver disease, Wilson's disease, cirrhosis due to viral hepatitis, and nonalcoholic fatty liver disease (NAFLD). While NAFLD is more commonly observed in obese patients with type 2 DM, GH is more common in patients with poorly controlled type 1 DM. However, the diagnostic dilemma continues as distinguishing GH from NAFLD is extremely difficult purely based on clinical presentation and laboratory work.

Various imaging modalities can be used to support or disprove the diagnosis of GH. Although occasionally normal, the hepatic ultrasonography of GH would reveal hepatomegaly with uniform echogenicity due to glycogen accumulation. While NAFLD occurs due to fat deposition in the liver, the findings of ultrasonography of the hepatic tissues of NAFLD are similar to those of GH. The ultrasound imaging in our patient revealed hepatomegaly with no evidence of steatosis and cirrhosis. Therefore, ultrasound is not a useful imaging modality to distinguish GH and NAFLD [9, 22].

An abdominal CT can provide clues to diagnose GH. The liver density on the abdominal CT helps differentiate GH from NAFLD. The glycogen accumulation in GH gives a hyperdense appearance to the liver while the fatty deposition gives a hypodense appearance in NAFLD. The difference in the liver density as a clue to GH has been reported by Sweetser and Kraichely [23]. In addition, Doppman et al. reported a dose-dependent increase in the liver density as the glycogen content increases and a decrease in the liver density as the fat content increases [24]. The CT imaging in our patient does reveal hyperdensity of the liver with an L/S HU ratio of >1, pointing against NAFLD [25]. However, further workup is indeed warranted to confirm the diagnosis of GH.

MRI scan provides a clear distinction between GH and NAFLD. T1-MRI is recorded with in-phase and opposed-phase conditions. Intrahepatic fat storage in NAFLD causes a significantly higher signal intensity in the in-phase than in the opposed-phase [23, 26]. However, no difference in the signal intensities between the two phases is noted in GH [8, 26]. Similar MRI findings were noted in our patient with no difference in the signal intensities between the in-phase and opposed-phased phases.

Liver biopsy is considered the gold standard for diagnosing GH. Histologically, GH reveals pale, swollen hepatocytes due to marked glycogen accumulation, and intact architecture with no significant fibrosis, necrosis, inflammation, or fatty change [8]. A hematoxylin and eosin stain of the biopsy specimen would show swollen hepatocytes with prominent plasma membranes, increased volume of cytoplasm, and numerous glycogenated nuclei [9]. Staining with Periodic-Acid Schiff (PAS) shows abundant cytoplasmic glycogen deposits, which disappear after the addition of diastase that causes an enzymatic breakdown of glycogen in the hepatocytes [16, 21].

While the liver biopsy is considered the gold standard, given the invasiveness of the intervention, it is recommended that intensive insulin therapy is tried before proceeding with the liver biopsy [9]. In addition, combining a gradient dual-echo MRI sequence with a thorough clinical evaluation, biochemical workup and other radiological modalities could confirm the diagnosis of GH [8]. Our patient was diagnosed with GH based on the constellation of imaging findings and ruling out other etiologies, without having to proceed with the invasive intervention of liver biopsy.

Improving glycemic control is considered the mainstay of treatment for GH, which usually results in clinical and biochemical amelioration in 2-14 weeks [27]. Repeated episodes of DKA could cause recurrence of GH; therefore, compliance with glycemic control stays as the main therapeutic goal [18].

4. Conclusion

GH is an under-recognized condition and physicians should consider it in the differential diagnoses of patients with uncontrolled T1DM presenting with elevated aminotransferases. Although considered the gold standard, a liver biopsy is not always necessary and GH can be considered a diagnosis of exclusion in the right clinical setting by ruling out other etiologies combined with imaging modalities.

References

[1] J. Mohamed, A. H. Nazratun Nafizah, A. H. Zariyantey, and S. B. Budin, "Mechanisms of diabetes-induced liver damage: the role of oxidative stress and inflammation," *Sultan Qaboos University Medical Journal*, vol. 16, no. 2, pp. e132–e141, 2016.

[2] P. Angulo, "Nonalcoholic fatty liver disease," *New England Journal of Medicine*, vol. 346, no. 16, pp. 1221–1231, 2002.

[3] P. Mauriac, "Gros ventre, hepatomegalie, troubles de las croissance chez les enfants diabetiques traits depuis plusieurs annes par l'insuline," *Gax Hebd Med Bordeaux*, vol. 26, pp. 402–410, 1930.

[4] J. M. Resnick, I. Zador, and D. L. Fish, "Dumping syndrome, a cause of acquired glycogenic hepatopathy," *Pediatric and Developmental Pathology*, vol. 14, no. 4, pp. 318–321, 2011.

[5] L. N. Kransdorf, D. Millstine, M. L. Smith, and B. A. Aqel, "Hepatic glycogen deposition in a patient with anorexia nervosa and persistently abnormal transaminase levels," *Clinics and Research in Hepatology and Gastroenterology*, vol. 40, no. 2, pp. e15–e18, 2016.

[6] T. C. Iancu, H. Shiloh, and L. Dembo, "Hepatomegaly following short-term high-dose steroid therapy," *Journal of Pediatric Gastroenterology and Nutrition*, vol. 5, no. 1, pp. 41–46, 1986.

[7] T. Tsujimoto, M. Takano, M. Nishiofuku et al., "Rapid onset of glycogen storage hepatomegaly in a type-2 diabetic patient

after a massive dose of long-acting insulin and large doses of glucose," *Internal Medicine*, vol. 45, no. 7, pp. 469–473, 2006.

[8] F. Murata, I. Horie, T. Ando et al., "A case of glycogenic hepatopathy developed in a patient with new-onset fulminant type 1 diabetes: the role of image modalities in diagnosing hepatic glycogen deposition including gradient-dual-echo MRI," *Endocrine Journal*, vol. 59, no. 8, pp. 669–676, 2012.

[9] J. M. Sherigar, J. de Castro, Y. M. Yin, D. Guss, and S. R. Mohanty, "Glycogenic hepatopathy: a narrative review," *World Journal of Hepatology*, vol. 10, no. 2, pp. 172–185, 2018.

[10] L. Carcione, F. Lombardo, M. F. Messina, M. Rosano, and F. de Luca, "Liver glycogenosis as early manifestation in type 1 diabetes mellitus," *Diabetes, Nutrition & Metabolism*, vol. 16, no. 3, pp. 182–184, 2003.

[11] M. Torres and D. López, "Liver glycogen storage associated with uncontrolled type 1 diabetes mellitus," *Journal of Hepatology*, vol. 35, no. 4, p. 538, 2001.

[12] A. Abaci, O. Bekem, T. Unuvar et al., "Hepatic glycogenosis: a rare cause of hepatomegaly in type 1 diabetes mellitus," *Journal of Diabetes and its Complications*, vol. 22, no. 5, pp. 325–328, 2008.

[13] R. Chatila and B. A. West, "Hepatomegaly and abnormal liver tests due to glycogenosis in adults with diabetes," *Medicine*, vol. 75, no. 6, pp. 327–333, 1996.

[14] J. C. Ferrer, C. Favre, R. R. Gomis et al., "Control of glycogen deposition," *FEBS Letters*, vol. 546, no. 1, pp. 127–132, 2003.

[15] B. G. Stone and D. H. van Thiel, "Diabetes mellitus and the liver," *Seminars in Liver Disease*, vol. 5, no. 1, pp. 8–28, 1985.

[16] M. Torbenson, Y. Y. Chen, E. Brunt et al., "Glycogenic hepatopathy: an underrecognized hepatic complication of diabetes mellitus," *The American Journal of Surgical Pathology*, vol. 30, no. 4, pp. 508–513, 2006.

[17] D. Brar, "The history of insulin," 2009, http://www.med.uni-giessen.de/itr/history/inshist.html.

[18] S. Messeri, L. Messerini, F. Vizzutti, G. Laffi, and F. Marra, "Glycogenic hepatopathy associated with type 1 diabetes mellitus as a cause of recurrent liver damage," *Annals of Hepatology*, vol. 11, no. 4, pp. 554–558, 2012.

[19] S. Haffar, M. Izzy, H. Habib et al., "Liver chemistries in glycogenic hepatopathy associated with type 1 diabetes mellitus: a systematic review and pooled analysis," *Liver International*, vol. 41, no. 7, pp. 1545–1555, 2021.

[20] R. M. Hudacko, A. v Manoukian, S. H. Schneider, and B. Fyfe, "Clinical resolution of glycogenic hepatopathy following improved glycemic control," *Journal of Diabetes and its Complications*, vol. 22, no. 5, pp. 329-330, 2008.

[21] T. Saadi, "Glycogenic hepatopathy: a rare disease that can appear and resolve rapidly in parallel with glycemic control," *The Israel Medical Association Journal*, vol. 14, no. 4, pp. 269-270, 2012.

[22] J. Khoury, Y. Zohar, N. Shehadeh, and T. Saadi, "Glycogenic hepatopathy," *Hepatobiliary and Pancreatic Diseases International*, vol. 17, no. 2, pp. 113–118, 2018.

[23] S. Sweetser and R. E. Kraichely, "The bright liver of glycogenic hepatopathy," *Hepatology*, vol. 51, no. 2, pp. 711-712, 2010.

[24] J. L. Doppman, M. Cornblath, A. J. Dwyer, A. J. Adams, M. E. Girton, and J. Sidbury, "Computed tomography of the liver and kidneys in glycogen storage disease," *Journal of Computer Assisted Tomography*, vol. 6, no. 1, pp. 67–71, 1982.

[25] I. Zeb, D. Li, K. Nasir, R. Katz, V. N. Larijani, and M. J. Budoff, "Computed tomography scans in the evaluation of fatty liver disease in a population based study: the multi-ethnic study of atherosclerosis," *Academic Radiology*, vol. 19, no. 7, pp. 811–818, 2012.

[26] M. Saikusa, S. Yatsuga, T. Tonan, and Y. Koga, "Glycogenic hepatopathy and non-alcoholic fatty liver disease in type 1 diabetes patients," *Pediatrics International*, vol. 55, no. 6, pp. 806-807, 2013.

[27] J. H. Cha, S. H. Ra, Y. M. Park et al., "Three cases of glycogenic hepatopathy mimicking acute and relapsing hepatitis in type I diabetes mellitus," *Clinical and Molecular Hepatology*, vol. 19, no. 4, pp. 421–425, 2013.

48

Type 1 Diabetes (T1D) and Latent Autoimmune Diabetes in Adults (LADA): The Difference Between a Honeymoon and a Holiday

Livia M. R. Marcon, Carmine G. Fanelli, and Riccardo Calafiore

Section of Endocrinology and Metabolism, Department of Medicine and Surgery, University of Perugia Medical School, Perugia, Italy

Correspondence should be addressed to Carmine G. Fanelli; carmine.fanelli@unipg.it

Academic Editor: Suat Simsek

Type 1 diabetes mellitus (T1D) is a chronic autoimmune disease in which destruction of the insulin-producing β-cells in the pancreatic islets requires regular lifelong insulin replacement therapy, the only lifesaving treatment available at this time. In young persons with a genetic predisposition, it usually manifests after being exposed to environmental triggers. A subtype of autoimmune diabetes mellitus (ADM) that typically occurs in adulthood is often referred to as latent autoimmune diabetes of adults (LADA). LADA is characterized by a milder process of β-cells destruction and less intensive insulin treatment, which may become necessary even many years after diagnosis. Genetic predisposition of T1D carries an increased risk for other autoimmune diseases, such as autoimmune thyroiditis, the most frequently associated condition, and pernicious anaemia (PA), present in approximately 4% of all individuals with T1D. Here, we describe the case of a 90-year-old woman with vitiligo and a mute medical history who was admitted to our University Hospital in Perugia with hyperglycaemia and severe anaemia due to vitamin B12 (VB12) depletion. A short time after setting the beginning treatment with a basal-bolus insulin regimen, her insulin requirement rapidly declined and treatment with sitagliptin, a dipeptidyl peptidase-4 inhibitor (DPP4), was started. A complete autoimmunity screening panel showed that GAD65 and intrinsic factor autoantibodies were positive.

1. Introduction

ADM is a chronic autoimmune disease affecting pancreatic insulin-producing β-cells that encompasses a wide spectrum of different clinical presentations. T1D is usually diagnosed at a young age; it manifests with ketoacidosis and requires lifelong insulin replacement therapy while LADA emerges later in life and insulin therapy can be postponed for years after diagnosis.

ADM is frequently accompanied by other autoimmune endocrine and nonendocrine diseases, the latter encompassing the so called "autoimmune polyglandular syndromes (APS)," more common in females. Among these is pernicious anaemia (PA), a form of autoimmune gastritis with impaired VB12 absorption.

In this report, we describe the unusual case of a polyautoimmune syndrome clinically emerging at an old age.

2. Case Presentation

The patient was a 90-year-old woman admitted to our clinical unit at the Perugia University Hospital, Perugia, Italy, for dyspnoea, anorexia, and agitation. Her body mass index was at the lower normal limit, she had a mute medical history, no family history of diabetes mellitus, and no history of smoking or other unhealthful habits. Relatives did not report previous episodes of anaemia or bleeding or recent viral infections. She was not on medications except furosemide prescribed a week earlier by the family doctor, due to worsening dyspnoea and peripheral oedema in the lower limbs.

The patient tested negative on the SARS-CoV-2 molecular test performed in the emergency department. Blood tests at admission showed a haemoglobin value of 5.4 g/dL with a high mean corpuscular volume (MCV) of 109.1 fl, platelets were 116,000 μL; fasting plasma glucose was 720 mg/dL (40 mmol/L) with a glycated haemoglobin (HbA1c) of 8.4% (68 mmol/mol), underestimated because of the presence of anaemia (Table 1). The arterial blood gas (ABG) analysis showed that the pH was normal (7.41), pCO_2 was considerably reduced (25 mmHg), plasma osmolarity was equal to 299.8 mmol/kg, and there was a marked increase of the anion gap equal to 19.8 mmol/L, likely due to high lactate levels (6 mmol/L) (Table 2). The latter could likely be explained by different concomitant factors such as severe anaemia-induced hypoxia, red blood cells haemolysis, and glucose toxicity. It has indeed been observed that a condition of hyperglycaemia can be associated with a higher lactate production due to the oversupply of glucose that pushes the glycolytic pathway [1].

Neither blood nor urine ketone bodies were dosed, and considering that the blood pH ranged normal levels, we could rule out with a reasonable degree of certainty the presence of diabetic ketoacidosis (DKA) [2]. Actually, the data did not match the diagnostic criteria of either two hyperglycaemic syndromes, DKA, and hyperosmolar hyperglycaemic state (HHS): we probably intercepted the pathologic process at a time when those diagnostic criteria were unmet.

The physical examination revealed a thin body with hands and face marked with well-defined milky patches of vitiligo. At the rectal examination stools appeared normochromic. Neuropathy was not detected based on clinical history and physical evaluation. Rehydration therapy was immediately started together with subcutaneous administration of fast-acting insulin and blood transfusions. Considering the haemoglobin values compatible with a diagnosis of severe anaemia and the general clinical conditions of the patient, we can assume the anaemia had developed slowly during the months preceding the admission.

Subsequent investigations showed that a process of haemolysis was present: LDH and bilirubin values were high, mostly the indirect form, and haptoglobin was consumed; a faecal occult blood test (FOBT) resulted slightly positive with normal serum iron levels.

We investigated all the major causes of haemolysis: direct and indirect Coombs tests were normal but the VB12 level was largely below the normal range. The presence of severe macrocytic anaemia and haemolysis led us to believe they were both related to VB12 deficiency resulting in ineffective erythropoiesis.

Connecting the dots, we decided to do a complete autoimmunity screening panel and the patient tested positive for GAD65 and intrinsic factor autoantibodies (Table 3). A supplemental therapy with once-weekly VB12 analogue subcutaneous injections was set up together with a basal-bolus insulin regimen. After few days, the daily insulin consumption started to decline until the complete withdrawal.

We concluded the clinical investigations with an abdominal echotomography that excluded hepatic and pancreatic alterations, and with an esophagogastroduodenoscopy that ruled out the presence of bleeding sites but showed chronic gastritis.

The patient was discharged with close outpatient monitoring for one month. At the one-month clinical evaluation, glycaemic control was still acceptable without insulin therapy. In order to prevent hypoglycaemic episodes and preserve the remaining β-cells function treatment with daily sitagliptin 100 mg, an oral glucose-lowering drug inhibiting the dipeptidyl peptidase-4 (DPP4) enzyme was started.

The subsequent follow-up visits confirmed the constant fair glycaemic control over time: the blood analysis one year later showed that haemoglobin was 13.7 g/dL, fasting plasma glucose was 92 mg/dL, and glycated haemoglobin was 5.9% (41 mmol/mol). The patient was still on daily sitagliptin 100 mg.

3. Discussion

The pathogenesis of T1D is well-known to involve both genetic and environmental factors [3]. Specific human leukocyte antigen (HLA) haplotypes, such as HLA-DR4-DQ8 and HLA-DR3-DQ2 [4], provide the immunological basis of the development of the disease once the subject has been exposed to external antigens. This exposure induces a T-lymphocyte-mediated reaction against pancreatic β-cells leading to their destruction and consequently to the loss of insulin production.

Shortly after a T1D diagnosis, a period occurs known as "diabetes honeymoon phase," or remission phase, lasting a variable length of time, usually from weeks to months; nevertheless, there have been some reported cases of this honeymoon lasting for years [5, 6].

The hallmarks of the honeymoon period are low or no insulin requirement together with a fair blood glucose control, with less glucose variability, less risk of hypoglycaemia, and lower overall average blood glucose levels [7]. In this phase, the remaining insulin-producing cells keep on working until they are finally killed off and the honeymoon comes to an end with insulin needs rising again.

In the case of LADA, the destruction of the insulin-producing cells by the self-reactive T lymphocytes proceeds at a slower speed and more mildly. Although questioned by some authors [8, 9], the criteria on which the diagnosis usually rests were proposed by the Immunology of Diabetes Society (IDS) in 2005: (1) onset age greater than 35 years, (2) islet autoantibodies as a marker of the autoimmune process, and (3) insulin independence for at least 6 months after diagnosis [10]. LADA shares genetic susceptibility and clinical phenotype both with T1D and T2D, thus suggesting it is a continuum between the two extremes [11].

Compared to patients with isolated T1D, those with T1D plus autoimmune diseases (AIDs) are older and exhibit a higher female: male ratio; average patient age and age at disease onset are higher in T1D plus AID vs T1D only [12]. Disease risk is associated with organ-specific autoantibodies, which can be used to screen subjects with T1D [13, 14]. Among these diseases, hypothyroidism occurs most frequently while adrenal gland insufficiency occurs the least. LADA has wide genetic overlap with T1D, actually sharing a great risk of other AID. Moreover, the risk seems to be

Table 1: Laboratory data.

Variable	Reference range, adults	Exams 7 years before admission	Exams 1 year before admission	Exams on admission	Exams at discharge	Exams 1 year after discharge
Haemoglobin (g/dL)	12–16	13	12.6	5.4	10	13.7
Haematocrit (%)	37–47	40.6	38.9	15.5	30	41.9
MCV (fl)	82–97	80.4	85.9	109.2	90.4	83.1
White cell count (per μL)	3,600–9,600	7,750	7,100	5,300	9,240	5,900
Platelets (μL)	140,000–440,000	382,000	340,000	116,000	650,000	248,000
Sodium (mEq/L)	136–146	143	139	130	145	142
Potassium (mEq/L)	3.5–5.1	4.5	4.5	4.4	3.4	4.6
Chloride (mEq/L)	101–109			102	111	
Urea nitrogen (mg/dL)	17–43	41	37	61	28	51
Creatinine (mg/dL)	0.55–1.12	0.57	0.71	0.80	0.89	0.87
Fasting blood	60–99	118	154	720		92
Glucose (mg/dL) (mmol/L)	3.9–5.5	6.55	8.55	40		5.1
HbA1c (%)	4.3–5.9		8.4			5.96
(mmol/mol)	23–41		68			42
Cholesterolemia (mg/dL)	70–190	258	246			240
Triglycerides (mg/dL)	<180	158	188			122
HDL cholesterol (mg/dL)	>40	82	70			56
Total bilirubin (mg/dL)	0.30–1.20	0.67	0.60	2	0.86	
Direct bilirubin (mg/dL)	0.00–0.20			0.43		
Alanine transaminase (UI/L)	0–35	13	9	9	5	7
Aspartate transaminase (UI/L)	0–35	16	17	13	11	13
Haptoglobine (mg/dL)	30–200			1	111	
Sideremia (mcg/dL)	60–180	90		207		
25-Hydroxyvitamin D (ng/mL)	>20		9.8	23.8		
Vitamin B12 (pg/mL)	180–914	203	160	44	>1,500	192
Folate (ng/mL)	3–20		10.3	5	>24.7	
TSH (uUI/mL)	0.34–5.60		1.250	1.180		

Table 2: Arterial blood gas analysis.

Variable	Reference range	On admission
pH	7.35–7.45	7.41
pCO_2 (mmHg)	35–45	25.7
pO_2 (mmHg)	75–100	70.4
HCO_3-std (mmol/L)	21–27	18.2
mOsm (mmol/kg)	275–295	299.8
AG (mmol/L)	4–12	19.8
Fasting blood glucose (mg/dL)	60–99	722
Lactate (mmol/L)	0.4–0.8	6

related to the GAD65 titre displayed by the subject at the moment of diagnosis [15], and, as in T1D, is maximum for hypothyroidism and minimum for adrenal gland insufficiency [15, 16].

In particular, in people with T1D, PA has a mean prevalence of 4.3% vs 0.2% in the general population [17], while no data are reported in the literature about the prevalence of PA in subjects with LADA. PA is marked by the presence of circulating antibodies to intrinsic factor which prevent VB12 absorption leading to a progressive decrease in vitamin storage, which is ten times more common in people with T1D than in nondiabetic persons [18, 19]. VB12 deficiency, in turn, leads to megaloblastic anaemia and neurological symptoms such as peripheral neuropathy and cerebral manifestations (confusion and psychosis) [20].

A Japanese report of people of all ages and both genders with concomitant PA and T1D showed that the subjects were mostly older women (the oldest was 87 years old) who exhibited T1D approximately 10 years prior to PA and had other AID, especially thyroiditis [21]. In the case of our 90-year-old female patient the association of vitiligo, ADM and PA matches the criteria of APS-4.

Differential diagnosis between T1D and LADA can sometimes be presumptive because rather than totally different pathological entities, they represent a seamless continuum. When the patient was initially referred to our clinical unit, we thought she could have T1D due to her phenotype (thin and with vitiligo) and the concomitant acute occurrence of another AID, PA. When her insulin

Table 3: Autoimmunity panel.

Variable	Reference range	Patient's value
IF Ab (U/ml)	<6	73.5
Anti-GAD65 Ab (U/ml)	<5	>250
21-OH Ab (U/ml)	<0.4	0.13
Parietal cell Ab	<1 : 140	<1 : 140
TPO Ab (UI/ml)	0–9	0.2
Tissue transglutaminase-IgA Ab (U/ml)$	<10.0	0.40

$Total IgA = 225 mg/dL. IF: intrinsic factor.

needs declined so quickly until the complete withdrawal, we wondered whether it was a honeymoon phase of T1D or a LADA, the two autoimmune conditions under which the insulin secretory capacity is preserved. The marked improvement in glycaemic control on sitagliptin treatment alone during the following months confirmed the second hypothesis and fully fulfilled the IDS LADA criteria [10].

After carrying out a comprehensive review of the currently available literature, we found no cases of APS diagnosed above 90 years old and only few cases of autoimmune diabetes emerged in very elderly individuals. Oriot et al. [22] reported the case of a 93-year-old woman whose diabetes was undoubtedly T1D as the onset was characterized by ketoacidosis proven by the presence of high levels of ketones in the urine sample together with metabolic acidosis. Moreover, the woman tested positive for more than one pancreatic islet autoantibody and immediately after the diagnosis insulin therapy became an irreplaceable treatment. A case of T1D in a 93-year-old woman with very akin clinical features has now been reported also by Ahmad et al. [23]. The oldest ultraelderly case of acute-onset autoimmune diabetes described so far by Yamaguchi et al. is instead of a 96-year-old Japanese woman who presented without ketoacidosis and in which insulin therapy became pleonastic few days after the diagnosis despite high anti-GAD antibody titre. She died few months after the discharge and whether she was experiencing a honeymoon phase or a LADA was impossible to ascertain [24].

The paucity of cases reporting newly diagnosed ADM in the elderly underlines the exceptionality of our case but could also be a warning of the risk of misclassification of adult-onset diabetes. Actually, there may be a latent proportion of adult-onset ADM misclassified as T2D due to the heterogeneous clinical features of LADA. Moreover, as the human average lifespan is lengthening, acute-onset autoimmune diabetes at an advanced age may be increasingly frequent in the close future.

In accordance with the current literature, our report demonstrates that a person may be born with a genetic pattern predisposed to autoimmunity, but this is not enough to make the disease surface. The time may come, however, when due to an external trigger such as an infection, the immune system reacts and misrecognizes its own genetic epitopes destroying the cells on which they are expressed. Contrary to the Japanese report cited above [21], we can see looking at our patient's laboratory data from the years before she came to our attention, VB12 depletion and the progressive increase in fasting plasma glucose began roughly at the same time. In 2013, seven years before the admission, fasting plasma glucose was slightly increased and VB12 was at the lower limit of normal with a haemoglobin amount related to the age of the patient, while in 2019, the year before admission, glycemia was far beyond a normal range and the VB12 pool was declining, but still no anaemia appeared. As far as we know, no treatment was initiated to correct both VB12 depletion and hyperglycaemia.

It is also important to underline that being a genetic predisposition the *sine qua non* for AID emergence, there is a high prevalence of autoimmunity recurrence in offspring. In fact, both sons of the patient have vitiligo: we invited them to perform a complete autoimmunity screening panel and to maintain longitudinal control with regular blood tests.

References

[1] J. Lund, D. M. Ouwens, M. Wettergreen, S. S. Bakke, G. H. Thoresen, and V. Aas, "Increased glycolysis and higher lactate production in hyperglycemic myotubes," *Cells*, vol. 8, no. 9, p. 1101, 2019.

[2] A. E. Kitabchi, G. E. Umpierrez, J. M. Miles, and J. N. Fisher, "Hyperglycemic crises in adult patients with diabetes," *Diabetes Care*, vol. 32, no. 7, pp. 1335–1343, 2009.

[3] D. M. Nyaga, M. H. Vickers, C. Jefferies, J. K. Perry, and J. M. O'Sullivan, "The genetic architecture of type 1 diabetes mellitus," *Molecular and Cellular Endocrinology*, vol. 477, pp. 70–80, 2018.

[4] C. C. Robertson and S. S. Rich, "Genetics of type 1 diabetes," *Current Opinion in Genetics & Development*, vol. 50, pp. 7–16, 2018.

[5] R. Shigemoto, T. Anno, F. Kawasaki, K. Kaku, and H. Kaneto, "Case report: markedly long-term preservation of pancreatic β-cell function in a subject with elderly onset of type 1 diabetes mellitus showing high-titer autoimmune antibodies for over 4 years," *Frontiers in Immunology*, vol. 12, Article ID 752423, 2021.

[6] M. M. Lima-Martínez, E. Guerra-Alcalá, M. Contreras, J. Nastasi, J. A. Noble, and C. Polychronakos, "One year remission of type 1 diabetes mellitus in a patient treated with sitagliptin," *Endocrinology, Diabetes & Metabolism Case Report*, vol. 2014, Article ID 140072, 6 pages, 2014.

[7] T. Zhong, R. Tang, S. Gong, J. Li, X. Li, and Z. Zhou, "The remission phase in type 1 diabetes: changing epidemiology, definitions, and emerging immuno-metabolic mechanisms," *Diabetes/Metabolism Research and Reviews*, vol. 36, no. 2, Article ID e3207, 2020.

[8] S. Brophy, K. Yderstræde, D. Mauricio et al., "Time to insulin initiation cannot be used in defining latent autoimmune diabetes in adults," *Diabetes Care*, vol. 31, no. 3, pp. 439–441, 2008.

[9] E. Maddaloni, C. Moretti, C. Mignogna, and R. Buzzetti, "Adult-onset autoimmune diabetes in 2020: an update," *Maturitas*, vol. 137, pp. 37–44, 2020.
[10] S. Fourlanos, F. Dotta, C. J. Greenbaum et al., "Latent autoimmune diabetes in adults (LADA) should be less latent," *Diabetologia*, vol. 48, no. 11, pp. 2206–2212, 2005.
[11] B. Liu, Y. Xiang, Z. Liu, and Z. Zhou, "Past, present and future of latent autoimmune diabetes in adults," *Diabetes/Metabolism Research and Reviews*, vol. 36, no. 1, Article ID e3205, 2020.
[12] L. Frommer and G. J. Kahaly, "Type 1 diabetes and associated autoimmune diseases," *World Journal of Diabetes*, vol. 11, no. 11, pp. 527–539, 2020.
[13] J. M. Barker, "Type 1 diabetes-associated autoimmunity: natural history, genetic associations, and screening," *Journal of Clinical Endocrinology & Metabolism*, vol. 91, no. 4, pp. 1210–1217, 2006.
[14] Y. K. Bao, L. G. Weide, V. C. Ganesan et al., "High prevalence of comorbid autoimmune diseases in adults with type 1 diabetes from the health facts database," *Journal of Diabetes*, vol. 11, no. 4, pp. 273–279, 2019.
[15] S. Zampetti, M. Capizzi, M. Spoletini et al., "GADA titer-related risk for organ-specific autoimmunity in LADA subjects subdivided according to gender (NIRAD study 6)," *Journal of Clinical Endocrinology & Metabolism*, vol. 97, no. 10, pp. 3759–3765, 2012.
[16] G. Gambelunghe, F. Forini, S. Laureti et al., "Increased risk for endocrine autoimmunity in Italian type 2 diabetic patients with GAD65 autoantibodies," *Clinical Endocrinology*, vol. 52, no. 5, pp. 565–573, 2000.
[17] C. Nederstigt, B. S. Uitbeijerse, L. G. M. Janssen, E. P. M. Corssmit, E. J. P. de Koning, and O. M. Dekkers, "Associated auto-immune disease in type 1 diabetes patients: a systematic review and meta-analysis," *European Journal of Endocrinology*, vol. 180, no. 2, pp. 135–144, 2019.
[18] C. E. M. De Block, I. H. De Leeuw, and L. F. Van Gaal, "High prevalence of manifestations of gastric autoimmunity in parietal cell antibody- positive type 1 (insulin-dependent) diabetic patients1," *Journal of Clinical Endocrinology & Metabolism*, vol. 84, no. 11, pp. 4062–4067, 1999.
[19] C. M. Rojas Hernandez and T. H. Oo, "Advances in mechanisms, diagnosis, and treatment of pernicious anemia," *Discovery Medicine*, vol. 19, no. 104, pp. 159–168, 2015.
[20] C. E. M. De Block, I. H. De Leeuw, and L. F. Van Gaal, "Autoimmune gastritis in type 1 diabetes: a clinically oriented review," *Journal of Clinical Endocrinology & Metabolism*, vol. 93, no. 2, pp. 363–371, 2008.
[21] N. Ohara, M. Kaneko, T. Yano et al., "Type 1 diabetes mellitus and pernicious anemia in an elderly Japanese patient: a case report and literature review," *Internal Medicine*, vol. 54, no. 18, pp. 2361–2365, 2015.
[22] P. Oriot, A. Louvet, G. Debugne, and I. Weets, "Sudden onset of immune-mediated type 1 diabetes mellitus in a 93-year-old woman: a case report," *Acta Diabetologica*, vol. 55, no. 12, pp. 1313–1315, 2018.
[23] W. Ahmad, C. Bates, L. Dale, and N. Siddaramaiah, "Newly diagnosed type 1 diabetes in a 93 year old," *BMJ Case Reports*, vol. 15, no. 1, Article ID e246799, 2022.
[24] H. Yamaguchi, T. Kanadani, M. Ohno, and A. Shirakami, "An ultra-elderly case of acute-onset autoimmune type 1 diabetes mellitus," *Journal of Endocrinology and Metabolism*, vol. 6, no. 2, pp. 71–74, 2016.

49

Combination Therapy with Empagliflozin and Insulin Results in Successful Glycemic Control: A Case Report of Uncontrolled Diabetes Caused by Autoimmune Pancreatitis and Subsequent Steroid Treatment

Miyako Kishimoto[1,2] **Kazuhide Yamaoki,**[1,2] **and Masayuki Adachi**[1,2]

[1]*Clinical Research Center, Department of Medicine, International University of Health and Welfare, Tochigi, Japan*
[2]*Department of Internal Medicine, Sanno Hospital, 8-10-16 Akasaka, Minato, Tokyo 107-0052, Japan*

Correspondence should be addressed to Miyako Kishimoto; mkishimoto@iuhw.ac.jp

Academic Editor: John Broom

Copyright © 2019 Miyako Kishimoto et al. This is an open access article distributed under the Creative Commons Attribution License, which permits unrestricted use, distribution, and reproduction in any medium, provided the original work is properly cited.

A 66-year-old Japanese male presented with thirst, polyuria, and hemoglobin A1c and postprandial glucose levels (13.1% and 529 mg/dL, respectively) that indicated severe hyperglycemia. Based on his high immunoglobulin G4 level and the results of magnetic resonance imaging and magnetic resonance cholangiopancreatography, we diagnosed him with autoimmune pancreatitis. Insulin was initiated to control his diabetes. One month later, the patient commenced on prednisolone therapy for the treatment of autoimmune pancreatitis, after which his total insulin dosage increased to a maximum of 52 units/day. When the prednisolone dosage was later tapered, the patient's total dosage of insulin was reduced to 42 units/day. However, he had gained 3.6 kg from the start of prednisolone therapy, and 42 units/day was insufficient for maintaining glycemic control. Thus, empagliflozin, a sodium-dependent glucose transporter 2 (SGLT2) inhibitor, was added. Thereafter, we were able to reduce the patient's total dosage of insulin; it was eventually discontinued with good glycemic control and weight loss. Such results suggest that the combination of insulin with an SGLT2 inhibitor may be a viable option for the treatment of diabetic patients on prednisolone therapy.

1. Introduction

Sodium-dependent glucose transporter 2 (SGLT2) is a protein in the early proximal tubule that reabsorbs the majority of filtered glucose. Inhibitors of SGLT2 enhance urinary glucose excretion, thereby lowering blood glucose levels in an insulin-independent manner. SGLT2 inhibitors have pleiotropic actions, including reduced glomerular hyperfiltration, hypertension, and weight loss [1], which may correlate with reduced cardiovascular risk. In a recent study of patients with type 2 diabetes who were at high risk for cardiovascular events, those who received empagliflozin (an SGLT2 inhibitor) in addition to standard care had lower rates of the primary composite cardiovascular outcome and death from any cause than did those on placebo [2, 3]. As a result of mounting evidence, the American Diabetes Association and the European Association for the Study of Diabetes recently updated their position statements on the management of type 2 diabetes in adults [4, 5]. In their statements, an SGLT2 inhibitor with proven benefit is recommended for the treatment of patients with chronic kidney disease or clinical heart failure and atherosclerotic cardiovascular disease.

Autoimmune pancreatitis (AIP) is a chronic and progressive inflammatory pancreatic disease that is uniquely characterized by diagnostic images of pancreatic enlargement and irregularly narrowed main pancreatic ducts. It is a condition that responds dramatically to corticosteroid therapy [6–8]. Corticosteroids are frequently used for the treatment of inflammatory conditions and autoimmune diseases, but are widely recognized to cause hyperglycemia and insulin resistance when used at high doses and for long durations [9, 10].

Table 1: Postprandial laboratory results on patient's first visit.

Hematology		**Auto-antibody tests**	
White blood cells	7400/μL	Antinuclear antibodies	< 40
Red blood cells	473×10^4/μL		
Hemoglobin	15.9 g/dL	**Immunoglobulin**	
Hematocrit	44.9%	Immunoglobulin A	186 mg/dL
Platelets	22.5×10^4/μL	Immunoglobulin M	90 mg/dL
		Immunoglobulin G	1104 mg/dL
Blood chemistry		Immunoglobulin G4	141 mg/dL
Albumin	4.9 g/dL		
T-bilirubin	0.8 mg/dL	**Tumor markers**	
Aspartate aminotransferase	18 IU/L	CEA	5.7 ng/mL
Alanine aminotransferase	20 IU/L	CA19-9	1.2 U/mL
Lactate dehydrogenase	162 IU/L	Span-1	< 1.0 U/mL
Alkaline phosphatase	448 IU/L	DUPAN-2	57 U/mL
γ-Glutamyl transpeptidase	47 IU/L		
Pancreatic amylase	13 IU/L	**Glycometabolism tests**	
Lipase	18 IU/L	Plasma glucose	529 mg/dL
Trypsin	111 ng/mL	HbA1c	13.1%
Elastase-1	93 IU/L	Glycoalbumin	43.2%
Cholinesterase	290 IU/L	C-peptide reactivity	1.15 ng/mL
Creatinine kinase	115 IU/L	Anti-GAD antibodies	< 5.0 U/mL
Uric acid	4.3 mg/dL		
Blood urea nitrogen	11.5 mg/dL	**Ketone body fractions**	
Creatinine	0.64 mg/dL	Total ketone bodies	895 μmol/L
eGFR	95 ml/min/1.73m^2	Acetoacetate	218 μmol/L
Sodium	135 mEq/L	β-Hydroxybutyrate	677 μmol/L
Potassium	4.1 mEq/L		
Chloride	98 mEq/L	**Urinalysis**	
Triglycerides	195 mg/dL	Protein	(–)
HDL cholesterol	65 mg/dL	Glucose	4+
LDL cholesterol	115 mg/dL	Occult blood	(–)
C-reactive protein	0.13 mg/dL	Ketones	(+/–)

Herein, we report the case of a patient in whom uncontrolled diabetes as a direct result of AIP and subsequent steroid treatment was successfully treated by the addition of empagliflozin to his insulin therapy.

2. Case Report

A 66-year-old Japanese man, 177 cm tall and weighing 66 kg (body mass index of 21.1), had been treated for hypertension for more than seven years. He had yearly medical evaluations but was never diagnosed with diabetes (postprandial glucose and hemoglobin A1c [HbA1c] levels in March 2017: 141 mg/dL and 5.4%, respectively). However, results of an annual medical check-up in March 2018 showed remarkable elevation of postprandial glucose and HbA1c levels (265 mg/dL and 11.4%, respectively). The following month (April), he reported symptoms of thirst and polyuria. His postprandial glucose and HbA1c levels on that day were 529 mg/dL and 13.1%, respectively. A high glycoalbumin level (43.2%) also suggested acute glucose elevation (Table 1). The patient's anti-glutamic acid decarboxylase antibody test was negative; however, because his postprandial C-peptide level was low (1.15 ng/mL), the patient's pancreas presumably had reduced insulin-secreting capacity. We noted that the patient's daily life had not changed in years; and he had no diabetic complications such as retinopathy, nephropathy, or neuropathy.

To identify the cause of hyperglycemia, we performed several imaging studies. Abdominal computed tomography, magnetic resonance imaging, and magnetic resonance cholangiopancreatography (MRCP) revealed diffuse swelling that extended from the pancreatic body to tail (Figures 1(a)–1(c)). In addition, MRCP showed narrowing of the associated main pancreatic duct (Figure 1(c)). The patient did not complain of any digestive symptoms such as upper abdominal pain; however, based on the imaging scans and elevation of serum immunoglobulin G4 (IgG4) levels (141.0 mg/dL), we diagnosed him with type 1 AIP.

To control diabetes, the patient began self-administering insulin injections: insulin aspart (Novo Nordisk) three times

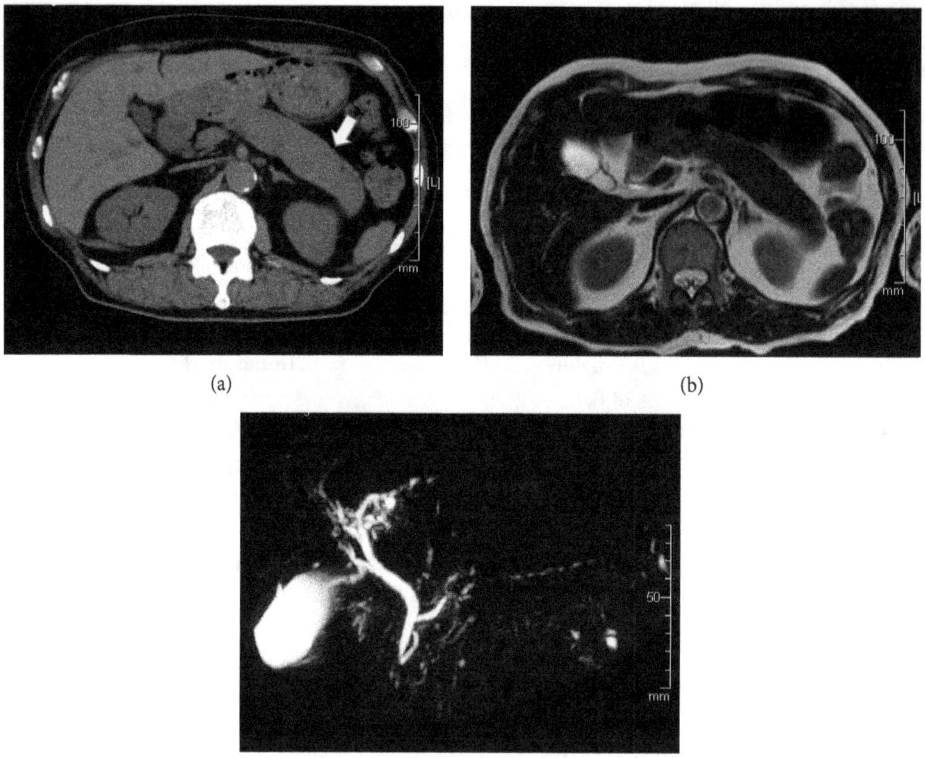

FIGURE 1: (a) An abdominal computed tomography scan performed on the patient's first visit shows diffuse swelling extending from the pancreatic body to tail. The arrow indicates the affected portion of the pancreas. (b) Magnetic resonance image (T2 weighted image) of the abdomen prior to prednisolone therapy reveals diffuse swelling extending from the pancreatic body to tail. (c) MRCP prior to prednisolone therapy shows narrowing of the main pancreatic duct extending from the pancreatic body to tail.

per day before each meal and insulin degludec (Novo Nordisk) before going to bed. Because tight adjustment of insulin dosage is required for achieving good glycemic control, the patient received a flash glucose monitoring system (Freestyle Libre™; Abbott Diabetes Care, Witney, UK) [11] upon initiation of insulin. He initially had considerable ketosis (Table 1), but, soon after, the levels of total ketone bodies, acetoacetate, and β-hydroxybutyrate declined to the normal range (36 μmol/L, 12 μmol/L, and 24 μmol/L, respectively). By the end of April, the patient's total insulin dosage was 36 units/day (Figure 2(a)). In May, prednisolone (35 mg/day) was initiated for the treatment of AIP. At that time, 42 units/day of insulin was not sufficient to control glucose elevation (Figure 2(b)); the patient required a maximum of 52 units/day (Figure 2(c)). One month later, IgG4 levels declined to 54.3 mg/dL. The dosage of prednisolone, which was being tapered by 5 mg/day every 2 weeks, was 20~25 mg/day; and the total dosage of insulin was also lower than that of the previous month. However, 42 units/day of insulin was required to maintain glycemic control (Figure 2(d)). In addition, the combination of high-dose insulin and prednisolone caused our patient to gain 3.6 kg weight from the start of prednisolone initiation.

To improve glycemic control, empagliflozin was added to insulin therapy. Because we expected empagliflozin to lower blood glucose levels, we reduced the dosage of insulin to 29 units/day beforehand. Nevertheless, the patient experienced hypoglycemia 1 hour after breakfast and 1 hour after dinner on the day of empagliflozin initiation (Figure 2(e)). By the end of June, 20 days after the addition of empagliflozin, the patient had lost 1.2 kg and his total insulin dosage had declined to 20 units/day (Figure 2(f)). In July, the prednisolone dosage was reduced to 10 mg/day. Because the patient had achieved good glycemic control (postprandial glucose, HbA1c, and glycoalbumin levels: 159 mg/dL, 6.9%, and 14.3%, respectively), the total dosage of insulin was further reduced and then eventually discontinued (Figure 2(g)). Thereafter, he maintained good glycemic control (postprandial glucose and HbA1c levels: 130–180mg/dL and 5.4–5.8%, respectively) despite receiving only empagliflozin for diabetes (Figure 3). However, his postprandial C-peptide level remained low (1.84 ng/mL), revealing that although the insulin-secreting capacity of his pancreas had slightly recovered, it remained insufficient.

In October, the patient's prednisolone dosage was 4 mg/day. His follow-up magnetic resonance imaging and MRCP showed that both the diffuse swelling of the pancreatic tail and narrowing of the associated main pancreatic duct had been ameliorated (Figures 4(a) and 4(b)). To date, the patient's AIP is well controlled and has not relapsed.

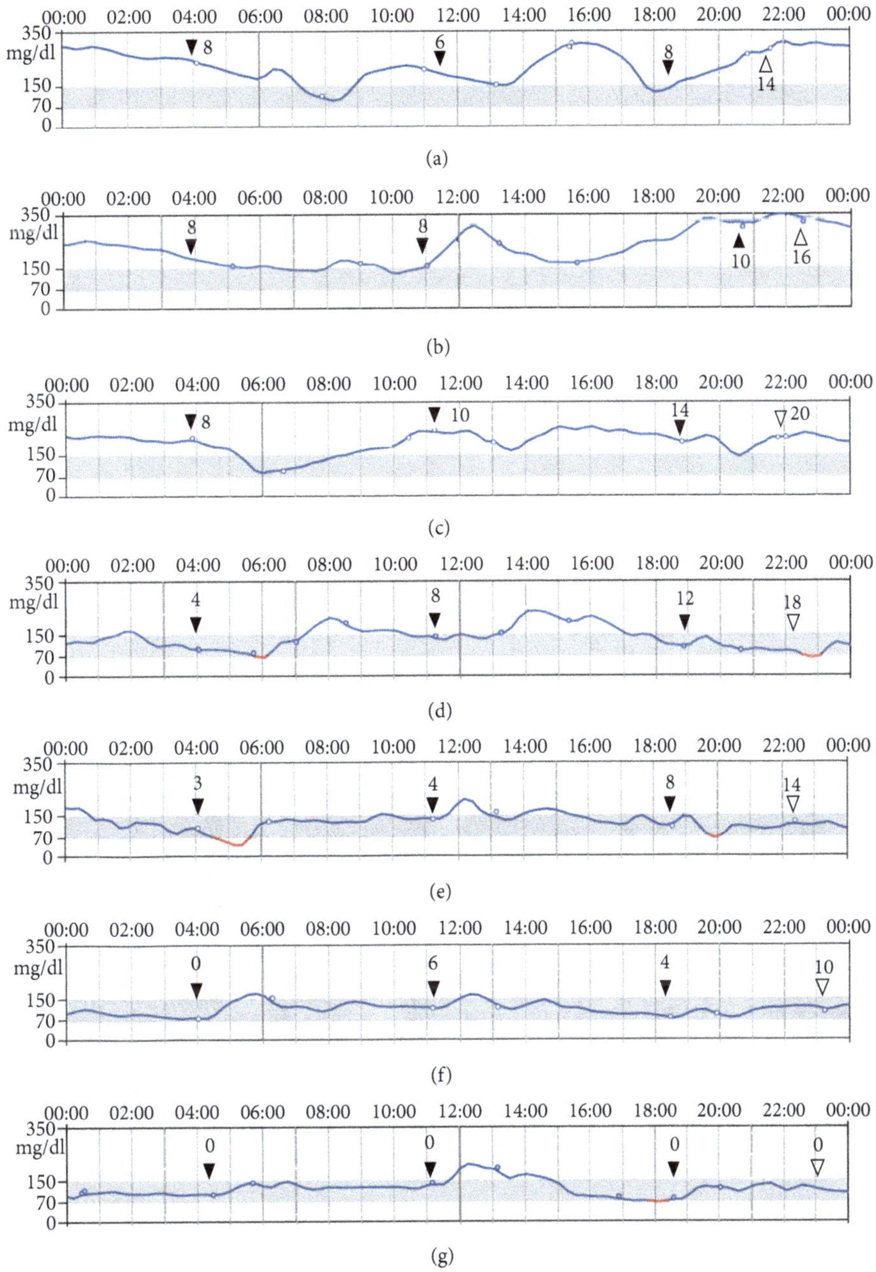

FIGURE 2: The results of continuous glucose monitoring (CGM) with the flash glucose monitoring system. Closed arrowheads indicate the timing of the patient's meals and insulin injections. Open arrowheads indicate the timing of the patient's insulin injections before sleep. Values adjacent to the arrowheads indicate the number of units of insulin injected. (a) One representative pattern of CGM prior to initiation of prednisolone. (b) Initiation of 35 mg/day of oral prednisolone. (c) Two days after initiation of prednisolone. Total dosage of insulin was increased to 52 units/day. (d) Because of the amelioration of AIP, prednisolone dosage was reduced to 25 mg/dL; however, 42 units/day of insulin was required to maintain glycemic control. (e) First day of empagliflozin administration. Hypoglycemia recorded at 5 AM to 6 AM and approximately 8 PM. (f) Twenty days after empagliflozin initiation. (g) CGM pattern of patient on empagliflozin only.

3. Discussion

The international consensus diagnostic criteria for AIP identify two subtypes: type 1 is characterized by serum IgG4 elevation and the classic histopathological patterns of lymphoplasmacytic sclerosing pancreatitis; type 2 is characterized by idiopathic duct-centric pancreatitis and is not associated with IgG4 levels [12–14]. Although the clinical findings in AIP are nonspecific, the most common presentation is obstructive jaundice and upper abdominal pain [6, 7]. Approximately 40–80% of patients with AIP reportedly also present with diabetes—some with simultaneous onset with AIP and some with exacerbation of preexisting diabetes [8, 14–21]. In addition, some patients develop diabetes after the start of steroid

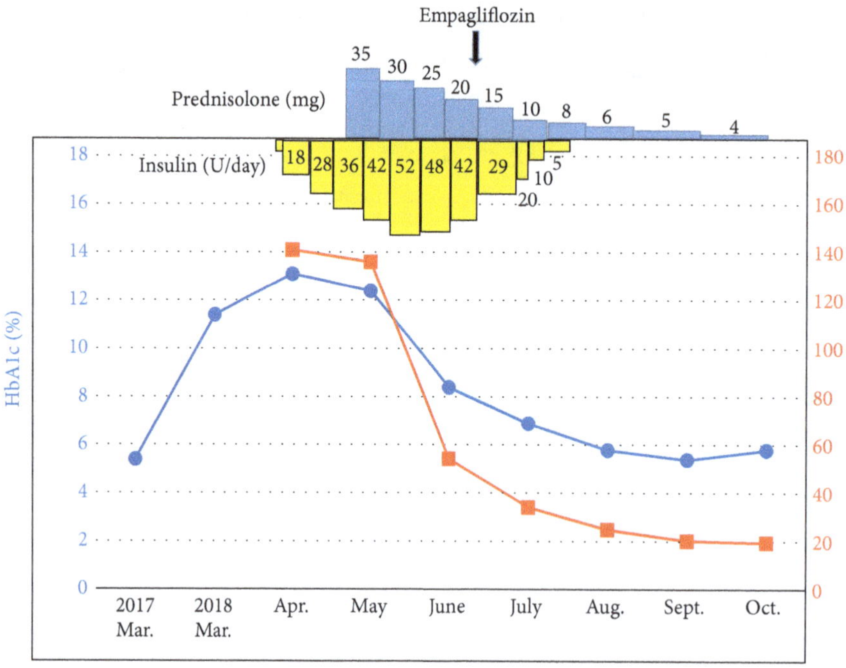

FIGURE 3: Changes in glycemic control and clinical course of AIP during prednisolone therapy. HbA1c levels (circles) and serum IgG4 levels (squares) declined over the course of treatment.

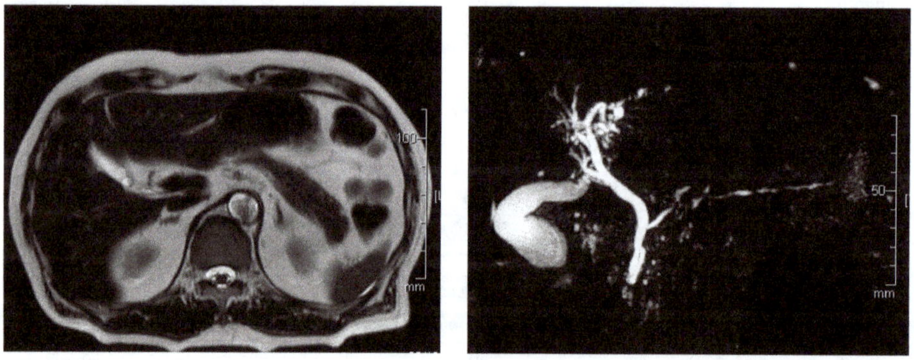

(a) (b)

FIGURE 4: (a) Magnetic resonance image (T2 weighted image) of the abdomen after prednisolone therapy reveals amelioration of the diffuse swelling that had affected the pancreas from body to tail. (b) MRCP after prednisolone therapy revealed amelioration of the narrowing of the main pancreatic duct.

therapy, the outcome of which varies with regard to glycemic control [17, 18, 20, 22–24].

The diabetes associated with AIP is assumed to be caused by a reduction in insulin secretion. This may be the result of various mechanisms. For one, AIP is characterized by infiltration of cluster of differentiation (CD)8 and CD4 T lymphocytes, which surround ductal cells and secrete cytokines to suppress and destroy β-islet cells of the pancreas [22, 23]. In addition, inflammation and fibrosis of exocrine glands is associated with the obstruction of blood flow in the endocrine glands, that results in ischemia of islet cells and dysfunctional insulin secretion. Furthermore, extensive destruction of the pancreatic islets caused by direct infiltration of inflammatory cells and fibroblasts proliferation also leads to dysfunctional insulin secretion [14, 16, 20, 23–27].

Glucocorticoids are counterhormones against insulin [9, 10], with mechanisms that include reduction of glucose uptake, induction of hepatic glucose production, and direct inhibition of insulin release [28–30]. Glucocorticoid-induced hyperglycemia is a common condition, which is often considered postprandial hyperglycemia [31, 32]. Prominent hyperglycemia is most often observed when individuals with known diabetes take high doses of glucocorticoids, but may also occur with intake of moderate and low doses in individuals without a known risk [29, 31, 33]. The odds ratio for new-onset diabetes mellitus in patients treated with glucocorticoids ranges from approximately 1.5 to 2.5, and the total glucocorticoid dose and duration of therapy are strong predictors of diabetes induction [32].

Thus, initiation of steroid therapy in patients with AIP may induce the onset of diabetes or worsen glycemic control in those with preexisting diabetes [34]. However, steroid therapy also inactivates inflammatory cells and fibroblast function, and may improve insulin secretion by controlling a series of autoimmune mechanisms, including cytokine production [16, 25]. It has been reported that pancreatic endocrine function improves after treatment with steroids in 25–45% of patients with AIP [20, 24, 35], with some patients eventually achieving a medication-free status [34]. Indeed, Miyamoto et al. reported that three months after the start of steroid therapy in patients with AIP and simultaneous onset of diabetes mellitus, 54% of patients experience improvement in diabetes, 36% do not have any change, and 9% have worsening of diabetes [16]. In addition, they noted that the long-term positive effect of corticosteroid therapy on glucose tolerance might be greater than its short-term negative effect on insulin [16].

Approximately half of patients with AIP-associated pancreatic diabetes are treated with insulin [35]. Such therapy is effective in lowering blood glucose. However, patients must be monitored for hypoglycemia and undesirable weight gain, especially when insulin dosage is increased. SGLT2 inhibitors may have glycemic benefits in patients with type 1 or type 2 diabetes who are on insulin therapy [36]. Accumulating reports indicate that SGLT2 inhibitors are well tolerated, and their addition to insulin therapy improves glycemic control and reduces body weight such that insulin dosages could sometimes be reduced [37–52]. The mechanism was explained by Ferrannini et al., who reported that empagliflozin lowers fasting and postprandial glycemia by inducing glycosuria, which improves β cell function and insulin sensitivity in patients with type 2 diabetes [53]. This was noted despite the fall in insulin secretion and tissue glucose disposal, and the rise in endogenous glucose production that occurs after a single dose of 25 mg empagliflozin [53]. We were able to reduce our patient's total insulin dosage upon initiation of empagliflozin. This lowered his risk of hypoglycemia and suppressed weight gain. Although improvement in glycemic control and reduction in total insulin dosage could have been the result of AIP amelioration alone, we believe that empagliflozin accelerated improvement of glycemic control in our patient.

One of the risks of SGLT2 inhibitors is diabetic ketoacidosis (DKA) [4, 5]. Similar to classic DKA, ketone accumulation in SGLT2 inhibitor-associated DKA is downstream of insulin deficiency and glucagon elevation, promoting lipolysis and hepatic ketogenesis. SGLT2 inhibitor-enhanced glucosuria effectively lowers plasma glucose levels, which decreases insulin secretion from pancreatic β cells. SGLT2 inhibitor-mediated glucosuria and attenuation of sodium reabsorption in the kidneys may also indirectly expand the ketone reservoir by enhancing renal ketone reabsorption [54–56]. Although our patient initially had prominent ketosis, the ketosis improved soon after initiation of insulin therapy. Although we rechecked for ketosis throughout his treatment with empagliflozin, no further signs of ketosis were detected.

In conclusion, this case report suggests that the combination of insulin and SGLT2 inhibitor can be effective for the treatment of secondary diabetes, such as prednisolone-induced diabetes associated with the treatment of AIP in our patient. Further studies on a larger scale are required to confirm the effectiveness of this combination for the treatment of diabetes in patients on corticosteroid therapy.

Ethical Approval

All procedures followed were in accordance with the ethical standards of the responsible committee on human experimentation (institutional and national) and the Helsinki Declaration of 1975, as revised in 2000 and 2008. In addition, this case report was approved by the Ethics Committee of Sanno Hospital.

Consent

The authors obtained written informed consent from the patient for publication.

References

[1] L. A. Gallo, E. M. Wright, and V. Vallon, "Probing SGLT2 as a therapeutic target for diabetes: Basic physiology and consequences," *Diabetes and Vascular Disease Research*, vol. 12, no. 2, pp. 78–89, 2015.

[2] B. Zinman, C. Wanner, J. M. Lachin et al., "Empagliflozin, cardiovascular outcomes, and mortality in type 2 diabetes," *The New England Journal of Medicine*, vol. 373, no. 22, pp. 2117–2128, 2015.

[3] K. Kaku, J. Lee, M. Mattheus, S. Kaspers, J. George, and H.-J. Woerle, "Empagliflozin and cardiovascular outcomes in Asian patients with type 2 diabetes and established cardiovascular disease — results from EMPA-REG OUTCOME®," *Circulation Journal: Official Journal of the Japanese Circulation Society*, vol. 81, no. 2, pp. 227–234, 2017.

[4] M. J. Davies, D. A. D'Alessio, J. Fradkin et al., "Management of hyperglycemia in type 2 diabetes, 2018. A consensus report by the american diabetes association (ADA) and the european association for the study of diabetes (EASD)," *Diabetes Care*, vol. 41, no. 12, pp. 2669–2701, 2018.

[5] M. J. Davies, D. A. D'Alessio, J. Fradkin et al., "Management of hyperglycaemia in type 2 diabetes, 2018. A consensus report by the american diabetes association (ADA) and the european association for the study of diabetes (EASD)," *Diabetologia*, vol. 61, no. 12, pp. 2461–2498, 2018.

[6] A. O. Omiyale, "Autoimmune pancreatitis," *Gland Surgery*, vol. 5, no. 3, pp. 318–326, 2016.

[7] O. Cai and S. Tan, "From pathogenesis, clinical manifestation, and diagnosis to treatment: an overview on autoimmune pancreatitis," *Gastroenterology Research and Practice*, vol. 2017, Article ID 3246459, 11 pages, 2017.

[8] T. Kamisawa, Y. Zen, S. Pillai, and J. H. Stone, "IgG4-related disease," *The Lancet*, vol. 385, article no. 9976, pp. 1460–1471, 2015.

[9] M.-Z. Liu, H.-Y. He, J.-Q. Luo et al., "Drug-induced hyperglycaemia and diabetes: pharmacogenomics perspectives," *Archives of Pharmacal Research*, vol. 41, no. 7, pp. 725–736, 2018.

[10] N. Fathallah, R. Slim, S. Larif, H. Hmouda, and C. Ben Salem, "Drug-induced hyperglycaemia and diabetes," *Drug Safety*, vol. 38, no. 12, pp. 1153–1168, 2015.

[11] "FreeStyle libre flash glucose monitoring system," https://www.freestylelibre.us/.

[12] T. Shimosegawa, S. T. Chari, and L. Frulloni, "International consensus diagnostic criteria for autoimmune pancreatitis: guidelines of the international association of pancreatology," *Pancreas*, vol. 40, no. 3, pp. 352–358, 2011.

[13] K. Okazaki, S. T. Chari, L. Frulloni et al., "International consensus for the treatment of autoimmune pancreatitis," *Pancreatology*, vol. 17, no. 1, pp. 1–6, 2017.

[14] K. Okazaki, S. Kawa, T. Kamisawa et al., "Amendment of the japanese consensus guidelines for autoimmune pancreatitis, 2013 I. Concept and diagnosis of autoimmune pancreatitis," *Journal of Gastroenterology*, vol. 49, no. 4, pp. 567–588, 2013.

[15] K. Takeshima, H. Ariyasu, H. Iwakura et al., "Predominant improvement of alpha cell function after steroid therapy in a patient with autoimmune pancreatitis: case report," *Diabetes Therapy*, vol. 9, no. 3, pp. 1385–1395, 2018.

[16] Y. Miyamoto, T. Kamisawa, T. Tabata et al., "Short and long-term outcomes of diabetes mellitus in patients with autoimmune pancreatitis after steroid therapy," *Gut and Liver*, vol. 6, no. 4, pp. 501–504, 2012.

[17] K. Hirano, A. Isogawa, M. Tada et al., "Long-term prognosis of autoimmune pancreatitis in terms of glucose tolerance," *Pancreas*, vol. 41, no. 5, pp. 691–695, 2012.

[18] I. Nishimori, A. Tamakoshi, S. Kawa et al., "Influence of steroid therapy on the course of diabetes mellitus in patients with autoimmune pancreatitis: Findings from a nationwide survey in Japan," *Pancreas*, vol. 32, no. 3, pp. 244–248, 2006.

[19] T. Kamisawa, N. Egawa, S. Inokuma et al., "Pancreatic endocrine and exocrine function and salivary gland function in autoimmune pancreatitis before and after steroid therapy," *Pancreas*, vol. 27, no. 3, pp. 235–238, 2003.

[20] T. Nishino, F. Toki, H. Oyama, K. Shimizu, and K. Shiratori, "Long-term outcome of autoimmune pancreatitis after oral prednisolone therapy," *Internal Medicine*, vol. 45, no. 8, pp. 497–501, 2006.

[21] F. Maire, Y. Le Baleur, V. Rebours et al., "Outcome of patients with type 1 or 2 autoimmune pancreatitis," *American Journal of Gastroenterology*, vol. 106, no. 1, pp. 151–156, 2011.

[22] I. G. Ketikoglou, I. S. Elefsiniotis, E. V. Vezali, and A. M. Moulakakis, "Diabetes mellitus responsive to corticosteroids in autoimmune pancreatitis," *Journal of Clinical Gastroenterology*, vol. 38, no. 10, p. 910, 2004.

[23] S. Tanaka, T. Kobayashi, K. Nakanishi et al., "Corticosteroid-responsive diabetes mellitus associated with autoimmune pancreatitis," *The Lancet*, vol. 356, no. 9233, pp. 910-911, 2000.

[24] T. Ito, I. Nishimori, N. Inoue et al., "Treatment for autoimmune pancreatitis: Consensus on the treatment for patients with autoimmune pancreatitis in Japan," *Journal of Gastroenterology*, vol. 42, Supplement 18, pp. 50–58, 2007.

[25] S. Tanaka, T. Kobayashi, K. Nakanishi et al., "Evidence of primary β-cell destruction by T-cells and β-cell differentiation from pancreatic ductal cells in diabetes associated with active autoimmune chronic pancreatitis," *Diabetes Care*, vol. 24, no. 9, pp. 1661–1667, 2001.

[26] T. Ito, K. Kawabe, Y. Arita et al., "Evaluation of pancreatic endocrine and exocrine function in patients with autoimmune pancreatitis," *Pancreas*, vol. 34, no. 2, pp. 254–259, 2007.

[27] S. Tanaka, T. Kobayashi, K. Nakanishi et al., "Corticosteroid-responsive diabetes mellitus associated with autoimmune pancreatitis: Pathological examinations of the endocrine and exocrine pancreas," *Annals of the New York Academy of Sciences*, vol. 958, pp. 152–159, 2002.

[28] F. Delaunay, A. Khan, A. Cintra et al., "Pancreatic β cells are important targets for the diabetogenic effects of glucocorticoids," *The Journal of Clinical Investigation*, vol. 100, no. 8, pp. 2094–2098, 1997.

[29] D. H. Van Raalte, M. Brands, N. J. Van Der Zijl et al., "Low-dose glucocorticoid treatment affects multiple aspects of intermediary metabolism in healthy humans: A randomised controlled trial," *Diabetologia*, vol. 54, no. 8, pp. 2103–2112, 2011.

[30] D. H. van Raalte, V. Nofrate, M. C. Bunck et al., "Acute and 2-week exposure to prednisolone impair different aspects of β-cell function in healthy men," *European Journal of Endocrinology*, vol. 162, no. 4, pp. 729–735, 2010.

[31] K. C. J. Yuen, P. A. McDaniel, and M. C. Riddle, "Twenty-four-hour profiles of plasma glucose, insulin, C-peptide and free fatty acid in subjects with varying degrees of glucose tolerance following short-term, medium-dose prednisone (20 mg/day) treatment: Evidence for differing effects on insulin secretion and action," *Clinical Endocrinology*, vol. 77, no. 2, pp. 224–232, 2012.

[32] J. N. Clore and L. Thurby-Hay, "Glucocorticoid-induced hyperglycemia," *Endocrine Practice*, vol. 15, no. 5, pp. 469–474, 2009.

[33] M. C. Gulliford, J. Charlton, and R. Latinovic, "Risk of diabetes associated with prescribed glucocorticoids in a large population," *Diabetes Care*, vol. 29, no. 12, pp. 2728-2729, 2006.

[34] M. Miyazawa, H. Takatori, T. Shimakami et al., "Prognosis of type 1 autoimmune pancreatitis after corticosteroid therapy-induced remission in terms of relapse and diabetes mellitus," *PLoS ONE*, vol. 12, no. 11, Article ID e0188549, 2017.

[35] T. Ito, T. Nakamura, N. Fujimori et al., "Characteristics of pancreatic diabetes in patients with autoimmune pancreatitis," *Journal of Digestive Diseases*, vol. 12, no. 3, pp. 210–216, 2011.

[36] Y. Yang, S. Chen, H. Pan et al., "Safety and efficiency of SGLT2 inhibitor combining with insulin in subjects with diabetes. Systematic review and meta-analysis of randomized controlled trials," *Medicine (Baltimore)*, vol. 96, no. 21, Article ID e6944, 2017.

[37] Y. Seino, D. Yabe, T. Sasaki et al., "Sodium-glucose cotransporter-2 inhibitor luseogliflozin added to glucagon-like peptide 1 receptor agonist liraglutide improves glycemic control with bodyweight and fat mass reductions in Japanese patients with type 2 diabetes: A 52-week, open-label, single-arm study," *Journal of Diabetes Investigation*, vol. 9, no. 2, pp. 332–340, 2018.

[38] H. Ishihara, S. Yamaguchi, I. Nakao, S. Asahina, and T. Sakatani, "Efficacy and safety of ipragliflozin as add-on therapy to insulin in Japanese patients with type 2 diabetes mellitus (IOLITE): a 36-week, open-label extension of a 16-week, randomized, placebo-controlled, double-blind study," *Diabetology International*, vol. 10, no. 1, pp. 37–50, 2019.

[39] H. Ishihara, S. Yamaguchi, I. Nakao, A. Okitsu, and S. Asahina, "Efficacy and safety of ipragliflozin as add-on therapy to insulin in Japanese patients with type 2 diabetes mellitus (IOLITE): a multi-centre, randomized, placebo-controlled, double-blind study," *Diabetes, Obesity and Metabolism*, vol. 18, no. 12, pp. 1207–1216, 2016.

[40] N. Inagaki, S.-I. Harashima, N. Maruyama, Y. Kawaguchi, M. Goda, and H. Iijima, "Efficacy and safety of canagliflozin

in combination with insulin: A double-blind, randomized, placebo-controlled study in Japanese patients with type 2 diabetes mellitus," *Cardiovascular Diabetology*, vol. 15, no. 1, 2016.

[41] N. Inagaki, S.-I. Harashima, K. Kaku et al., "Long-term efficacy and safety of canagliflozin in combination with insulin in Japanese patients with type 2 diabetes mellitus," *Diabetes, Obesity and Metabolism*, vol. 20, no. 4, pp. 812–820, 2018.

[42] J. P. H. Wilding, V. Woo, K. Rohwedder, J. Sugg, and S. Parikh, "Dapagliflozin in patients with type 2 diabetes receiving high doses of insulin: efficacy and safety over 2 years," *Diabetes, Obesity and Metabolism*, vol. 16, no. 2, pp. 124–136, 2014.

[43] J. Rosenstock, A. Jelaska, G. Frappin et al., "Improved glucose control with weight loss, lower insulin doses, and no increased hypoglycemia with empagliflozin added to titrated multiple daily injections of insulin in obese inadequately controlled type 2 diabetes," *Diabetes Care*, vol. 37, no. 7, pp. 1815–1823, 2014.

[44] J. Rosenstock, A. Jelaska, C. Zeller, G. Kim, U. C. Broedl, and H. J. Woerle, "Impact of empagliflozin added on to basal insulin in type 2 diabetes inadequately controlled on basal insulin: A 78-week randomized, double-blind, placebo-controlled trial," *Diabetes, Obesity and Metabolism*, vol. 17, no. 10, pp. 936–948, 2015.

[45] T. R. Pieber, S. Famulla, J. Eilbracht et al., "Empagliflozin as adjunct to insulin in patients with type 1 diabetes: A 4-week, randomized, placebo-controlled trial (EASE-1)," *Diabetes, Obesity and Metabolism*, vol. 17, no. 10, pp. 928–935, 2015.

[46] E. Araki, Y. Onishi, M. Asano, H. Kim, and T. Yajima, "Efficacy and safety of dapagliflozin over 1 year as add-on to insulin therapy in Japanese patients with type 2 diabetes: the DAISY (Dapagliflozin Added to patients under InSulin therapY) trial," *Diabetes, Obesity and Metabolism*, vol. 19, no. 4, pp. 562–570, 2017.

[47] G. Das, A. Surya, and H. Abusahmin, "Use of dapagliflozin as an add-on to insulin therapy in patients with suboptimally controlled type 2 diabetes," *Therapeutic Advances in Endocrinology and Metabolism*, vol. 9, no. 8, pp. 269-270, 2018.

[48] Y. Terauchi, M. Tamura, M. Senda, R. Gunji, and K. Kaku, "Long-term safety and efficacy of tofogliflozin as add-on to insulin in patients with type 2 diabetes: Results from a 52-week, multicentre, randomized, double-blind, open-label extension, Phase 4 study in Japan (J-STEP/INS)," *Diabetes, Obesity and Metabolism*, vol. 20, no. 5, pp. 1176–1185, 2018.

[49] B. Neal, V. Perkovic, D. De Zeeuw et al., "Efficacy and safety of canagliflozin, an inhibitor of sodium-glucose cotransporter 2, when used in conjunction with insulin therapy in patients with type 2 diabetes," *Diabetes Care*, vol. 38, no. 3, pp. 403–411, 2015.

[50] E. Araki, Y. Onishi, M. Asano et al., "Efficacy and safety of dapagliflozin in addition to insulin therapy in Japanese patients with type 2 diabetes: Results of the interim analysis of 16-week double-blind treatment period," *Journal of Diabetes Investigation*, vol. 7, no. 4, pp. 555–564, 2016.

[51] K. Suzuki, Y. Mitsuma, T. Sato, T. Anraku, and M. Hatta, "Comparison of combined tofogliflozin and glargine, tofogliflozin added to insulin, and insulin dose-increase therapy in uncontrolled type 2 diabetes," *Journal of Clinical Medicine Research*, vol. 8, no. 11, pp. 805–814, 2016.

[52] C. Mathieu, P. Dandona, P. Gillard et al., "Efficacy and safety of dapagliflozin in patients with inadequately controlled type 1 diabetes (the depict-2 study): 24-week results from a randomized controlled trial," *Diabetes Care*, vol. 41, no. 9, pp. 1938–1946, 2018.

[53] E. Ferrannini, E. Muscelli, S. Frascerra et al., "Metabolic response to sodium-glucose cotransporter 2 inhibition in type 2 diabetic patients," *The Journal of Clinical Investigation*, vol. 124, no. 2, pp. 499–508, 2014.

[54] W. Ogawa and K. Sakaguchi, "Euglycemic diabetic ketoacidosis induced by SGLT2 inhibitors: Possible mechanism and contributing factors," *Journal of Diabetes Investigation*, vol. 7, no. 2, pp. 135–138, 2016.

[55] R. M. Goldenberg, L. D. Berard, A. Y. Cheng et al., "SGLT2 inhibitor–associated diabetic ketoacidosis: clinical review and recommendations for prevention and diagnosis," *Clinical Therapeutics*, vol. 38, no. 12, pp. 2654–2664.e1, 2016.

[56] J. Rosenstock and E. Ferrannini, "Euglycemic diabetic ketoacidosis: a predictable, detectable, and preventable safety concern with SGLT2 inhibitors," *Diabetes Care*, vol. 38, no. 9, pp. 1638–1642, 2015.

50

Overcoming Barriers to Diabetes Technology in Youth with Type 1 Diabetes and Public Insurance: Cases and Call to Action

Ming Yeh Lee, Molly L. Tanenbaum, David M. Maahs, and Priya Prahalad

Division of Pediatric Endocrinology, Stanford University School of Medicine, Standford, CA, USA

Correspondence should be addressed to Priya Prahalad; prahalad@stanford.edu

Academic Editor: Wayne V. Moore

Advancements in diabetes technology such as continuous glucose monitoring (CGM), insulin pumps, and automated insulin delivery provide opportunities to improve glycemic control for youth with type 1 diabetes (T1D). However, diabetes technology use is lower in youth on public insurance, and this technology use gap is widening in the US. There is a significant need to develop effective interventions and policies to promote equitable care. The dual purpose of this case series is as follows: (1) describe success stories of the CGM Time in Range Program (CGM TIPs), which removed barriers for initiating CGM and provided asynchronous remote glucose monitoring for youth on public insurance, and (2) advocate for improving CGM coverage by public insurance. We describe a series of six youths with T1D and public insurance who obtained and sustained use of CGM with assistance from the program. Three youths had improved engagement with the care team while on CGM and the remote monitoring protocol, and three youths were able to leverage sustained CGM wear to obtain insurance coverage for automated insulin delivery systems. CGM TIPs helped these youths achieve lower hemoglobin A1c and improved time in range (TIR). Despite the successes, expansion of CGM TIPs is limited by stringent barriers for CGM approval and difficult postapproval patient workflows to receive shipments. These cases highlight the potential for combining diabetes technology and asynchronous remote monitoring to support continued use and provide education to improve glycemic control for youth with T1D on public insurance and the need to reduce barriers for obtaining CGM coverage by public insurance.

1. Introduction

Sustained use of diabetes technology, such as continuous glucose monitoring (CGM) and insulin pumps, improves glycemic outcomes in youth with type 1 diabetes (T1D), thereby reducing the risk for short-term and long-term complications [1–10]. The 2021 American Diabetes Association (ADA) standards of care expanded recommendation of CGM use to all people with diabetes on rapid-acting insulin [11], and the International Society of Pediatric and Adolescent Diabetes (ISPAD) 2018 guidelines encourage CGM use [8]. Additionally, social determinants of health (SDOH) are increasingly acknowledged as an important target to achieve equity in diabetes care [12]. In the United States, diabetes technology use is lower in youth of lower socioeconomic status (SES), and the gap of technology use between the highest and lowest SES groups has widened in the past decade [13–16]. The disparity may be, at least in part, due to restrictions in coverage for CGM by public insurance [17]. Our study focuses on public insurance coverage by California Children's Services (CCS), a Medicaid supplement for children in California with certain chronic health conditions, including diabetes. Youth with CCS need to demonstrate four or more self-monitored blood glucose (SMBG) checks daily for a month for CGM approval, a requirement that does not exist for privately insured youth. Insulin pump approval requires four SMBG checks daily or consistent CGM use, which is typically ≥70% wear based on our experience. These requirements present systemic barriers to technology adoption in youth on public insurance and contribute to the disparity. The purpose of this case series is as follows: (1) describe success stories of the CGM Time in Range Program (CGM TIPs), which removed barriers for initiating diabetes technology and provided asynchronous remote glucose monitoring for youth on public insurance, and (2) advocate for improving CGM coverage by public insurance to improve diabetes care and as a gateway to automated insulin delivery (AID). Specifically, this case series highlights an urgent need to remove systemic barriers causing disparity to access diabetes technology, while larger scale studies on this topic are ongoing.

2. Methods

The six youths in this case series were identified by pediatric endocrinologists and clinical diabetes care and education specialists (CDCES) as having CCS and being unable to meet CCS criteria for CGM coverage or having inconsistent CGM coverage. The youths were enrolled in an IRB-approved clinical research program called CGM TIPs, which supports youth with T1D and public insurance to initiate and sustain CGM use. Philanthropic funding for this program allowed us to provide CGM supplies for initial weeks, while clinic staff assisted families to obtain insurance coverage for further supplies. For interested families who have met the CCS requirement to qualify for an insulin pump, which includes CGM wear for at least one month, the program also assisted families in obtaining insurance coverage for insulin pumps and AID systems. CDCES remotely reviewed youths' CGM data monthly and provided diabetes education and dose adjustments as needed according to previously published protocol from the 4T study [18]. Hemoglobin A1c (HbA1c) was also monitored quarterly per routine care.

3. Case

Youth 1 is a 14-year-old male with a four-year history of T1D on SMBG and multiple daily injection (MDI) insulin. His HbA1c was 12.1% prior to CGM TIPs. Barriers to diabetes management included that his family is primarily Spanish-speaking, had limited understanding of diabetes, and were not comfortable using smartphones. He did not like checking fingerstick glucoses, and the team was concerned that he was bolusing insulin without checking his blood glucose. In addition, his mother aimed to keep bedtime glucose above target range (>200 mg/dL) due to her worry about overnight hypoglycemia.

Outcome: with CGM TIPs, he obtained and sustained on CGM. He preferred using the sensor compared to SMBG and began taking insulin more consistently. The CGM data provided reassurance for his mother's fear of hypoglycemia, leading to increased time in target range. Seven months into CGM TIPs, his HbA1c improved to 7.1% with CGM TIR 65.

Youth 2 is a 20-year-old female with T1D for five years and Hashimoto thyroiditis. She did not like SMBG checks and struggled with consistent insulin injections. Her HbA1c was in the range of 9.3–14% prior to CGM TIPs. She lives with her father, who has not been involved with her diabetes care. As a high school student, she benefitted from school nurse support to ensure consistent insulin injections. Since graduating from high school, she no longer has a school nurse as a resource. She experiences difficulty obtaining diabetes supplies consistently from the pharmacy and reports challenges with bolusing consistently. She is successful at consistent delivery of long-acting insulin.

Outcome: since enrollment in CGM TIPs, she is more engaged in her diabetes care and discusses CGM data and diabetes management frequently with CDCES through the remote monitoring program. Six months into CGM TIPs, her HbA1c improved to 7.1% with CGM TIR 53%. As she transitions off CCS insurance after 21 years of age, continuing CGM coverage will likely be challenging.

Youth 3 is an 18-year-old female with T1D for four years with HbA1c persistently >14% prior to CGM TIPs. The youth's mother had a history of substance abuse and homelessness; she died soon after the youth's T1D diagnosis. This youth's family is primarily Spanish-speaking, so she manages calls with insurance and medical equipment suppliers. Since graduating high school, she no longer has access to school nurse support to promote consistent SMBG and boluses.

Outcome: nine months since enrolling in CGMTIPs, her HbA1c improved steadily to 6.3% with CGM TIR 82%. She was briefly off CGM due to device malfunction and running out of supplies early. The program bridged the gap with supplies until she received new supplies.

Youth 4 is a 17-year-old female with T1D for nine years and a history of disordered eating. For the past several years, she has lacked support and supervision at home for diabetes management. She had sole responsibility for SMBG, dosing insulin and obtaining diabetes supplies. She was on CGM with an AID system intermittently prior to CGM TIPs, but had several lapses in her supplies due to difficulty navigating the healthcare system to obtain refills. Her HbA1c ranged 12–13% when she was off CGM and reverted to open loop and improved to 9–10% on the AID system prior to CGM TIPs. Her CGM TIR varied widely from 19% to 65%.

Outcome: with coaching from CDCES through CGM TIPs, she gained healthcare navigation skills such as knowing when and how to contact device companies when devices malfunction, which enabled her to maintain access to supplies. She now consistently uses her AID system, and her latest HbA1c was 7.7% and CGM TIR was 62%.

Youth 5 is a 15-year-old male with a five-year history of T1D, as well as asthma, eosinophilic esophagitis, and celiac disease. Prior to CGM TIPs, his HbA1c was >14%, and he had nine intensive care admissions for diabetic ketoacidosis (DKA) in the past 2 years. Lack of stable housing and co-occurring anxiety and depression presented major challenges to this youth's diabetes management. Based on assessment from the clinical team, family barriers included limited health literacy and communication skills to navigate the healthcare system. SMBG, insulin doses, and clinic appointments occurred less frequently than recommended.

Outcome: through CGM TIPs, he initiated CGM and subsequently an AID system. He became more engaged in his diabetes care, including responding to high glucose alerts on his CGM with correction doses, bolusing for carbohydrates, and responding to CDCES messages to adjust insulin pump settings. His HbA1c improved to 11.5% with CGM TIR 32%. He has had no DKA admissions in the seven months since enrollment in CGM TIPs, despite having

COVID-19. His family developed a strong therapeutic alliance with the care team and continues to have frequent contact with his primary CDCES and social worker.

Youth 6 is a 14-year-old male with T1D for five years and attention deficit hyperactivity disorder. He had three DKA admissions in the past year, during which he did not attend any clinic appointments. Prior to CGM TIPs, his HbA1c ranged 9.7–12%. Family was interested in CGM, but he was unable to meet CCS criteria of four SMBG checks daily. He was resistant to wearing CGM sensors and removed them due to discomfort.

Outcome: after CDCES worked closely with him to discuss benefits of CGM and optimize comfort, he has worn the sensor consistently for 10 months. He subsequently obtained an AID system through CCS. His HbA1c improved to 8.3%, with CGM TIR 39%, and he had no additional DKA admissions. Although CGM TIPs facilitated initiation of technology, the family continues to have difficulty navigating the healthcare system to sustain supplies, such as responding to supplier phone calls. The program has bridged the gaps by providing supplies and coaching the family on communication skills to maintain supplies.

4. Discussion

This case series demonstrates how six youths on public insurance with suboptimal management of T1D benefitted from CGM TIPs, a program that reduced barriers to CGM access and use, provided asynchronous remote glucose monitoring, and increased multidisciplinary team support for troubleshooting diabetes management. These cases identify how the program supported them to initiate and sustain diabetes technology with subsequent improvements in glycemic control. Based on our experience with CGM TIPs and in alignment with the most recent ADA Standards of Care [11] and ISPAD guidelines [8], we recommend changes in the US public insurance policies to cover CGM for youths with diabetes and without unrealistic barriers for initiation, similar to many other countries [10, 19–21].

CGM TIPs removed barriers to CGM initiation for youths with public insurance by providing CGM and CDCES support. We found associated improvement in engagement with care, reduction in HbA1c, sustained CGM use, and decrease in DKA admissions. In this case series, we observed reduction in fear of hypoglycemia, which is a previously described benefit of CGM technology [22]. The remote monitoring program provided frequent short touchpoints for CDCES to help families troubleshoot diabetes management issues and learn to navigate the health system, such as calling suppliers monthly to reorder supplies, reaching out to suppliers for replacements, and contacting the diabetes team for medical issues. We also observed reduction in gaps in CGM supplies. Interruptions in CGM use in youth with public insurance is primarily due to gaps in insurance coverage and is associated with increased HbA1c [9]. CGM TIPs addressed this barrier by bridging gaps in supplies with philanthropic funding. All youths in this case series demonstrated reduction in HbA1c after enrollment in CGM TIPs, including impressive reductions from >14% to 7%. Two youths with prior frequent DKA admissions have had no admissions since CGM TIPs initiation.

SDOH are essential intervention targets to achieve equity in diabetes care [12]. Financial cost is a major obstacle to diabetes technology use [23]. In the US, youths of lower SES on public insurance are unlikely to afford CGM and insulin pumps without insurance coverage. They are also especially at risk for having low health literacy and technology literacy [24, 25]. Many of these youths also come from non-English speaking families or lack resources such as stable housing, transportation, and Internet connection. These factors contribute to challenges engaging with care and obtaining diabetes technology. Currently, CCS coverage for CGM requires demonstration of >4 SMBG checks daily for a month. This is an outdated policy given the most recent ADA [11] and ISPAD guidelines [8] and an unnecessary hurdle as CGM provides more data and safety without requiring finger sticks. The process of navigating the insurance system is especially challenging for non-English speaking families and youth without adequate family support. Currently, CGM TIPs has philanthropic support to supply CGMs for families until insurance coverage is approved and to bridge supplies during gaps in insurance coverage. Scalability of this program depends on removal of outdated criteria for CGM coverage by public insurance, reducing friction for obtaining supplies, and adequate support for youths and their families.

CGM use is a gateway to an AID system, a technology that can help youths achieve even better glycemic control with less burden of care [5, 26–28]. Real-world data evaluating youths on an AID system demonstrated decreased HbA1c over six months, with the greatest HbA1c decrease in participants with the highest baseline HbA1c [29]. Historically, many practices restricted access to diabetes technology to youths who were not checking SMBG regularly or who had elevated HbA1c due to concerns of risk of DKA. However, more recent data suggest lower rates of severe hypoglycemia and DKA with CGM and pumps [30, 31]. Unrestricted CGM coverage for youths with T1D on public insurance improves engagement and provides a gateway to obtaining AID systems to improve their diabetes management.

Authors' Contributions

Ming Yeh Lee drafted the initial manuscript and reviewed and revised the manuscript. Molly L Tanenbaum and Jeannine Leverenz reviewed and revised the manuscript. Priya Prahalad and David M Maahs designed the study and reviewed and revised the manuscript. The 4T study group CDCES identified and started youths on CGMs. Jeannine Leverenz, Piper Sagan, and Anjoli Martinez-Singh performed CGM data remote monitoring. Brianna Leverenz coordinated youth recruitment to the 4T study.

Acknowledgments

The authors would like to thank the other members of the 4T Study Group (David Scheinker, PhD, Manisha Desai, PhD,

Korey Hood, PhD, Ananta Addala, DO, Ramesh Johari, PhD, Dessi Zaharieva, PhD, Franziska Bishop, MS, CDCES, Brianna Leverenz, BS, Julie Hooper MPH, RD, Ana Cortes, BS, Alex Freeman, NP, Natalie Pageler, MD, Jeannine Leverenz, RN, CDCES, Piper Sagan, RN, CDCES, Anjoli Martinez-Singh, RD, CDCES, Barry Conrad RD, CDCES, Annette Chmielewski, RD, CDCES, Julie Senaldi RN, CDCES, Nora Arrizon-Ruiz, Erica Pang, BS, Carolyn Herrera, BS, Victoria Ding, MS, Rebecca Gardner, MS, Simrat Ghuman, PhD, and Esli Osmanlliu, MD) for their help with this project. The authors thank the numerous SURF team (David Scheinker, Oseas Oyardi, Angela Gu, Josh Grossman, Jacqualine Jil Valon, Anastasiya Vitko, Dianelys Perez Morales, Daniel Jun, Ryan Leonard, Michael Zikai Gao, Annie Chang, Prashant Yadav, Isha Thapa, and Johannes Opsahl Ferstad) that contributed to the development and deployment of the technology that facilitated remote data review. This study was funded in part by the Stanford Diabetes Research Center (P30DK116074 and R18 DK122422) and by a grant through the Lucile Packard Children's Hospital Auxiliaries Endowment for CGM supplies.

References

[1] K. K. Hood, C. M. Peterson, J. M. Rohan, and D. Drotar, "Association between adherence and glycemic control in pediatric type 1 diabetes: a meta-analysis," *Pediatrics*, vol. 124, no. 6, pp. e1171–e1179, 2009.

[2] H.-C. Yeh, T. T. Brown, N. Maruthur et al., "Comparative effectiveness and safety of methods of insulin delivery and glucose monitoring for diabetes mellitus," *Annals of Internal Medicine*, vol. 157, no. 5, pp. 336–347, 2012.

[3] A. L. Brorsson, G. Viklund, E. Örtqvist, and A. Lindholm Olinder, "Does treatment with an insulin pump improve glycaemic control in children and adolescents with type 1 diabetes? a retrospective case-control study," *Pediatric Diabetes*, vol. 16, no. 7, pp. 546–553, 2015.

[4] S. Rosenlund, T. W. Hansen, S. Andersen, and P. Rossing, "Effect of 4 years subcutaneous insulin infusion treatment on albuminuria, kidney function and HbA1ccompared with multiple daily injections: a longitudinal follow-up study," *Diabetic Medicine*, vol. 32, no. 11, pp. 1445–1452, 2015.

[5] A. Weisman, J.-W. Bai, M. Cardinez, C. K. Kramer, and B. A. Perkins, "Effect of artificial pancreas systems on glycaemic control in patients with type 1 diabetes: a systematic review and meta-analysis of outpatient randomised controlled trials," *Lancet Diabetes & Endocrinology*, vol. 5, no. 7, pp. 501–512, 2017.

[6] L. M. Laffel, L. G. Kanapka, R. W. Beck et al., "Effect of continuous glucose monitoring on glycemic control in adolescents and young adults with type 1 diabetes," *JAMA*, vol. 323, no. 23, pp. 2388–2396, 2020.

[7] A. Szypowska, A. Schwandt, J. Svensson et al., "Insulin pump therapy in children with type 1 diabetes: analysis of data from the SWEET registry," *Pediatric Diabetes*, vol. 17, no. S23, pp. 38–45, 2016.

[8] J. L. Sherr, M. Tauschmann, T. Battelino et al., "ISPAD clinical practice consensus guidelines 2018: diabetes technologies," *Pediatric Diabetes*, vol. 19, no. 27, pp. 302–325, 2018.

[9] A. Addala, D. M. Maahs, D. Scheinker, S. Chertow, B. Leverenz, and P. Prahalad, "Uninterrupted continuous glucose monitoring access is associated with a decrease in HbA1c in youth with type 1 diabetes and public insurance," *Pediatric Diabetes*, vol. 21, no. 7, pp. 1301–1309, 2020.

[10] Z. Šumník, M. Pavlíková, R. Pomahačová et al., "Use of continuous glucose monitoring and its association with type 1 diabetes control in children over the first 3 years of reimbursement approval: population data from the ČENDA registry," *Pediatric Diabetes*, vol. 22, no. 3, pp. 439–447, 2021.

[11] American Diabetes Association, "7. Diabetes technology: standards of medical care in diabetes-2021," *Diabetes Care*, vol. 44, pp. S85–S99, 2021.

[12] F. Hill-Briggs, N. E. Adler, S. A. Berkowitz et al., "Social determinants of health and diabetes: a scientific review," *Diabetes Care*, vol. 44, no. 1, pp. 258–279, 2021.

[13] N. C. Foster, R. W. Beck, K. M. Miller et al., "State of type 1 diabetes management and outcomes from the T1D exchange in 2016-2018," *Diabetes Technology & Therapeutics*, vol. 21, no. 2, pp. 66–72, 2019.

[14] M. H. Lin, C. G. Connor, K. J. Ruedy et al., "Race, socioeconomic status, and treatment center are associated with insulin pump therapy in youth in the first year following diagnosis of type 1 diabetes," *Diabetes Technology & Therapeutics*, vol. 15, no. 11, pp. 929–934, 2013.

[15] A. Addala, M. Auzanneau, K. Miller et al., "A decade of disparities in diabetes technology use and HbA1c in pediatric type 1 diabetes: a transatlantic comparison," *Diabetes Care*, vol. 44, no. 1, pp. 133–140, 2021.

[16] K. M. Miller, R. W. Beck, N. C. Foster, and D. M. Maahs, "HbA1c levels in type 1 diabetes from early childhood to older adults: a deeper dive into the influence of technology and socioeconomic status on HbA1c in the T1D exchange clinic registry findings," *Diabetes Technology & Therapeutics*, vol. 22, no. 9, pp. 645–650, 2020.

[17] J. E. Anderson, J. R. Gavin, and D. F. Kruger, "Current eligibility requirements for CGM coverage are harmful, costly, and unjustified," *Diabetes Technology & Therapeutics*, vol. 22, no. 3, pp. 169–173, 2020.

[18] P. Prahalad, D. P. Zaharieva, A. Addala et al., "Improving clinical outcomes in newly diagnosed pediatric type 1 diabetes: teamwork, targets, technology, and tight control-the 4T study," *Frontiers Endocrinology*, vol. 11, p. 360, 2020.

[19] Health and Aged Care, "58,000 type 1 diabetics to have free access to new glucose monitoring device," 2020, https://www.health.gov.au/ministers/the-hon-greg-hunt-mp/media/58000-type-1-diabetics-to-have-free-access-to-new-glucose-monitoring-device.

[20] *Continuous Glucose Monitoring (CGM)*, Diabetes UK, London, UK, 2021, https://www.diabetes.org.uk/guide-to-diabetes/managing-your-diabetes/testing/continuous-glucose-monitoring-cgm.

[21] C. Graham, "Continuous glucose monitoring and global reimbursement: an update," *Diabetes Technology & Therapeutics*, vol. 19, no. S3, pp. S60–S66, 2017.

[22] T. C. Walker and C. B. Yucha, "Continuous glucose monitors," *Journal of Diabetes Science and Technology*, vol. 8, no. 3, pp. 488–493, 2014.

[23] A. F. Walker, K. K. Hood, M. J. Gurka et al., "Barriers to technology use and endocrinology care for underserved communities with type 1 diabetes," *Diabetes Care*, vol. 44, no. 7, pp. 1480–1490, 2021.

[24] R. V. Rikard, M. S. Thompson, J. McKinney, and A. Beauchamp, "Examining health literacy disparities in the United States: a third look at the national assessment of adult literacy (NAAL)," *BMC Public Health*, vol. 16, no. 1, p. 975, 2016.

[25] C. R. Lyles, R. M. Wachter, and U. Sarkar, "Focusing on digital health equity," *JAMA*, vol. 326, no. 18, pp. 1795-1796, 2021.

[26] L. Ekhlaspour, G. P. Forlenza, D. Chernavvsky et al., "Closed loop control in adolescents and children during winter sports: use of the tandem control-IQ AP system," *Pediatric Diabetes*, vol. 20, no. 6, pp. 759–768, 2019.

[27] E. Bekiari, K. Kitsios, H. Thabit et al., "Artificial pancreas treatment for outpatients with type 1 diabetes: systematic review and meta-analysis," *BMJ*, vol. 361, Article ID k1310, 2018.

[28] X. Dai, Z.-C. Luo, L. Zhai, W.-P. Zhao, and F. Huang, "Artificial pancreas as an effective and safe alternative in patients with type 1 diabetes mellitus: a systematic review and meta-analysis," *Diabetes Therapy*, vol. 9, no. 3, pp. 1269–1277, 2018.

[29] C. Berget, L. H. Messer, T. Vigers et al., "Six months of hybrid closed loop in the real-world: an evaluation of children and young adults using the 670G system," *Pediatric Diabetes*, vol. 21, no. 2, pp. 310–318, 2020.

[30] B. Karges, A. Schwandt, B. Heidtmann et al., "Association of insulin pump therapy vs insulin injection therapy with severe hypoglycemia, ketoacidosis, and glycemic control among children, adolescents, and young adults with type 1 diabetes," *JAMA*, vol. 318, no. 14, pp. 1358–1366, 2017.

[31] M. Tauschmann, J. M. Hermann, C. Freiberg et al., "Reduction in diabetic ketoacidosis and severe hypoglycemia in pediatric type 1 diabetes during the first year of continuous glucose monitoring: a multicenter analysis of 3,553 subjects from the dpv registry," *Diabetes Care*, vol. 43, no. 3, pp. e40–e42, 2020.

Permissions

All chapters in this book were first published by Hindawi Publishing Corporation; hereby published with permission under the Creative Commons Attribution License or equivalent. Every chapter published in this book has been scrutinized by our experts. Their significance has been extensively debated. The topics covered herein carry significant findings which will fuel the growth of the discipline. They may even be implemented as practical applications or may be referred to as a beginning point for another development.

The contributors of this book come from diverse backgrounds, making this book a truly international effort. This book will bring forth new frontiers with its revolutionizing research information and detailed analysis of the nascent developments around the world.

We would like to thank all the contributing authors for lending their expertise to make the book truly unique. They have played a crucial role in the development of this book. Without their invaluable contributions this book wouldn't have been possible. They have made vital efforts to compile up to date information on the varied aspects of this subject to make this book a valuable addition to the collection of many professionals and students.

This book was conceptualized with the vision of imparting up-to-date information and advanced data in this field. To ensure the same, a matchless editorial board was set up. Every individual on the board went through rigorous rounds of assessment to prove their worth. After which they invested a large part of their time researching and compiling the most relevant data for our readers.

The editorial board has been involved in producing this book since its inception. They have spent rigorous hours researching and exploring the diverse topics which have resulted in the successful publishing of this book. They have passed on their knowledge of decades through this book. To expedite this challenging task, the publisher supported the team at every step. A small team of assistant editors was also appointed to further simplify the editing procedure and attain best results for the readers.

Apart from the editorial board, the designing team has also invested a significant amount of their time in understanding the subject and creating the most relevant covers. They scrutinized every image to scout for the most suitable representation of the subject and create an appropriate cover for the book.

The publishing team has been an ardent support to the editorial, designing and production team. Their endless efforts to recruit the best for this project, has resulted in the accomplishment of this book. They are a veteran in the field of academics and their pool of knowledge is as vast as their experience in printing. Their expertise and guidance has proved useful at every step. Their uncompromising quality standards have made this book an exceptional effort. Their encouragement from time to time has been an inspiration for everyone.

The publisher and the editorial board hope that this book will prove to be a valuable piece of knowledge for researchers, students, practitioners and scholars across the globe.

List of Contributors

Mathilde Sollier, Marine Halbron, Olivier Bourron, Marie Bastin, Héléna Mosbah, Agnès Hartemann, Fabrizio Andreelli and Chloé Amouyal
Diabetology-Metabolism Dpt, Sorbonne Université, APHP, Institut Hospitalo-Universitaire de Cardiometabolisme et Nutrition (ICAN), Pitié-Salpêtrière-Charles Foix Hospital, 75013 Paris, France

Jean Donadieu
Hemato-Oncology Dpt, Trousseau Hospital, APHP, 75012 Paris, France

Ahmed Idbaih
Sorbonne Université, Inserm, CNRS, UMRS 1127, Institut du Cerveau et de la Moelle épinière, ICM, AP-HP, Hôpitaux Universitaires La Pitié Salpêtrière -Charles Foix, Service de Neurologie 2, Mazarin, 75013 Paris, France

Fleur Cohen Aubart
Department of Internal Medicine 2, Sorbonne Université, APHP, Institut Hospitalo-Universitaire de Cardiometabolisme et Nutrition (ICAN), Pitié-Salpêtrière-Charles Foix Hospital, 75013 Paris, France

Corinne Vigouroux and Martine Auclair
Inserm UMRS 938, Centre de Recherche Saint-Antoine, Sorbonne Université, Reference Center for Rare Diseases of Insulin Secretion and Insulin Sensitivity, Institut Hospitalo-Universitaire de Cardiometabolisme et Nutrition (ICAN), Paris, APHP, Saint Antoine Hospital, Paris, France

Géraldine Béra
Nuclear Medicine Dpt, Sorbonne Université, APHP, Pitié-Salpêtrière-Charles Foix Hospital, 75013 Paris, France

Philippe Touraine
Department of Endocrinology and Reproductive Medicine, Pitié-Salpêtrière Hospital, APHP, Reference Center for Rare Endocrine Diseases of Growth, Reference Center for Rare Gynecological Pathologies, Institut Hospitalo-Universitaire de Cardiometabolisme et Nutrition (ICAN), Sorbonne University, 75013 Paris, France
Pitié-Salpêtrière-Charles Foix Hospital, 75013 Paris, France

Jacques Young
Reproductive Endocrinology Department, Paris Sud University, APHP, Le Kremlin-Bicêtre, 94275, France

Soheila Torabiyan, Behnam Dalfardi and Mojgan Sanjari
Endocrinology and Metabolism Research Center, Institute of Basic and Clinical Physiology Sciences, Kerman University of Medical Sciences, Kerman, Iran

Yotsapon Thewjitcharoen, Ekgaluck Wanothayaroj, Haruethai Jaita, Soontaree Nakasatien, Siriwan Butadej, Waralee Chatchomchuan, Sirinate Krittiyawong and Thep Himathongkam
Diabetes and Thyroid Center, Theptarin Hospital, Bangkok, Thailand

Ishant Khurana and Scott Maxwell
Epigenetics in Human Health and Disease Laboratory, Department of Diabetes, Central Clinical School, Faculty of Medicine Nursing and Health Sciences, Monash University, Melbourne, Australia

Assam El-Osta
Epigenetics in Human Health and Disease Laboratory, Department of Diabetes, Central Clinical School, Faculty of Medicine Nursing and Health Sciences, Monash University, Melbourne, Australia
Hong Kong Institute of Diabetes and Obesity, Prince of Wales Hospital, The Chinese University of Hong Kong, Hong Kong, China
University College Copenhagen, Faculty of Health, Department of Technology, Biomedical Laboratory Science, Copenhagen, Denmark

Zeinab Alnahas
Department of Internal Medicine, Cairo University, Giza, Egypt

Mohamad H. Horani
Chandler Regional Medical Center, AZ 1955 W Frye Rd, Chandler, AZ 85224, USA

Wanling Zeng and Joan Khoo
Department of Endocrinology, Changi General Hospital, 2 Simei Street 3 529889, Singapore

Eleni Papadokostaki
Emergency Department, General Hospital of Heraklion "Venizeleio-Pananeio," Heraklion, 71409, Greece

Evangelos Liberopoulos
Department of Internal Medicine, Faculty of Medicine, University of Ioannina, Ioannina, 45110, Greece

Soji Toda, Hiroyuki Iwasaki, Nobuyasu Suganuma and Daisuke Murayama
Department of Breast and Endocrine Surgery, Kanagawa Cancer Center, Yokohama, Japan

Yoichiro Okubo and Tomoyuki Yokose
Department of Pathology, Kanagawa Cancer Center, Yokohama, Japan

Katsuhiko Masudo
Department of Breast and Thyroid Surgery, Yokohama City University Medical Center, Yokohama, Japan

Hirotaka Nakayama and Munetaka Masuda
Department of Surgery, Yokohama City University School of Medicine, Yokohama, Japan

Prachi Rana
Department of Internal Medicine, Los Angeles County Hospital/University of Southern California, USA

Brian Kim
Department of Gastroenterology and Liver Diseases, Los Angeles County Hospital/University of Southern California, USA

Michelle N. Lee, WingYee Wan and Maria I. Kravchenko
Department of Medicine, Department of Endocrinology, San Antonio Military Medical Center, 3551 Roger Brooke Drive, JBSA Fort Sam Houston, San Antonio, TX 78234, USA

Dianna C. Chormanski
Department of Pathology, San Antonio Military Medical Center, 3551 Roger Brooke Drive, JBSA Fort Sam Houston, San Antonio, TX 78234, USA

N. Messaoudi, N. Bouichrat, M. Karrou, I. Assarrar and S. Rouf
Department of Endocrinology-Diabetology and Nutrition, Mohammed VI University Hospital Center, Faculty of Medicine and Pharmacy, University of Mohammed 1st, Oujda, Morocco

S. Malki and N. Karich
Department of Anatomical Pathology, Mohammed VI University Hospital Center, Faculty of Medicine and Pharmacy, University of Mohammed 1st, Oujda, Morocco

S. Elmahjoubi and A. Lachkar
Department of Orthopedic Surgery B, Mohammed VI University Hospital Center, Faculty of Medicine and Pharmacy, University of Mohammed 1st, Oujda, Morocco

S. Sefiani
AGDAL Anatomical Pathology Center, Rabat, Morocco

M. Bouziane
Department of General Surgery, Mohammed VI University Hospital Center, Faculty of Medicine and Pharmacy, University of Mohammed 1st, Oujda, Morocco

I. Kamaoui
Department of Radiology, Mohammed VI University Hospital Center, Faculty of Medicine and Pharmacy, University of Mohammed 1st, Oujda, Morocco

Firas Warda and Marilu Jurado-Flores
Division of Endocrinology, Diabetes, and Metabolism, University of Florida College of Medicine-Jacksonville, Jacksonville, FL 32209, USA
Department of Medicine, University of Florida College of Medicine-Jacksonville, Jacksonville, FL 32209, USA

Sam Ho and Enoch Kuo
Department of Pathology, Immunology and Laboratory Medicine, University of Florida College of Medicine-Gainesville, Gainesville, FL 32610, USA

Dinesh Rao
Department of Radiology, University of Florida College of Medicine-Jacksonville, Jacksonville, FL 32209, USA

W. Benothman, G. Saad, M. Kacem and K. Ach
Endocrinology Unit, Department of Endocrinology, Farhat Hached University Hospital, Avenue Ibn El Jazzar, Sousse 4000, Tunisia

Gerdi Tuli, Jessica Munarin, Daniele Tessaris, Raffaele Buganza, Patrizia Matarazzo and Luisa De Sanctis
Department of Pediatric Endocrinology, Regina Margherita Children's Hospital of Turin, Turin, Italy
Department of Sciences of Public Health and Pediatrics, University of Turin, Turin, Italy

Ibtissem Oueslati, Marwa Ben Jemaa, Meriem Yazidi, Fatma Chaker and Melika Chihaoui
Department of Endocrinology, La Rabta University Hospital, University of Tunis-El Manar, Faculty of Medicine, Tunis, Tunisia

Dinuka S. Warapitiya, W. A. H. P. Sanjeewa and Kushalee Poornima Jayawickreme
Postgraduate Institute of Medicine, University of Colombo, Colombo, Sri Lanka

Dimuthu Muthukuda
Diabetes and Endocrinology Unit, Sri Jayewardenepura General Hospital, Nugegoda, Colombo, Sri Lanka

Shyama Subasinghe
Sri Jayewardenepura General Hospital, Nugegoda, Colombo, Sri Lanka

Toru Sugiyama, Yuriko Sasahara and Eri Hayakawa
Division of Endocrinology and Metabolism, Japanese Red Cross Musashino Hospital, Tokyo, Japan

Hironobu Sasano
Department of Pathology, Tohoku University School of Medicine, Sendai, Miyagi, Japan

R. Daya, F. Seedat, S. Bulbulia and Z. Bayat
Division of Endocrinology and Metabolism, Department of Internal Medicine, Helen Joseph Hospital, 1 Perth Road, Rossmore, Johannesburg, South Africa
Division of Endocrinology and Metabolism, Department of Internal Medicine, Faculty of Health Sciences, School of Clinical Medicine, University of the Witwatersrand, Johannesburg, South Africa

C. Wingfield and P. Sotshononda
Division of Endocrinology and Metabolism, Department of Internal Medicine, Helen Joseph Hospital, 1 Perth Road, Rossmore, Johannesburg, South Africa

M. D. Simmons and M. Louw
Department of Anatomical Pathology, School of Pathology, University of the Witwatersrand, Johannesburg, South Africa

Hiroshi Nomoto, Tatyana Gurlo, Madeline Rosenberger and Peter C. Butler
David Geffen School of Medicine at UCLA, Larry L. Hillblom Islet Research Center, Los Angeles, CA, USA

Mark D. Girgis
David Geffen School of Medicine at UCLA, Department of Surgery, Los Angeles, CA, USA

Sarah Dry
David Geffen School of Medicine at UCLA, Department of Pathology, Los Angeles, CA, USA

Jennifer Apsan and Zoltan Antal
Department of Pediatrics, Division of Endocrinology Weill Cornell Medicine, New York Presbyterian Hospital, New York, NY, USA

Phan Tuong Quynh Le and Thi Minh Thi Ha
Department of Medical Genetics, University of Medicine and Pharmacy, Hue University, Hue, Vietnam
Center of Prenatal and Neonatal Screening-Diagnosis, University of Medicine and Pharmacy Hospital, Hue University, Hue, Vietnam

Thanh Nha Uyen Le
Department of Medical Genetics, University of Medicine and Pharmacy, Hue University, Hue, Vietnam

Thi Thanh Binh Nguyen
Department of Pediatrics, University of Medicine and Pharmacy, Hue University, Hue, Vietnam

Minh Thao Nguyen
Department of Anatomy and Surgical Training, University of Medicine and Pharmacy, Hue University, Hue, Vietnam

Laura Y. Sue
VA Greater Los Angeles Healthcare System and Division of Endocrinology, Diabetes and Hypertension, Department of Medicine, UCLA David Geffen School of Medicine, 900 Veteran Avenue, 24-130 Warren Hall, Los Angeles, CA 90095, USA

Anna Milanesi
Department of Medicine, Veterans Affairs Greater Los Angeles Healthcare System and Division of Endocrinology, Departments of Medicine and Physiology, UCLA David Geffen School of Medicine, 11301 Wilshire Boulevard, Los Angeles, CA 90073, USA

R. El Qadiry, A. Ouayad, H. Nassih, A. Bourrahouat and I. Ait Sab
Pediatric B Department, Mother-Child Pole, Mohammed VI University Hospital, Marrakesh, Morocco

Anika Toor, Amit Toor and Mahesh Krishnamurthy
Department of Internal Medicine, Easton Hospital, Easton, PA 18045, USA

Koroush Khalighi
Drexel University, EP Lab, Easton Hospital, Easton, PA 18045, USA

Hiroyuki Ito and Daiji Nemoto
Department of Respiratory Surgery, Kanagawa Cancer Center, Yokohama, Japan

Hiroyuki Hayashi
Department of Pathology, Yokohama City Hospital, Yokohama, Japan
Department of Pathology, Kanagawa Cancer Center, Yokohama, Japan

Suranut Charoensri, Jin Sothornwit and Chatlert Pongchaiyakul
Division of Endocrinology and Metabolism, Department of Medicine, Faculty of Medicine, Khon Kaen University, Khon Kaen, Thailand

Akeatit Trirattanapikul
Department of Medicine, Faculty of Medicine, Khon Kaen University, Khon Kaen, Thailand

Michelle Romijn and Martijn J. J. Finken
Department of Pediatric Endocrinology, Emma Children's Hospital, Amsterdam UMC, Amsterdam, Netherlands

Leo M. G. Geeraedts Jr.
Department of Surgery, Section Trauma Surgery Amsterdam UMC, Location VUmc, Amsterdam, Netherlands

Jonathan I. M. L. Verbeke
Department of Radiology and Nuclear Medicine, Amsterdam UMC, Location VUmc, Amsterdam, Netherlands

M. Aabdi, O. Es-Saad, K. Malki, H. Bkiyar and B. Housni
Anesthesiology and Intensive Care Unit Department, MOHAMMED VI University Hospital Center, Oujda, Morocco

A. Aarab
Laboratory Unit Department, MOHAMMED VI University Hospital Center, Oujda, Morocco

A. Tahri, W. Abdellaoui, S. Benyakhlef, K. Boujtat, I. Mahroug and S. Rouf
Department of Endocrinology-Diabetology, Mohammed VIth University Hospital, Faculty of Medicine and Pharmacy of Oujda, Mohammed the First University, Oujda, Morocco

I. Kamaoui
Department of Urology, Mohammed VIth University Hospital, Faculty of Medicine and Pharmacy of Oujda, Mohammed the First University, Oujda, Morocco

A. Barki
Department of Radiology, Mohammed VIth University Hospital, Faculty of Medicine and Pharmacy of Oujda, Mohammed the First University, Oujda, Morocco

F. Kellani
United Nations Center of Cytopathology, Rabat, Morocco

H. Latrech
Department of Endocrinology-Diabetology, Mohammed VIth University Hospital, Faculty of Medicine and Pharmacy of Oujda, Mohammed the First University, Oujda, Morocco
Laboratory of Epidemiology, Clinical Research and Public Health, Faculty of Medicine and Pharmacy of Oujda, Mohammed the First University, Oujda, Morocco

Aida Al Jabri
Department of Pediatrics, King Abdulaziz Hospital, Ministry of the National Guard-Health Affairs, King Abdullah International Medical Research Center, King Saud Bin Abdulaziz University for Health Sciences, Al-Ahasa, Saudi Arabia

Nusaybah Al Naim and Abeer Al Dossari
Department of Pediatrics, King Abdulaziz Hospital, Ministry of National Guard-Health Affairs, Al-Ahasa, Saudi Arabia

Valeria Calcaterra
Pediatric and Adolescent Unit, Department of Internal Medicine University of Pavia, Pavia, Italy
Department of Pediatrics, Children' Hospital "Vittore Buzzi", Milan, Italy

Francesco Bassanese, Andrea Martina Clemente and Corrado Regalbuto
Pediatric Unit, Department of the Mother and Child Health Fondazione IRCCS Policlinico San Matteo and University of Pavia, Pavia, Italy

Rossella Amariti
Pediatric and Adolescent Unit, Department of Internal Medicine University of Pavia, Pavia, Italy
Pediatric Unit, Department of the Mother and Child Health Fondazione IRCCS Policlinico San Matteo and University of Pavia, Pavia, Italy

Anna Sala and Gian Vincenzo Zuccotti
Department of Pediatrics, Children' Hospital "Vittore Buzzi", Milan, Italy
Department of Biomedical and Clinical Science "L. Sacco", University of Milano, Milano, Italy

Sunam M. Sujanani, Mohanad M. Elfishawi, Paria Zarghamravanbaksh, Francisco J. Cuevas Castillo and David M. Reich
Department of Medicine, Icahn School of Medicine at Mount Sinai, NYC Health and Hospitals/Queens, Jamaica, NY 11432, USA

Rami Salameh, Mumtaheena Miah and Catherine Anastasopoulou
Endocrinology Department, Albert Einstein Medical Center-Philadelphia, Philadelphia, PA, USA

Guillermo E. Guzmán Gómez
Fundación Clínica Valle del Lili, Department of Endocrinology, Universidad Icesi, Cali, Colombia

Julian A. Viggiano
PGY3 Internal Medicine Resident, Fundación Clínica Valle del Lili, Universidad Icesi, Cali, Colombia

A. Silva-De Las Salas
Universidad Icesi, Cali, Colombia

Veline Martínez
Fundación Clínica Valle del Lili, Department of Internal Medicine, Universidad Icesi, Cali, Colombia

María A. Urbano Bonilla
Fundación Clínica Valle del Lili, Clinical Investigations Center, Cali, Colombia

Jessica S. Thomas
Weill Cornell Medicine, New York, NY, USA
Department of Pathology and Genomic Medicine, Houston Methodist Hospital, Houston, TX, USA

Jawairia Shakil
Division of Endocrinology, Diabetes, and Metabolism, Department of Medicine, Houston Methodist Hospital, Houston, TX, USA

Richard J. Robbins and Patricia Mejia Osuna
Weill Cornell Medicine, New York, NY, USA

Emir Tas, Vildan Tas and Juan D. Mejia-Otero
Department of Pediatrics, University of Arkansas for Medical Sciences, Little Rock, AR, USA

Serife E. Uzun
College of Osteopathic Medicine, New York Institute of Technology, Glen Head, Long Island, NY, USA

Nelson Carvalho Cunha, Leonor Gomes, Joana Saraiva and Isabel Paiva
Department of Endocrinology, Hospitais da Universidade de Coimbra, Centro Hospitalar e Universitário de Coimbra, 3075 Coimbra, Portugal

Francisco Barrera and Natia Murvelashvili
Amita Health Saint Francis Hospital, 355 Ridge Avenue, Evanston, IL 60202, USA

L. Paschke
Division of Endocrinology, Department of Endocrinology and Nephrology, University Clinic Leipzig, Germany

T. Lincke
Division of Nuclear Medicine, Department of Radiology, University Clinic Leipzig, Germany

K. Mühlberg
Department of Angiology, University Clinic Leipzig, Germany

Tom H. Lindner
Division of Nephrology, Department of Endocrinology and Nephrology, University Clinic Leipzig, Germany

R. Paschke
Department of Medicine, Division of Endocrinology, Departments of Oncology, Pathology and Biochemistry and Molecular Biology & Arnie Charbonneau Cancer Institute Cumming School of Medicine, University of Calgary, Canada

Mussa H. AlMalki
Obesity, Endocrine and Metabolism Center, King Fahad Medical City, Riyadh, Saudi Arabia
King Fahad Medical City, College of Medicine, King Saud Bin Abdul Aziz University for Health Science, Riyadh, Saudi Arabia

Metib Alotaibi and Mohammad Maswood Ahmad
Obesity, Endocrine and Metabolism Center, King Fahad Medical City, Riyadh, Saudi Arabia

Muhammad Amin ur Rahman
Department of Pathology and Laboratory Medicine Administration, King Fahad Medical City, Riyadh, Saudi Arabia

Turki Alharthi
Department of Endocrinology, Military Hospital, Jeddah, Saudi Arabia

Adnan Haider, Oksana Symczyk and Dylan Holland
600 Suncrest Towne Center, Morgantown, WV 26505, USA
Department of Endocrinology Department of Medicine, West Virginia University, Morgantown, WV, USA

Ayesha Hassan
Department of Internal Medicine, West Virginia University, Morgantown, WV, USA

Muhammad Atif Khan
Ohio State University, 281 W Lane Avenue, Columbus, OH 43210, USA

Inderpreet Madahar
West Virginia School of Medicine, Morgantown, WV 26506, USA

Martin Litzel and Stefan Fischli
Division of Endocrinology, Diabetes and Clinical Nutrition, Luzerner Kantonsspital, Luzern 6000, Switzerland

Gianluca Caridi and Francesca Lugani
Laboratory of Molecular Nephrology, Istituto Giannina Gaslini, IRCCS, Genoa 16147, Italy

Monica Campagnoli and Lorenzo Minchiotti
Department of Molecular Medicine, University of Pavia, Pavia 27100, Italy

Tina Mosaferi
Department of Medicine, David Geffen School of Medicine, University of California Los Angeles, Los Angeles, CA, USA

Sahar Sherf, Laura Y. Sue and Ines Donangelo
Division of Endocrinology, David Geffen School of Medicine, University of California Los Angeles, Los Angeles, CA, USA

Anna Delamerced
The Warren Alpert Medical School of Brown University, Providence, RI, USA

Lauren J. Massingham and Jose Bernardo Quintos
The Warren Alpert Medical School of Brown University, Rhode Island Hospital, Hasbro Children's Hospital, 593 Eddy Street, Providence, Rhode Island 02903, USA

Samantha Steinmetz-Wood, Matthew Gilbert and Katherine Menson
Department of Medicine, Larner College of Medicine at the University of Vermont, 111 Colchester Ave, Burlington, VT, USA

Rashi Sandooja and Monisha Priyadarshini Kumar
Department of Internal Medicine, Cleveland Clinic Akron General, Akron, OH, USA

John M. Moorman
Department of Pharmacy Practice, Northeast Ohio Medical University, Rootstown, OH, USA

Karla Detoya
Department of Endocrinology, Cleveland Clinic Akron General, Akron, OH, USA

Einas Alrashidi
Department of Internal Medicine, Al-Farwaniya Hospital, Kuwait

Thamer Alessa
Division of Endocrinology, Diabetes and Metabolism, Jaber Al-Ahmad Hospital, Kuwait

Samhitha Munugoti, Vamsee Reddy, Gaurav Patel and Triveni Abburi
Department of Internal Medicine, Prime Health Care Consortium at St. Mary's and St. Clare Denville Hospital Program, Denville, NJ, USA

Maneesh Gaddam
Division of Pulmonary, Critical Care, and Sleep Medicine, Tufts Medical Center, Boston, MA, USA

Livia M. R. Marcon, Carmine G. Fanelli and Riccardo Calafiore
Section of Endocrinology and Metabolism, Department of Medicine and Surgery, University of Perugia Medical School, Perugia, Italy

Miyako Kishimoto, Kazuhide Yamaoki and Masayuki Adachi
Clinical Research Center, Department of Medicine, International University of Health and Welfare, Tochigi, Japan
Department of Internal Medicine, Sanno Hospital, 8-10-16 Akasaka, Minato, Tokyo 107-0052, Japan

Ming Yeh Lee, Molly L. Tanenbaum, David M. Maahs and Priya Prahalad
Division of Pediatric Endocrinology, Stanford University School of Medicine, Standford, CA, USA

Index

www.ingramcontent.com/pod-product-compliance
Lightning Source LLC
LaVergne TN
LVHW082147200926
848484LV00008B/2119